Stress,
Stress Hormones
and the Immune System

Stress, Stress Hormones and the Immune System

Edited by

Julia C. Buckingham
Glenda E. Gillies

and

Anne-Marie Cowell

Imperial College School of Medicine
London, UK

JOHN WILEY & SONS

Chichester • New York • Weinheim • Brisbane • Singapore • Toronto

Copyright © 1997 by John Wiley & Sons Ltd,
Baffins Lane, Chichester,
West Sussex PO19 1UD, England

National   01243 779777
International (+44) 1243 779777
e-mail (for orders and customer service enquiries): cs-books@wiley.co.uk
Visit our Home Page on http://www.wiley.co.uk
or http://www.wiley.com

Other Wiley Editorial Offices

John Wiley & Sons, Inc., 605 Third Avenue,
New York, NY 10158-0012, USA

WILEY-VCH Verlag GmbH, Pappelallee 3,
D-69469 Weinheim, Germany

Jacaranda Wiley Ltd, 33 Park Road, Milton,
Queensland 4064, Australia

John Wiley & Sons (Asia) Pte Ltd, 2 Clementi Loop #02-01,
Jin Xing Distripark, Singapore 129809

John Wiley & Sons (Canada) Ltd, 22 Worcester Road,
Rexdale, Ontario M9W 1L1, Canada

Library of Congress Cataloging-in-Publication Data

Stress, stress hormones, and the immune system / edited by Julia C. Buckingham, Glenda E. Gillies, and
Anne-Marie Cowell.
     p.   cm.
   Includes bibliographical references and index.
   ISBN 0-471-95886-7 (cased : alk. paper)
   1. Stress (Physiology)   2. Psychoneuroendocrinology.
3. Neuroimmunology.   I. Buckingham, Julia C.   II. Gillies, Glenda E.   III. Cowell, Anne-Marie.
   [DNLM: 1. Neuroimmunomodulation.   2. Stress, Psychological–immunology.   3. Neurosecretory
Systems—immunology.   4. Hormones–immunology.   5. Immune System—physiology.   WL 103.7
S915 1997]
QP88.2.S8S77   1997
616.98—dc21
DNLM/DC   97–5380
for Library of Congress   CIP

British Library Cataloguing in Publication Data
A catalogue record for this book is available from the British Library

ISBN 0-471-95886-7

Typeset in 10/12pt Times from the author's disks
Printed and bound in Great Britain by Biddles Ltd, Guildford and King's Lynn
This book is printed on acid-free paper responsibly manufactured from sustainable forestation,
for which at least two trees are planted for each one used for paper production.

Contents

Contributors

Dr R. Aspinall, Division of Diagnostic and Investigative Services, Imperial College School of Medicine, Chelsea and Westminster Hospital Hospital, 369 Fulham Road, London SW10 9NH, UK

Dr S. M. Baigent, School of Animal and Microbial Sciences, Department of Biochemistry and Physiology, The University of Reading, Whiteknights, PO Box 228, Reading RG6 2AG, UK

Prof. I. Berczi, Department of Immunology, Faculty of Medicine, University of Manitoba, 795 McDermot Avenue, Winnipeg, Manitoba, Canada R3E 0W3

Prof. J. C. Buckingham, Department of Neuroendocrinology, Division of Neuroscience and Psychological Medicine, Imperial College School of Medicine, Charing Cross Hospital, Fulham Palace Road, London W6 8RF, UK

Dr A.-M. Cowell, Department of Neuroendocrinology, Division of Neuroscience and Psychological Medicine, Imperial College School of Medicine, Charing Cross Hospital, Fulham Palace Road, London W6 8RF, UK

Dr E. B. De Souza, Neurocrine Biosciences Inc., 3050 Science Park Road, San Diego, CA 92121, USA

Dr J. E. G. Downing, Department of Biology, Imperial College of Science, Technology and Medicine, Prince Consort Road, London SW7 2BB, UK

Prof. R. J. Flower, Department of Biochemical Pharmacology, The William Harvey Institute, St. Bartholomew's and the Royal London Hospital School of Medicine and Dentistry at Queen Mary and Westfield College, Charterhouse Square, London EC1M 6BQ, UK

Dr G. E. Gillies, Department of Neuroendocrinology, Division of Neuroscience and Psychological Medicine, Imperial College School of Medicine, Charing Cross Hospital, Fulham Palace Road, London W6 8RF, UK

Dr. W. C. Gorospe, Department of Cell Biology and Anatomy, 171 Ashley Avenue, Medical University of South Carolina, Charleston, SC 29425, USA

Dr N. J. Goulding, Department of Rheumatology, The William Harvey Institute, St. Bartholomew's and the Royal London Hospital School of Medicine and Dentistry at Queen Mary and Westfield College, Charterhouse Square, London EC1M 6BQ, UK

Dr D. Grammatopoulos, Division of Molecular Medicine, The Department of Biological Sciences, The University of Warwick, Coventry CV4 7AL, UK

Prof. A. B. Grossman, Department of Endocrinology, St. Bartholomew's Hospital, West Smithfield, London EC1A 7BE, UK

Dr M. S. Harbuz, University Department of Medicine, Bristol Royal Infirmary, Marlborough Street, Bristol, BS2 8HW, UK

Dr A. E. Herbison, Laboratory of Neuroendocrinology, The Babraham Institute, Cambridge CB2 4AT, UK

Prof. E. W. Hillhouse, Division of Molecular Medicine, The Department of Biological Sciences, The University of Warwick, Coventry CV4 7AL, UK

Dr D. S. Jessop, University Department of Medicine, Bristol Royal Infirmary, Marlborough Street, Bristol BS2 8HW, UK

Prof. M. D. Kendall, The Thymus Laboratory, The Babraham Institute, Cambridge CB2 4AT, UK

Prof. S. L. Lightman, University Department of Medicine, Bristol Royal Infirmary, Marlborough Street, Bristol BS2 8HW, UK

Prof. P. J. Lowry, School of Animal and Microbial Sciences, Department of Biochemistry and Physiology, The University of Reading, Whiteknights, PO Box 228, Reading RG6 2AG, UK

Dr. P. Navarra, Institute of Pharmacology, Catholic University Medical School, Rome, Italy

Dr. P. J. Neveu, Neurobiologie Intégrative, INSERM- U. 394, rue Camille Saint-Sans, 33077 Bordeaux cedex, France

Prof. N. J. Rothwell, Division of Neuroscience, School of Biological Sciences, University of Manchester, Manchester M13 9PT, UK

Dr G. Schettini, Institute of Pharmacology, School of Medicine, University of Genoa, Via De Toni, Genoa 16132, Italy

Prof. Emeritus G. F. Solomon, University of California, Los Angeles, 19054 Pacific Coast Highway, Malibu, CA 90265, USA

Dr B. L. Spangelo, Department of Chemistry, University of Nevada Las Vegas, 4505 Maryland Parkway, Las Vegas, NV 89154-4003, USA

Dr J. H. Steel, Histopathology Unit, Imperial Cancer Research Fund, 35–43 Lincoln's Inn Fields, London WC2 3PN, UK

Dr T. Takao, Second Department of Internal Medicine, Kochi Medical School, Nankoku 783, Japan

Dr A. V. Turnbull, Peptide Laboratory, Salk Institute, PO Box 85800, San Diego, CA 92037, USA

Dr S. V. Vellucci, The Babraham Institute, Babraham Hall, Babraham, Cambridge CB2 4AT, UK

Prof. G. P. Vinson, Department of Biochemistry, Queen Mary and Westfield College, Mile End Road, London E1 4NS, UK

Dr R. J. Woods, School of Animal and Microbial Sciences, Department of Biochemistry and Physiology, The University of Reading, Whiteknights, PO Box 228, Reading RG6 2AG, UK

Preface

More than two thousand years ago, Galen observed that tumour growth was more pronounced in sanguine women than in melancholy women. Thus, the seeds of the idea that mental processes and emotional status are linked with physical health and disease have long been planted. However, apart from the somewhat intangible "humours", the means whereby processes in the brain could impinge either positively or negatively on the health status of an individual remained elusive for many centuries. An important advance in constructing a scientific framework for understanding the pathways of communication came with Hans Selye's descriptions of the body's responses to and defences against a variety of stressful stimuli. Indeed, we are grateful to Professor Istvan Berczi for providing a Prologue to this book describing Hans Selye's influential contributions to the field which, as a student and colleague of Selye's, he came to know at first hand. Thus, we know that the anterior pituitary gland and its control centre in the brain (the hypothalamus), which together constitute the classical neuroendocrine system, play a critical role in controlling the release of stress hormones, especially the powerfully immunosuppressive glucocorticoids, which can then "talk" to the cells of the immune system whether they be moving within the circulation or static in the primary and secondary lymphoid tissues. Equally, we now know that products of the immune system can "talk" to the neuroendocrine tissues. The hypothalamus is also a critical modulator of the behavioural responses to stress and of the autonomic nervous system which is activated by stress and which innervates tissues of the immune system. Stress hormones and the cells and secretory products of the immune system therefore emerge as the cellular and molecular links between brain processes, health and disease. A further understanding of the biochemical, immunological, neurobiological and psychological implications of the cross-talk between the stress–neuroendocrine and immune systems thus offers exciting alternative approaches to, and more effective therapies for, the management of a range of conditions such as immune deficiencies and autoimmune states which have proven notoriously difficult to control. With growing resistance to antibiotics, it is not inconceivable that in the future new approaches may have to be sought for dealing with bacterial infections.

With this background, we believe that research into the interactions between the neuroendocrine and immune systems could result in better maintenance of physical and mental health. Such work requires a certain depth of understanding of two relatively complex fields, namely neuroendocrinology and immunology. Therefore, this volume aims to provide final year honours students, graduate scientists or researchers in mainstream (neuro)endocrinology, immunology or the clinical sciences with the basic understanding needed to embark on what might be called neuroendocrine–immunological research. To our knowledge, this is the first book in the field to cater for such a readership. Section I deals with concepts concerning the neuroendocrine, autonomic and immune systems while Section II sets out the principal methods currently used to assess the function of each system. Various aspects of the functional interplay between stress hormones and the immune system are covered in Section III. This volume is not intended to be an exhaustive coverage of the literature, which is growing fast, but to serve to illustrate the breadth and implications of the work.

We are indebted to the experts in immunology, cell biology, behavioural science and the emerging field of psychoneuroimmunology for making their excellent contributions to this book and for providing the counterpoint to our own neuroendocrinological backgrounds. As editors, we have aimed to adopt a uniform structure to the chapters within each section so that the reader, whether student, researcher, clinician or teacher, may easily find the required information. Sections for further reading are detailed at the end of each chapter. In addition, the contributors themselves have published many seminal papers which will undoubtedly inform and fire future research.

J. C. B.
G. E. G.
A.-M. C.

The Stress Concept: An Historical Perspective of Hans Selye's Contributions

Istvan Berczi

University of Manitoba, Canada

The terms "stress" and "stress syndrome" were first adopted some 60 years ago by the late Hans Selye who, in a seminal article in *Nature*, described a series of pathophysiological changes which typically develop in the rat following exposure to noxious stimuli as diverse as physical (cold, surgery), chemical (formaldehyde, morphine, adrenaline) or emotional challenges (1). These responses encompass an initial shock–counter-shock phase, termed the "general alarm reaction", which occurs irrespective of the nature of the stimulus and which is characterised by enlargement of the adrenal glands and profound shrinkage of the thymus and other lymphoid organs together with haemorrhage, especially in the gastrointestinal tract. The alarm reaction is followed by a period of resistance, the "general adaptation syndrome", during which the organs return to their normal state provided that the stimulus is withdrawn or its intensity reduced; if, however, the stimulus is sustained or its intensity enhanced, the symptoms of the alarm reaction return and exhaustion or even death may ensue. The development of resistance, unlike the general alarm reaction, may be stimulus-specific although in many instances "cross tolerance" may develop between certain stimuli, i.e. resistance may be non-specific (2).

By 1946 Selye had accumulated a considerable body of data on the general adaptation syndrome. This is embodied in the first comprehensive account of the stress concept published in the *Journal of Clinical Endocrinology* (Fig. 1) where he also predicted that diseases may develop as a result of maladaptation to stressful stimuli (2). Most notably, he described the stress response in terms of:

(a) changes in blood sugar and electrolytes,
(b) elevations in the white blood cell count,

Stress, Stress Hormones and the Immune System. Edited by J. C. Buckingham, G. E. Gillies and A.-M. Cowell
© 1997 John Wiley & Sons, Ltd.

(c) adrenocortical hypertrophy (widening of the cortex, loss of lipid granules and delineation between the fasciculata and reticularis), and

(d) involution of the thymus (depletion of cortical thymocytes, pyknotic nuclei, nuclear debris, intense macrophage activity to eliminate dead thymic cells, de-differentiation of thymic reticulum) lymph nodes, spleen and other lymphoid organs and tissues.

He noted that the involution of the thymus parallelled the growth of the adrenal cortices and also that it was prevented by adrenalectomy as, too, was the atrophy of the other lymphoid organs, albeit to a lesser extent. Although Selye's pioneering work was done at a time when the functions of the thymus and lymphoid organs were unknown, it was nonetheless fundamental in establishing sensitivity of these tissues to glucocorticoid hormones (3). The emergence in the late 1940s of the concept that the hypothalamo–pituitary axis fulfils a critical role in controlling the secretory activity of the peripheral endocrine glands (4) led Selye to propose a fundamental role for the pituitary hormones in the aetiology of the stress response (2, 5)—see Fig. 1; this, he considered, was effected in part through the release of adrenocorticotrophic hormone (ACTH), which increases adrenocortical size and hormone production with ensuing metabolic changes

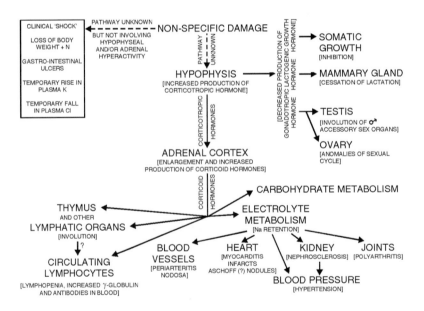

Figure 1 Summary of the consequences of non-specific damage. (See text and (2) for further explanation.) Reproduced with permission from Selye H. *J Clin Endocrinol*, 1946, **6**, 117. © 1946 The Endocrine Society

(carbohydrates, electrolytes), thymic atrophy etc., but also by inhibition of the secretion of the gonadotrophins, prolactin and growth hormone. This may now be recognised as a fairly accurate outline of the primary features of the relatively recently defined "acute phase response", with its characteristic alterations in neuroendocrine, metabolic and immune function (6).

Selye went on to demonstrate that administration of cortisone or ACTH suppresses the inflammatory reaction evoked by the injection of egg whites into rats, whereas mineralocorticoids (e.g. deoxycorticosterone acetate) have opposing actions. This important observation led first to the demonstration that glucocorticoids (cortisone and cortisol) exhibit powerful anti-inflammatory activity in a variety of animal models and, ultimately, that they quell the inflammatory responses in patients with diseases such as rheumatoid arthritis, rheumatic fever and allergic inflammation (7), an advance for which Hench and his co-workers were later awarded the Nobel Prize. In 1955, Selye set out a basis for the relationship between stress and disease (7) or, more specifically, between stress and inflammation, which supported his earlier prediction that maladaptation to stressful stimuli may be a key factor in the pathogenesis of inflammatory disease (2). In this he proposed that, while glucocorticoids suppress inflammatory responses, growth hormone and the mineralocorticoids exert pro-inflammatory actions (Fig. 2) and that a critical balance between these adaptive hormones

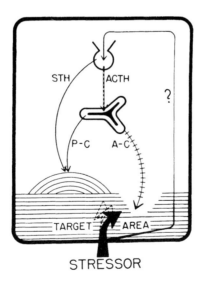

Figure 2 Schematic representation of the relationship between stress and inflammation. Selye proposed that growth hormone (somatotrophic hormone, STH), released from the anterior pituitary gland, and mineralocorticoids (termed flogistic corticoids, P-C), released from the adrenal cortex, are pro-inflammatory whereas glucocorticoids are anti-flogistic (A-C) or anti-inflammatory (7). Reproduced with permission from Selye H. *Science*, 1955, **122**, 625. © 1955 American Association for the Advancement of Science

is essential for health. This theory placed the pituitary gland in a prime position for regulating inflammation and underscored Selye's subsequent life-long fascination with the relevance of specific neuroendocrine mechanisms to the pathogenesis of diseases. This subject has attracted much renewed interest today, as evidenced by the contents of this volume.

In addition to diseases more obviously related to inflammatory conditions, Selye also recognised that disturbances in the balance of adaptive hormones, such as those apparent in stress, may lead to metabolic derangements, altered responsiveness and ultimately abnormal function of target organs; this in turn may lead to disease in many tissues such as the liver, kidneys and even the nervous system, with the latter contributing especially to the possible psychiatric effects of steroid hormones. Indeed, although Selye faced many criticisms from his contemporaries in the basic sciences, his novel ideas were received warmly by psychologists who took interest in examining the relationship between pathological processes and the neuroendocrine system.

When I took up a post in Selye's laboratory at McGill University in 1967, the functions of the lymphoid organs were newly discovered and the theory of neurogenic inflammation had only just been put forward (8). During my time in his laboratory, I was privileged to take part in many discussions on problems such as "Why should the immune system be affected by noxious stimuli as diverse as an immunological challenge (bacterial, viral) or an emotional, physical or chemical insult? What does the immune system have to do with the response to non-specific injury? If glucocorticoids suppress the immune system, which other hormones serve to antagonise this effect and how do they act?" Many of these questions remain to be fully answered. The fundamental role of the immune system in providing specific defence against potentially harmful pathogenic micro-organisms and other foreign agents has long been recognised. However, only now are we beginning to realise that the immune system also fulfils a broader role in the maintenance of homeostasis. For example, its activation by non-specific stimuli, such as physical injury, is fundamental to the elimination of damaged cells and tissues and to the control of tissue regeneration and repair (6). Moreover, both the competence and the level of activity in the immune system are intricately interwoven with the psychological state of the host and from such recognitions new disciplines, such as psychoneuroimmunology (see Chapter 19), have emerged.

Selye became aware progressively that the stress response is barely, if at all, distinguishable from the exacerbated physiological responses to overstimulation and, consequently, he referred to two subgroups of stress, namely eustress (a pleasurable impulse) and distress (an unpleasant or dangerous impulse). He also recognised that the line of demarcation between these stimuli is difficult to define as individual susceptibility to stress varies greatly; hence, a stimulus which is pleasant to one individual may be very stressful to another. Indeed, Selye himself described the, now well-recognised, overburdened businessman who experiences severe stress because he is forced by his family to take a holiday. The variation among individuals in their responses often frustrated Selye in his attempt to find the perfect definition of stress which, even today, we find elusive.

As already alluded to, Selye's thinking was often not appreciated by his contemporaries who favoured the scientific ethos of strict definitions, the isolation and characterisation of molecules and a general preoccupation with details. In fact, for much of his life, Selye's ideas preceded the knowledge and the methodologies required for the experimental validation of his hypotheses. It is only now that his concepts and predictions can be tested by rigorous scientific analysis with powerful modern tools that make commonplace experiments which were inconceivable only a few years ago. As we progress in our understanding of psychoneurobiology, Selye's originality, wisdom and foresight are increasingly understood and appreciated. For example, his original concept that the pathogenesis of disease is often not attributable to a single cause but rather the coincident emergence of several factors, an hypothesis from which he accurately predicted the fail-safe and redundant nature of biological regulatory and defence mechanisms, is now supported by compelling evidence (9–11). His interest in his twilight years in the ability of certain steroid hormones, which he termed "catatoxic steroids", to provide protection against toxins and other noxious agents (12, 13) is the focus of much current research. Moreover, like many contemporary researchers, he recognised the importance of adopting a multi-disciplinary approach to the study of biological problems. "You can never learn what a mouse is like by carefully examining each of its cells separately under the electron microscope any more than you could appreciate the beauty of a cathedral by chemical analysis of each stone which went into its construction" (14) is, perhaps, one of his most poignant quotations.

Selye was not only well ahead of his time in science but also in his views on politics and science. Indeed, in addition to his prolific contributions to the scientific press, Selye served as a grand ambassador for science by writing books and articles on the processes of scientific research and on stress and related subjects which appealed to a wider public audience (15–18). As his career progressed, his desire to popularise science and to promote its future development by training enthusiastic young scientists assumed an importance which equalled his passion for scientific endeavours and for which he will long be remembered.

ACKNOWLEDGEMENTS

I am much obliged to Madame Louis Dreve Selye and to Dr Beatrice Tuchweber-Farbstein, President of the Hans Selye Foundation for providing material and valuable information for this historical overview and I also thank Mrs Jean Sylweter for her devoted work during its preparation.

REFERENCES

1. Selye H. A syndrome produced by diverse nocuous agents. *Nature*, 1936, **138**: 32.
2. Selye H. The general adaptation syndrome and the diseases of adaptation. *J Clin Endocrinol*, 1946, **6**: 117–230.
3. Selye H. Thymus and adrenals in the response of the organism to injuries and intoxication. *Brit J Exp Path*, 1936, **17**: 234–48.
4. Harris G. W. Neural control of the pituitary gland. *Physiol Rev*, 1948, **28**: 139–79.
5. Selye H. Effects of ACTH and cortisone upon an "anaphalactyoid reaction". *Can Med Assoc J*, 1949, **61**: 553–6.
6. Berczi I. and Nagy E. Neurohormonal control of cytokines during injury. In: N. J. Rothwell and F. Berkenbosch (eds). *Brain control of the response to injury*. Cambridge University Press, Cambridge, 1994, pp. 96–144.
7. Selye H. Stress and disease. *Science*, 1955, **122**: 625–31.
8. Jancso N., Jancso-Gabor A. and Szolcsanyi J. Direct evidence for neurogenic inflammation and its prevention by denervation and by pretreatment with capsaicin. *Br J Pharmacol*, 1967, **31**: 138–51.
9. Selye H. *The Pluricausal Cardiopathies*, Springfield, Charles C Thomas Pub., 1961.
10. Berczi I., Baragar F. D., Chalmers I. M., Keystone E. C., Nagy E. and Warrington R.J. Hormones in self tolerance and autoimmunity: a role in the pathogenesis of rheumatoid arthritis. *Autoimmunity*, 1993, **16**: 45–56.
11. Klein G. *Tumor Suppressor Genes*. New York, Dekker, 1990.
12. Selye H. *Hormones and resistance*. New York, Springer-Verlag, 1970.
13. Selye H. Catatoxic steroids. *Can Med Assoc J*, 1969, **101**: 51–2.
14. Selye H. *In Vivo: The Case for Supramolecular Biology*. New York, Livesight Pub Co, 1967.
15. Selye H. *The Story of the Adaptation Syndrome*. Montreal, Acta Inc Med Pub, 1952.
16. Selye H. *The Stress of Life*. New York, McGraw Hill, 1956.
17. Selye H. *From Dream to Discovery*. New York, McGraw Hill, 1964.
18. Selye H. *The Stress of My Life: A Scientist's Memory*. New York, Van Nostrand Reinhold, 1979.

Basic Concepts

Chapter 1

The Neuroendocrine System: Anatomy, Physiology and Responses to Stress

Julia C. Buckingham, Anne-Marie Cowell, Glenda E. Gillies

Imperial College School of Medicine, London, UK

Allan E. Herbison

The Babraham Institute, Cambridge, UK and

Jennifer H. Steel

Imperial Cancer Research Fund, London, UK

Stress, Stress Hormones and the Immune System. Edited by J. C. Buckingham, G. E. Gillies and A.-M. Cowell
© 1997 John Wiley & Sons, Ltd.

1.1   INTRODUCTION

Exposure of an individual to a noxious stimulus (i.e. a stress), whether it be cognitive (e.g. emotional distress) or non-cognitive (e.g. immune insults such as infections), precipitates a co-ordinated series of responses which typically includes alterations in neuroendocrine and autonomic function together with complex changes in behaviour. The purpose of these diverse responses is to protect the host and to restore homeostasis; not surprisingly therefore, the pattern of responses is dependent on the nature of the stress, its intensity and its duration (acute, chronic, intermittent) as well as the nature and the current state of health of the individual. Failure to mount an appropriate response to stress is potentially hazardous and is now considered to be a significant factor in the pathogenesis of a wide range of diseases including disorders of the cardiovascular system (e.g. hypertension) and gastrointestinal tract (e.g. gastric and duodenal ulcers, the irritable bowel syndrome), psychiatric conditions (e.g. depression, anorexia nervosa) and disturbances in immune function, which, in turn, may predispose the individual to other diseases (e.g. infections, inflammatory disease). The autonomic and behavioural responses to stress are described in Chapter 2 and various aspects of the interactions between stress hormones and the immune system, along with the possible consequences for health and disease, are considered from Chapter 8 onwards. This chapter will discuss the role of the hypothalamo–pituitary axis in mounting the neuroendocrine responses to stress, with particular reference to the hypothalamo–pituitary–adrenal (HPA) axis and its critical function in the maintenance of homeostasis.

1.2   THE HYPOTHALAMO–PITUITARY AXIS

The pituitary gland is responsible for the production of a number of hormones which, directly or indirectly, exert powerful regulatory effects over a wide array of bodily functions including growth, development, metabolism, osmotic balance, reproductive function, behaviour and host defence processes. For many years the pituitary gland was termed the "master gland". However, the elegant studies of the late Geoffrey Harris (1) led us to realise that the secretory activity of the pituitary gland is orchestrated by the hypothalamus which lies in close proximity to the pituitary gland and provides the final common pathway whereby the central nervous system (CNS) exerts control over the endocrine system. The "common pathway" which is critical to pituitary function involves two classes of neurosecretory cells, termed the *parvocellular* and *magnocellular* cells or neurones, which can be distinguished on both anatomical and functional grounds. The parvocellular cells are concerned with the regulation of anterior pituitary function; their axons terminate in the median eminence region of the hypothalamus and the neurohormones they release are delivered to the anterior pituitary gland via the hypophysial portal vessels. The magnocellular neurones by contrast extend to the posterior pituitary gland and secrete their products directly into the systemic circulation. The major anatomical features of the hypothalamo–pituitary axis are summarised schematically in Fig. 1.1 and are considered in greater detail below.

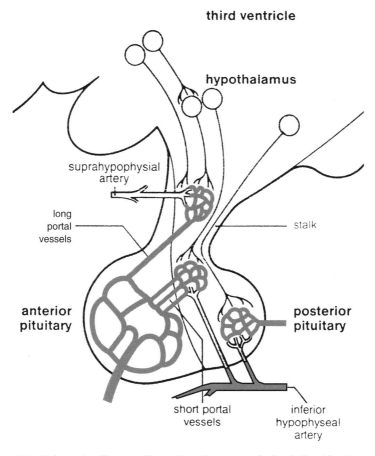

Figure 1.1 Schematic diagram illustrating the anatomical relationships between the hypothalamus and the pituitary gland. Redrawn and modified from Reichlin S., Neuroendocrine control of pituitary function. In: G. M. Besser and M. O. Thorner (eds) *Clinical Endocrinology,* London, Mosby-Wolfe, 1994, with permission of authors and the publishers

1.2.1   Anatomy and Function of the Pituitary Gland

General Structure

The pituitary gland is a small, bilobed structure which lies in a bony cavity, termed the sella turcica, immediately below the median eminence area of the hypothalamus to which it is connected by the pituitary stalk (Fig. 1.1). The two lobes of the pituitary gland, the adenohypophysis and neurohypophysis, are distinct anatomically and physiologically, having different embryological origins and separate control mechanisms. The adenohypophysis, which is the larger of the two, is derived from ectodermal tissue of the oral epithelium. In most species it is clearly differentiated into three distinct zones, *viz.* the pars distalis and pars intermedia which fulfil classical endocrine functions and the pars tuberalis, which forms a tube of glandular cells in the pituitary stalk surrounding the infundibulum (neural stalk) and portal blood vessels (see Fig. 1.1). In man, however, only two zones of the adenohypophysis are normally apparent as the pars intermedia regresses perinatally, leaving only a few islets of glandular cells which persist into adulthood and, paradoxically, reside in the neurohypophysis. The adenohypophysis is highly vascularised. It receives arterial blood from the superior hypophysial artery (a branch of the internal carotid artery) and venous blood from the hypothalamus via a portal system which arises from a capillary plexus in the median eminence (the primary plexus) and comprises "long vessels" which pass through the pituitary stalk and empty into sinusoidal vessels in the anterior lobe. This portal system plays an essential role in transporting neurohormones from the hypothalamus to the pars distalis (see Section 1.2.3). The innervation of the adenohypophysis is sparse; however, fine nerve fibres have recently been identified amongst the secretory cells (2) and autonomic neurones supply the blood vessels.

Unlike the adenohypophysis, the neurohypophysis (also called the pars nervosa) is derived from neural tissues of the diencephalon and is in fact a downgrowth of the hypothalamus. It comprises the axons and terminals of magnocellular neurosecretory cells, the perikarya of which are located in discrete nuclei in the hypothalamus, together with glial cells called pituicytes. The neurohypophysis receives its blood from the inferior hypophysial arteries which form a capillary plexus in the gland and into which the neurosecretory cells release their products. Although the blood supplies of the adenohypophysis and neurohypophysis are largely separate, there are vascular connections between the two lobes (short portal vessels) which permit a degree of chemical intercommunication. The precise nature and physiological significance of this intercommunication remains to be determined.

The adenohypophysis and neurohypophysis are often referred to respectively as the anterior and posterior lobes of the pituitary gland. Strictly speaking, however, the anterior lobe comprises only the pars distalis and pars tuberalis while the posterior lobe includes the pars nervosa and the pars intermedia and is sometimes termed the neurointermediate lobe.

The Adenohypophysis

The endocrine function of the adenohypophysis is located primarily within the pars distalis, which secretes at least seven hormones whose physiological functions are generally well understood. These include growth hormone (GH, normal growth and development), thyrotrophin (TSH, control of thyroid function), corticotrophin (ACTH, regulation of adrenocortical function), β-lipotrophin (β-LPH) and β-endorphin (functions unknown but may include regulation of duodenal bicarbonate secretion), prolactin (PRL, regulation of lactation) and the gonadotrophins (luteinising hormone, LH, and follicle stimulating hormone, FSH; regulation of gonadal function). The pars intermedia produces α-melanocyte stimulating hormone (α-MSH, camouflage, pigmentation, regulation of the fetal adrenal) and β-endorphin. Most, if not all, of these hormones have been shown to exert direct effects on immune cell function and many are also synthesised within the immune system (see Chapters 3, 10, 11, 15 and 16 for further details).

The endocrine cells in the pars distalis have been classified into five major types according to the hormones they produce:

(a) somatotrophs (GH),
(b) thyrotrophs (TSH),
(c) corticotrophs (ACTH, β-LPH/β-endorphin),
(d) lactotrophs (PRL), and
(e) gonadotrophs (LH/FSH).

Modified corticotrophs, responsible for the production of α-MSH, β-endorphin and related peptides are also found in the pars intermedia.

The secretory cells may be differentiated by light microscopy either by classical histological methods that distinguish acidophils (somatotrophs, lactotrophs), basophils (thyrotrophs, gonadotrophs) and chromophobes (corticotrophs) or, more precisely, by immunohistochemistry which, using specific antibody probes, permits identification of the cells on the basis of the hormones they secrete (3). Alternatively, cells may be identified at the electron microscope level either on ultrastructural criteria (size, shape and distribution of the secretory granules they contain (4)) or by immunohistochemistry using immunogold probes. The latter methods have also led to the identification of further subdivisions of the secretory cell populations (e.g. small- and mixed-granule gonadotrophs) and shown conversely that some cells express more than one hormone (e.g. somatomammotrophs, which produce GH and PRL (4)). The distribution of secretory cells within the pars distalis normally follows a distinct, species specific pattern, which is likely to facilitate cell–cell communication; for example, in man the somatotrophs are concentrated typically in the lateral wings, while the corticotrophs are found mainly in the median wedge and the lacto-trophs and gonadotrophs have a more general distribution. However, the cell population may change according to the endocrine environment, with an increase in one cell type occurring at the expense of another. For example, in the rat thyroidectomy produces an increased number of thyrotrophs while the somatotroph population all but disappears, a phenomenon which may reflect "transdifferentia-tion" of one cell type into another (5).

In addition to the endocrine cells, the pars distalis also includes significant resident populations of glial-related cells, termed folliculostellate cells, and macrophages. The folliculostellate cells are slender and stellate in appearance and lack the secretory granules which are abundant in the endocrine cells; they tend to form follicles around a central lumen but also surround and make close contact with the endocrine cells. Like glial cells, the folliculostellate cells were regarded originally merely as supporting cells. Current evidence, however, suggests that they fulfil a wider brief which includes participation in intercellular communication, a view which is supported by evidence that they express a number of regulatory substances (e.g. cytokines and other regulatory peptides) which may be released locally to act on neighbouring cells (6). Rather less is known of the functional biology of the resident macrophage population. These cells are located in the perivascular spaces in close apposition to the endocrine cells; they are thus well positioned both to remove local cell debris and to release factors which may exert local (paracrine) regulatory actions. A recent study has also identified a distinct population of dendritic cells in the adenohypophysis; their function is unknown but, since dendritic cells are potent antigen presenting cells of myeloid origin, it seems likely that they may play a role in immune–endocrine communication (7).

The Neurohypophysis

The neurohypophysis is primarily responsible for the secretion of two neurohor-mones, each of which is a nonapeptide: vasopressin (also known as antidiuretic hormone, ADH) is concerned with the maintenance of osmotic balance and the regulation of blood pressure, particularly in conditions of haemorrhage; oxytocin regulates uterine contractility and milk ejection. In the majority of mammalian species, including the rat and man, vasopressin exists as 8-arginine vasopressin (AVP) but in some species (e.g. the pig) it is present as 8-lysine vasopressin (LVP). For simplicity we will refer subsequently only to AVP but the activities of the two peptides are essentially the same. Vasopressin and oxytocin are produced by separate populations of hypothalamic magnocellular neurosecretory cells and are subject to independent control mechanisms (see Section 1.2.5).

1.2.2 Chemistry and Biosynthesis of the Pituitary Hormones

All of the hormones produced by the pituitary gland are polypeptide in nature. ACTH, β-LPH, β-endorphin, PRL, GH, AVP and oxytocin each comprise single peptide chains, which are formed from precursor molecules (called prohormones) by proteolytic cleavage and, in some instances, further modified (e.g. acetylation). For example, ACTH and related peptides (β-LPH, β-endorphin) are synthesised in the corticotrophs from a prohormone, pro-opiomelanocortin (POMC), which is the product of a well-characterised gene (8); see Fig. 1.2. Following gene transcription and translation, newly formed pre-POMC is translocated via the endoplasmic reticulum (where the signal peptide is removed) to the Golgi apparatus where it is packaged into secretory vesicles together with the enzymes required to process the molecule. Proteolytic cleavage occurs between paired basic amino acids (normally lysine and arginine) and results in the generation of ACTH together with three other peptides (N-POMC$_{1-76}$, β-LPH and a 31 amino acid peptide located between N-POMC$_{1-76}$ and ACTH— J-peptide) which, dependent on circumstances, may undergo further cleavage; for review see Buckingham and Gillies (8). The mature peptides are stored in the vesicles and released when required into the systemic circulation by a process of Ca^{2+}-dependent exocytosis. It is important to note that the POMC gene is expressed in several tissues other than the pars distalis (e.g. pars intermedia, hypothalamus, placenta) where tissue-specific, generally more extensive, processing results in the formation of a different spectrum of peptides including, for example, α-MSH, Fig. 1.2 (8). Of particular relevance to this volume is the expression of ACTH and other POMC-derived peptides (e.g. β-endorphin) by activated immune cells, which is considered in Chapter 10.

The synthesis of LH, FSH and TSH, which each comprise two glycosylated polypeptide chains (α and β), is more complex and invokes the activation of two genes. The α-chain or subunit is common to all three hormones and is encoded by a single gene expressed by both thyrotrophs and gonadotrophs. Hormone specificity is conferred by the respective β-subunits each of which is encoded by a single gene which is expressed only by the appropriate cell type. Following post-translational processing, the two subunits are united and stored in a glycosylated form. Further modification of the sugar residues may occur immediately before release and the small changes occurring, for example at the mid-cycle, influence markedly the biological potency of the molecule.

1.2.3 The Control of Adenohypophysial Function

The adenohypophysial hormones play a vital role in the maintenance of homeostasis. Abnormalities in their secretion invariably result in the manifestation of a variety of pathologies which, dependent on the lesion, may include disorders of

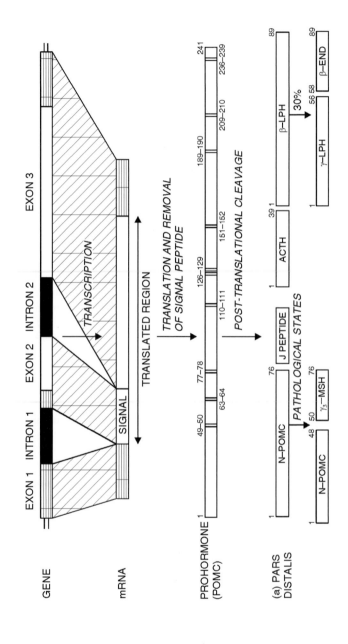

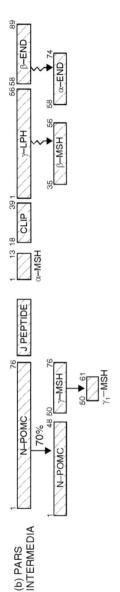

Figure 1.2 Steps in the biosynthesis and post translational processing of pro-opiomelanocortin (POMC) in (a) the pars distalis and (b) the pars intermedia of the pituitary gland.

Hatched bars, untranslated sequences; ACTH, adrenocorticotrophic hormone; LPH, lipotrophin; END, endorphin; MSH, melanocyte stimulating hormone; J. PEPTIDE, joining peptide; ||, sites of paired basic amino acids (i.e. potential cleavage sites) in the pro-hormone; ⇢, incomplete processing; ⤳, species specific incomplete processing. Redrawn and modified from J. C. Buckingham and G. E. Gillies, Hypothalamus and pituitary gland—xenobiotic induced toxicity and models for its investigation. In C. K. Atterwill and J. D. Flack (eds) *Endocrine Toxicology*, Cambridge University Press, Cambridge, 1992, by permission of Cambridge University Press

growth, development, metabolism, reproductive function and host defence processes. It is not, therefore, surprising that the secretion of each of these hormones is subject to very fine control. *In vivo*, the pituitary cells exhibit bursts of secretory activity that result in the characteristic "episodic" patterns of hormone release. The frequency and amplitude of pulses shown by various cell types may be age dependent and/or sexually dimorphic (e.g. somatotrophs) or both; they may also vary according to a circadian pattern (e.g. corticotrophs, somatotrophs) and to the reproductive cycle (e.g. gonadotrophs and, in some species, lactotrophs). Superimposed on these phasic patterns of activity are cell specific responses to a wide spectrum of stimuli including, for example, environmental changes, emotional or physical trauma, auditory or visual stimuli, pain, alterations in body temperature, metabolic factors (e.g. alterations in blood glucose or amino acids) and osmotic changes.

The Role of the Hypothalamus

The secretion of the anterior pituitary hormones is controlled primarily by chemical transmitter substances which are liberated from hypothalamic neurones into the primary capillary plexus in the median eminence region of the hypothalamus (see Fig. 1.1) and transported to their target cells via the hypophysial portal vessels (1). These neurohormones are termed variously the "hypophysiotrophic hormones", the "releasing hormones" or, if their actions are inhibitory, the "release inhibiting hormones". Hypothalamic hormones also control the secretory activity of the pars intermedia; some may be conveyed via the portal vessels but others may be released from neurones terminating in the vicinity of the secretory cells.

It was assumed originally that each anterior pituitary hormone would be controlled by one hypothalamic factor (i.e. there would be five releasing factors initiating the secretion of ACTH, GH, TSH, LH and FSH respectively and a release inhibiting factor effecting the tonic inhibition of PRL release). This view, however, proved to be over-simplistic. It is now evident that most of the pituitary hormones are subject to regulation by two or more hypothalamic hormones whose actions may be complementary (e.g. corticotrophin releasing hormone, CRH, and AVP, on the corticotrophs) or antagonistic (e.g. growth hormone releasing hormone, GHRH, and somatostatin, SRIH, on the somatotrophs). Furthermore, one hypothalamic hormone may regulate the secretion of two (and possibly more) anterior pituitary hormones (e.g. gonadotrophin releasing hormone, GnRH, stimulates the secretion of both LH and FSH). Table 1.1 provides details of the major releasing factors and release inhibiting factors identified to date (8). As can be seen, the majority are small peptides, with sequences ranging in length from three (thyrotrophin releasing hormone, TRH) to 44 (GHRH) amino acids, but some "classical" transmitter substances are also involved (e.g. dopamine, the major PRL release inhibiting hormone). Each of these substances

Table 1.1 Hypothalamic hormones controlling the secretory activity of the adenohypophysis: principal sites of synthesis, receptors, signal transduction systems and effects on hormone release. PVN, paraventricular nucleus; PeVN, periventricular nucleus; Arc, arcuate nucleus; VMN, ventromedial nucleus; cAMP, cyclic 3'5'-adenosine monophosphate; cGMP, cyclic 3'5'-guanosine monophosphate; PI, phosphoinositol metabolism; DA, dopamine; AA, amino acids. Redrawn and modified from J. C. Buckingham and G. E. Gillies, Hypothalamus and pituitary gland—xenobiotic induced toxicity and models for its investigation, in C. K. Atterwill and J. D. Flack (eds) *Endocrine Toxicology*, Cambridge University Press, Cambridge, 1992, with permission of Cambridge University Press

	Hypothalamic hormone	Chemical nature	Locus of cell body	Pituitary second messenger	Effects on pituitary hormone secretion
Thyrotrophs	TRH	Peptide (3AA)	PVN, PeVN	PI ($\uparrow$)	Increase
	Somatostatin	Peptide (14AA)	PeVN	cAMP ($\downarrow$)	Decrease
Gonadotrophs	GnRH	Peptide (14AA)	Preoptic or Arc (species dependent)	PI ($\uparrow$)	Increase
Somatotrophs	GHRH	Peptide (44AA)	Arc, VMN	cAMP ($\uparrow$)	Increase
	Somatostatin	Peptide (14AA)	PeVN	cAMP ($\downarrow$)	Decrease
	Dopamine	Catecholamine	Arc	cAMP ($\downarrow$) K$^+$ efflux ($\uparrow$) (DA$_2$ receptor)	Decrease
Lactotrophs	Dopamine	Catecholamine	Arc	cAMP ($\downarrow$) K$^+$ efflux ($\uparrow$) (DA$_2$ receptor)	Decrease
	GABA	Amino acid	? Ubiquitous	Cl-influx ($\uparrow$) GABA$_A$ receptor	Predominantly decrease
	TRH	Peptide (3AA)	PVN, PeVN	PI ($\uparrow$)	Increase
	VIP	Peptide (28AA)	PVN, PeVN	cAMP ($\uparrow$)	Increase
Corticotrophs (pars distalis)	CRH-41	Peptide (41AA)	PVN	cAMP ($\uparrow$)	Increase
	Vasopressin	Peptide (9AA)	PVN	PI ($\uparrow$)	Increase
	Atriopeptin III	Peptide (24AA)	PVN, PeVN	cGMP ($\uparrow$)	Decrease
	Substance P	Peptide (11AA)	PVN	cAMP ($\downarrow$)	Decrease
Corticotrophs (pars intermedia)	Dopamine	Catecholamine	Arc	cAMP ($\downarrow$) (DA$_{2B}$ receptor)	Decrease

has been shown to exert specific, concentration or dose dependent effects on the secretory activity of the adenohypophysis *in vitro* and *in vivo*. Moreover, inhibition of their activity by administration of specific antagonists or neutralising antisera causes significant alterations in pituitary activity. The physiological importance of the neurohormones is further substantiated by reports that they are present in high concentrations in both hypophysial portal blood and in nerve terminals that impinge on the capillary plexus in the external zone of the median eminence where their respective concentrations are modified specifically by appropriate physiological stimuli.

Molecular Basis of Hypothalamic Hormone Action

The actions of the hypothalamic hormones on their respective target cells in the anterior pituitary gland are complex and may involve not only stimulation or inhibition of hormone release but also regulation of hormone synthesis (transcription and translation), post-translational processing (proteolysis, glycosylation etc.) and margination of the secretory granules. In addition, some hypothalamic hormones promote target cell mitogenesis (e.g. CRH on the corticotrophs and GHRH on the somatotrophs). The effects on hormone release occur rapidly and are normally maximal within one minute of stimulation. The other effects occur more slowly and normally are apparent only after repeated stimulation of the cells. The responses to each of the hypothalamic hormones are mediated by specific membrane-bound receptors on the target cells, see Table 1.1 (8). Some of the receptors (e.g. gamma-amino-butyric acid, GABA) are linked to ion channels and thus, when stimulated, alter the excitability of the membrane. The majority however are G-protein linked and thereby utilise second messenger systems. Of particular importance in this respect are cyclic adenosine monophosphate (cAMP) formed from AMP by the action of adenylyl cyclase and inositol trisphosphate (IP_3) and diacyglycerol (DAG) liberated from membrane phospholipids by the actions of phospholipase C. Other second messenger systems may also be involved including arachidonic acid and its metabolites (prostanoids, leukotrienes and epoxides which are known collectively as eicosanoids), which may be derived either from membrane phospholipids by the actions of phospholipase A_2 (PLA_2) or from DAG by lipase degradation, and cyclic guanosine monophosphate (cGMP). In addition, increasing evidence points to a role for cytokine-like receptors which use tyrosine kinases of the janus kinase (JAK) family to activate transduction systems. Further information on receptors and signal transduction systems is provided in Chapter 4. Stimulation of the membrane-bound receptor may culminate in phosphorylation and internalization of the receptor-ligand complex. The receptor may be degraded, a process important in the regulation of receptor number and turnover, or recycled. The internalised ligand is also likely to be metabolised rapidly although, in some instances, it may exert further regulatory actions via an intracellular target receptor; for example, TRH is translocated to the nuclei of thyrotrophs where it may modulate genomic function.

Factors Influencing the Pituitary Responses to the Hypothalamic Hormones

The ability of pituitary cells to respond to their respective hypophysiotrophic hormones is modulated by a number of factors. The pattern of stimulation is particularly important. Adenohypophysial hormones are normally released in short pulses, the frequency and amplitude of which may vary according to physiological or pathological state. The episodic mode of secretion is dependent on complementary pulsatile secretion of appropriate hypothalamic hormones. The frequency of pulses is critical because continuous or over repeated exposure to the hypothalamic hormone may render the cells refractory to stimulation (i.e. they become tolerant) while a marked reduction in pulse frequency may be insufficient to maintain pituitary function. For example, prolonged infusion of GnRH or administration of long acting GnRH analogues renders the gonado-trophs unresponsive to further stimulation with the releasing hormone. By contrast, when given in a pulsatile manner (1 pulse/90 min, s.c.) so as to mimic the physiological pattern of secretion, GnRH effectively maintains gonadal function in laboratory animals in which the GnRH neurones have been ablated experimentally and in human subjects with infertility or hypogonadism of hypothalamic origin. The desensitisation evoked by GnRH was originally ascribed simply to a reduction in the number of pituitary receptors; other data however suggest that other factors, which lead to disruption of the intracellular signalling mechanisms, may be more important (9).

In the case of pituitary cells under the influence of mutually antagonistic hypothalamic hormones (e.g. somatotrophs), the magnitude of the response to one factor will depend not only on its mode of delivery (pulsatile or sustained) but also on the prevailing tone exerted by the other. For example, a single injection of GHRH may precipitate a marked rise in serum GH; however, a second injection, administered two hours later, may be relatively ineffective not because the cells are refractory to the releasing hormone but because SRIH secretion is increased. Much remains to be learnt about the profiles of GHRH and SRIH release *in vivo*. It seems unlikely that the two peptides are released simultaneously but rather that their secretion is co-ordinated so as to ensure optimal somatotroph function (10). Interactions may also occur between releas-ing factors whose actions on the target cells are complementary. For example, the stimulatory actions of CRH and AVP on the corticotrophs are not additive but powerfully synergistic; thus, the secretory responses to CRH depend largely on the degree of vasopressinergic tone to the corticotrophs and *vice versa* (8, 11).

Secretion of pituitary hormones is also modulated by a variety of blood borne factors (8). Feedback effects, negative and positive, exerted by hormones released from the peripheral endocrine glands in response to pituitary stimulation are particularly important. For example, the thyroid hormones (thyroxine, T_4 and tri-iodothyronine, T_3) exert powerful inhibitory actions on the thyrotrophs and thereby suppress the secretory responses to TRH. Similarly, the adrenocortical steroids (cortisol and corticosterone) and the gonadal hormones (androgens, oestrogens, progestogens, inhibin and related peptides) attenuate the functional activity of the corticotrophs and gonadotrophs respectively. In some instances however oestradiol exerts a positive influence on the gonadotrophs thereby augmenting the actions of GnRH, a phenomenon which is particularly important in initiating the mid-cycle LH surge which triggers ovulation. Similarly, oestrogen may facilitate PRL secretion. Other systemic factors also play a significant role in the regulation of pituitary hormone release, in particular the army of mediators (termed immunokines) released from activated immune cells (see Chapter 13 for further details). In addition, pituitary hormone secretion may be fine-tuned by substances produced locally within the pituitary gland. These may arise from the endocrine cells themselves and thus exert autocrine or paracrine actions (e.g. galanin which is released from a specific cohort of lactotrophs and appears to augment PRL release). Alternatively, they may emanate from the folliculostellate, resident macrophage or dendritic cell populations and thereby exert paracrine influences on the endocrine cells. Particular interest is currently centred on the role of the folliculostellate cells in this regard as these cells not only express "classical endocrine peptides" but also growth factors and cytokines which are likely to exert significant effects on the growth and secretory activity of the endocrine cells. Indeed, recent reports that cytokine expression is increased in conditions of immune challenge point to a role for the folliculostellate cells in the complex interplay between the immune and endocrine systems.

1.2.4   Synthesis and Secretion of the Hypophysiotrophic Hormones

Anatomical Considerations: the Parvocellular System

Anatomical studies have revealed that the hypophysiotrophic hormones are synthesised by parvocellular neurones which originate in the medial hypothalamus and adjacent pre-optic areas; see Table 1.1 and (12) for review. The cell bodies of these neurones are concentrated in four main centres, *viz.* the arcuate, periventricular, paraventricular and ventromedial nuclei although, in some instances, they may be found elsewhere. For example, in the guinea pig and primates the GnRH perikarya are concentrated caudally in the arcuate nucleus while in the rat and the sheep they are located mainly rostrally in the septum and preoptic area. The axons may follow a direct, midline periventricular route to the median eminence (e.g. the majority of the SRIH and TRH neurones which arise in the periventricular nucleus); alternatively, they may project laterally to pursue the lateral retrochiasmatic path, passing caudally via the medial forebrain bundle and turning medially past the optic chiasma to reach the lateral zone of the external median eminence (e.g. the TRH and CRH neurones, which arise in the parvocellular division of the paraventricular nucleus, PVN, and the majority of GnRH neurones). The terminals of the parvocellular neurones lie in close apposition to the capillaries of the hypothalamo-hypophysial portal system into which they release their products for direct transportation to the anterior pituitary gland. It is important to note that the parvocellular AVP neurones, which arise in the PVN and project to the median eminence, are concerned with the regulation of anterior pituitary function, in particular ACTH secretion (see Section 1.3.2). These neurones are functionally and anatomically distinct from the *magnocellular* AVP neurones, which arise both in the PVN and in the supraoptic nucleus (SON) and project to the posterior lobe of the pituitary gland, releasing AVP into the systemic circulation to fulfil its classical role as an antidiuretic and pressor agent (see Section 1.2.5).

Many of the parvocellular neurones also send projections to other sites within the hypothalamus and elsewhere in the brain where the neurohormones they release are likely to subserve other physiological functions. Examples include the SRIH fibres, which pass from the periventricular nucleus to the arcuate nucleus and may thereby modulate the activity of the GHRH cells, and the CRH neurones, which project to sites in the limbic system and brainstem and are strongly implicated in the co-ordination of behavioural and autonomic responses to stress (see also Chapter 2). Studies based on immunohistochemistry and *in situ* hybridisation have shown that the majority of hypophysiotrophic neurones express more than one peptide or transmitter. For example AVP, neurotensin and enkephalin are expressed in abundance in CRH neurones together with smaller amounts of cholecystokinin, vasoactive intestinal polypeptide (VIP) and galanin; however, not all CRH neurones contain AVP and others express GABA. In most instances the physiological significance of the high degree of co-expression is poorly understood although it is widely considered to be associated either with the fine control of hormone release from the nerve terminal or with modulation of hormone action on the target cells. Such arguments are supported by evidence that both GABA and enkephalin depress the release of CRH while AVP acts synergistically with CRH on the corticotrophs (see Section 1.3.2).

Attempts to characterise the neural inputs to the parvocellular neurones have involved a variety of experimental approaches including anatomical investigations at the light and electron microscope levels, electrophysiological studies, biochemical correlations of transmitter turnover with hypothalamo–pituitary activity, functional studies following surgical or pharmacological manipulation of "specific" nervous pathways and *in vitro* studies on acutely removed or cultured hypothalamic tissue. The picture is far from complete but the data accrued advocate significant roles for a number of ascending and descending pathways. A detailed discussion is beyond the scope of this article—for review see (13)—but it is pertinent to note that there are significant inputs from the ascending noradrenergic tracts which originate in the A1 and A6 (locus coeruleus) nuclei, the 5-hydroxytryptaminergic pathways arising in the raphe nuclei and the descending pathways from the limbic system and cortex. In addition, numerous interneurones within the hypothalamus which produce transmitters as diverse as GABA, dopamine, opioid peptides, neuropeptide Y and excitatory amino acids connect with the parvocellular neurones as also do the glial cell population.

Mechanisms of Synthesis and Release

The neuropeptides (e.g. CRH), like the adenohypophysial hormones (see Section 1.2.2), are derived from large precursor molecules; these are formed by gene transcription and translation in the cell body of the neurone and packaged into storage vesicles for transportation down the nerve axon by axoplasmic flow. Post-translational processing of the prohormones occurs within the vesicles during transit and the mature peptides are stored in vesicles in the nerve terminal until required. The non-peptide neurohormones (e.g. dopamine) by contrast are synthesised and packaged primarily in the nerve terminal, using enzymes that are synthesised in the cell body and transported to the terminal by axoplasmic flow.

Release of the mature neurohormones into the portal circulation occurs by a process of Ca^{2+}-dependent exocytosis which is triggered by specific stimuli. Primary control is effected by the complex array of ascending and descending nervous pathways which converge upon the hypothalamus and relay essential information to the parvocellular neurones regarding the circadian periodicity, metabolic and osmotic status, environmental factors, emotional trauma, immune status etc. Secretion is also subject to control by a number of humoral factors which include:

(a) adrenocortical, thyroid and gonadal hormones, which exert feedback effects that are essentially analogous to those they exert at the pituitary level,
(b) pituitary hormones, which exert predominantly negative regulatory influences on the secretion of their respective hypophysiotrophic hormones,
(c) dietary and osmotic factors (e.g. glucose, amino acids, Na^+), and
(d) immunokines released from activated immune cells (see Chapters 9 and 13 for further details).

A further level of control is brought about by local regulatory factors which may originate from the parvocellular neurones themselves or, more probably, from adjacent interneurones or glial cells.

1.2.5   The Control of the Neurohypophysis

The neurohypophysial hormones, AVP and oxytocin, are synthesised in the magnocellular neurones, which arise in the paraventricular and supraoptic hypothalamic nuclei (SON). Although the two neuropeptides are structurally very similar, they are products of different genes and they are synthesised in separate neurones, which can be distinguished on electrophysiological and immunohistochemical grounds and which are subject to different control mechanisms— reviewed in (14). Vasopressin release is triggered by a number of physiological stimuli including:

(a) volume depletion detected by the baroreceptors in the left atrium and pulmonary vein along with those in the carotid sinus and aortic arch (which are also sensitive to chemical stimulants, e.g. hypoxia) and relayed via the nucleus tractus solitarius and the dorsal vagal nuclei to the hypothalamus, and

(b) increases in serum osmolarity, which are detected by osmoreceptors located on the circumventricular organs (subfornical organ, organ vasculosum of the lamina terminalis) and cell bodies of the vasopressinergic neurones.

Vasopressin may also be considered as a stress hormone as it is released into the general circulation in response to emotional trauma, nociceptive factors and other stressful stimuli, apparently via mechanisms dependent on limbic afferents originating mainly in the amygdala and septum (see Section 1.4.5). Numerous neurotransmitter substances have been implicated in the control of vasopressin release including noradrenaline (from the ascending noradrenergic tracts), acetylcholine (mainly via nicotinic receptors), excitatory amino acids and GABA, which exerts powerful inhibitory actions on both the brain stem nuclei and the hypothalamus. Release may be further modulated by humoral substances (e.g. glucocorticoids, immunokines) and by local factors (e.g. opioid peptides) produced by the pituicytes which lie in close proximity to the nerve terminals in the pituitary gland. Oxytocin is produced primarily in labour and in lactation but is also released in response to certain stressors. Its release in lactation is provoked by suckling, which initiates a series of nerve impulses which pass via spinal afferents and the brain stem to the hypothalamus. The mechanisms controlling its release during labour are poorly understood but may involve sensory stimuli arising from the vagina and cervix and, possibly, a reduction in circulating relaxin, a polypeptide reputed to depress oxytocin release in the third trimester of pregnancy. Oxytocin release is also provoked by gastric distension and, like vasopressin, it is sensitive to osmotic stimuli and depressed by alcohol.

1.3   STRESS AND THE HYPOTHALAMO–PITUITARY–ADRENAL (HPA) AXIS

The HPA axis (Fig. 1.3) is responsible for the production of the glucocorticoids (cortisol or corticosterone or both, dependent on species) by the adrenal cortex. In normal circumstances, the activity of the axis is contained within narrow limits with marked excursions in glucocorticoid secretion occurring only in accord with the well established circadian rhythm; serum glucocorticoid levels are thus normally maximal at the end of the sleep phase (i.e. in the morning in diurnal species, e.g. man, and in the evening in nocturnal animals, e.g. the rat) and reach a nadir some hours after waking. However, the HPA axis is readily activated by cognitive and non-cognitive stressful stimuli and the substantial quantities of glucocorticoids which are consequently released into the systemic circulation play a vital role in the maintenance of homeostasis. The HPA axis thus provides an essential interface between the internal and external environment and enables the organism to adapt to diverse noxious stimuli.

Perhaps not surprisingly, the onset, magnitude and duration of the adrenocortical responses to stress are each tailored precisely according to the nature, intensity and duration of the stimulus. For example, insulin-induced hypoglycaemia produces a rapid, dose-dependent rise in serum glucocorticoid concentration which attains a maximum within 20–30 min and declines promptly to base line values when the blood sugar level is restored to normal. By contrast, the adrenocortical response to injection of endotoxin (bacterial lipopolysaccharide, LPS) is delayed, emerging after 1–2 h, and is likely to persist for 24 h or longer. Significant interspecies variations in the responses may also occur; for example, humans are particularly susceptible to emotional trauma whereas the rat and other rodents respond more readily to physical stimuli, such as cold. Failure to mount an appropriate adrenocortical response to stress is potentially hazardous and indeed disturbances in HPA function are now considered to be a significant contributory factor in the aetiology of a variety of disease processes. For example, excessive glucocorticoid secretion (which may arise from a primary disorder of the HPA axis or from causes as diverse as e.g. ectopic ACTH-producing tumours, depression, stress, alcoholism, anorexia) causes diverse metabolic and behavioural disturbances together with immunosuppression which, in turn, may predispose the individual to other diseases, such as infections. Conversely, adrenocortical insufficiency (which may reflect primary or secondary adrenal failure or steroid resistance in the target tissues) precipitates a vulnerability to stress and is increasingly implicated in the pathogenesis of autoimmune, inflammatory and allergic disorders (e.g. rheumatoid arthritis, multiple sclerosis, systemic lupus erythematosus, see Chapter 9).

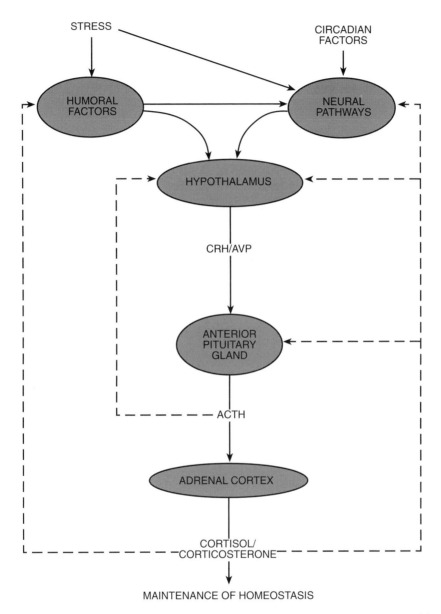

Figure 1.3 The hypothalamo–pituitary–adrenal axis. Solid lines represent positive stimuli; dotted lines represent negative (inhibitory) influences

1.3.1 Stress Protective Properties of the Glucocorticoids

The glucocorticoids exert widespread actions in the body, which together serve to restore homeostasis and thus to protect the organism from stress (15, 16). They are powerful catabolic agents and promote the breakdown of carbohydrate, protein and lipid; they thus mobilise energy reserves and serve as physiological antagonists of insulin. They also play a key role in the regulation of immune and inflammatory cell responses and are required for numerous processes associated with host defence. In general, glucocorticoids are powerfully immunosuppressive, particularly with regard to cell-mediated immune events, although evidence has now emerged to indicate that they augment antibody production. Importantly, glucocorticoids prevent the pathophysiological responses to stresses (such as injury, inflammation and infection) proceeding to a point where they threaten the survival of the host. (Further details of the actions of the steroids on immune and inflammatory cell function are provided in Chapter 8). Glucocorticoids also possess a spectrum of other properties. They have complex effects on bone (in excess leading to osteoporosis) and exert both positive and negative effects on cell growth. They also exhibit significant aldosterone-like actions and may thus modulate salt and water balance. Within the CNS, glucocorticoids target both neuronal and glial cells; they exert important organisational effects pre- and post-natally while in adult life they contribute to neuronal plasticity and are implicated in the processes of neural degeneration. Other central effects of the glucocorticoids include complex changes of mood and behaviour, stimulation of feeding, antipyresis and modulation of neuroendocrine function—for review see (16).

The actions of the glucocorticoids are mediated primarily by the "classical pathway of steroid action", i.e. the free steroid enters the target cell by passive diffusion and binds to an intracellular cytoplasmic receptor which is subsequently translocated to the nucleus where it initiates specific changes in DNA transcription and hence in protein generation (see Chapter 4 for further details). Two distinct subtypes of corticosteroid receptor have been identified, namely the mineralocorticoid receptor (MR) and the glucocorticoid receptor (GR). The MR has a high and approximately equal affinity for aldosterone and the endogenous glucocorticoids, cortisol and corticosterone (K_d ~1–2 nM). The GR, by contrast, is of low affinity (K_d for cortisol/corticosterone ~10–20 nM) but does not bind aldosterone readily and is thus glucocorticoid selective. MRs in epithelial cells are effectively protected from endogenous glucocorticoids by the enzyme 11β-hydroxysteroid dehydrogenase which rapidly inactivates cortisol/corticosterone and thus permits selective access of aldosterone to its receptors. In some cells however (notably in the CNS) MRs are not protected in this way and may therefore be fully occupied at low physiological concentrations of glucocorticoids. MRs may thus contribute to several facets of glucocorticoid action, particularly in the CNS. However, the majority of the actions of the glucocorticoids, particularly those concerned with the suppression of immune or inflammatory responses, are effected by GRs; indeed, MR stimulation appears to oppose at least some of the actions of the glucocorticoids within the immune system (for further details see Chapter 8 and also the Prologue).

GRs are widely distributed throughout the body; the biological responses to receptor stimulation are highly sensitive to receptor concentration, which is known to fluctuate during development, the cell cycle and following disturbances in endocrine status. The level of GR expression may also be altered in other pathological conditions and may contribute to the phenomenon of "steroid resistance" as also may the expression of mutant GRs which bind the ligand but fail to transmit the signal—see Chapter 8 and (17). Increasingly, evidence suggests that, in the short term, the activated glucocorticoid-receptor complex may also exert significant regulatory actions via "non-classical" mechanisms. For example, in some instances activated GR represses genes by interacting with and blocking the activity of transcription factors such as activating protein-1 (AP-1). In addition, the activated receptor complex may regulate post-translational events including mRNA stability and translation, post-translational processing and secretion. These actions are particularly relevant to steroid effects manifest before the full transcriptional effects of the "classical" genomic actions are apparent, for example in the feedback inhibition of ACTH secretion (see Section 1.3.3.). It is also important to note that some aspects of glucocorticoid action may be mediated via interactions of the steroids with cell membranes, thus bypassing intracellular receptors; such actions may involve stimulation of specific membrane bound receptors or, alternatively, allosteric modulation of receptors for other substances (e.g. GABA) by interactions with specific steroid-binding domains within the receptor complex—see also Chapters 4 and 8 and (16).

1.3.2   The Control of Glucocorticoid Secretion

The increases in glucocorticoid secretion that occur in stress are triggered primarily by stimuli which converge upon the hypothalamus and precipitate the release of the corticotrophin releasing hormones, CRH and AVP, into the hypophysial portal vessels—reviewed in (16, 18). These peptides act synergistically on the corticotrophs to augment the episodic secretion of ACTH (see Section 1.2.3), with CRH increasing the amplitude although not the frequency of the pulses and AVP augmenting both parameters. CRH also stimulates the biosynthesis of ACTH and, in the longer term, promotes corticotroph mitogenesis but AVP does not. ACTH is transported in the systemic circulation to target cells in the zona fasciculata of the adrenal cortex where it acts via specific membrane bound receptors to activate the rate limiting enzyme in the steroidogenic pathway; it thereby promotes the conversion of cholesterol to pregnenolone from which cortisol/corticosterone are synthesised rapidly. The newly synthesised hormones are released immediately into the systemic circulation and, dependent on the stress, increases in the serum concentration of the steroids may be apparent within 10 min of the onset of the stimulus. Once in the circulation, approximately 95% of cortisol/corticosterone is bound to a carrier protein called transcortin. The half-life of the endogenous glucocorticoids is approximately 90 min; metabolism occurs in the liver and the resulting conjugated metabolites are excreted in the urine and the bile.

The parvocellular CRH/AVP neurones in the hypothalamus are well positioned to monitor, integrate and respond to emotional insults and physical changes in the internal and external environment which threaten homeostasis. Importantly, these neurones receive inputs from many ascending and descending nervous pathways (16, 18–20). In addition, they are sensitive to a variety of substances which may be relayed via the blood stream or the cerebrospinal fluid (e.g. glucose, immunokines, steroids) and to local factors released from glial cells and/or interneurones. Anatomical, electrophysiological, biochemical and pharmacological studies have identified major roles for the ventral and dorsal ascending noradrenergic bundles and for pathways originating in the raphe nuclei, the hippocampus and the amygdala but other tracts (arising, for example, elsewhere in the limbic system and in the cortex) probably also fulfil significant roles. Many neurotransmitter systems have been implicated in these systems including acetylcholine, 5-hydroxytryptamine (5-HT) and noradrenaline, all of which exert stimulatory influences, GABA which powerfully inhibits CRH/AVP release and various neuropeptides (e.g. opioids, neuropeptide Y, VIP). Not surprisingly, the complement of neural pathways, humoral substances and local mediators which orchestrates the release of CRH/AVP in stress depends on the nature of the stimulus. Thus, for example, the HPA responses to hypotension (caused by haemorrhage or by injection of sodium nitroprusside) depend on the integrity of the noradrenergic pathways which project from the brain stem to the PVN. On the other hand, the increases in glucocorticoid secretion provoked by certain emotional trauma require inputs from the limbic system, while those to cold depend on connections between peripheral C-fibres and the PVN. Furthermore, since in normal subjects AVP appears not to be expressed by all of the CRH fibres, the ratio of CRH:AVP released may vary in a stimulus specific manner according to the subpopulation of CRH neurones stimulated; moreover, further fine tuning of the CRH:AVP ratio may be brought about by differential release of the peptides from individual neurones.

Since the mid 1980s, innumerable studies have focused on the mechanisms by which immune insults activate the HPA axis (18). This work is considered in Chapters 9–13 and only a brief overview will be provided here. The evidence available argues strongly that the neuroendocrine responses to stimuli such as infections and inflammatory lesions are driven primarily by the battery of mediators (immunokines) released from activated immune or inflammatory cells. Many of these substances have been shown to be potent activators of the HPA axis; these include certain interleukins (e.g. IL-1β and IL-6), interferons, phospholipid metabolites (notably eicosanoids), peptides (e.g. bradykinin, angiotensin II, thymic peptides) and amines (e.g. histamine, 5-HT) together with enzymes such as PLA$_2$ which are released into the systemic circulation in conditions such as septicaemia. Some of these agents (e.g. IL-1β, IL-6, PLA$_2$, eicosanoids) appear to target the HPA axis directly, acting mainly within the CNS (notably at the hypothalamus) but also on the anterior pituitary gland and the adrenal cortex to trigger hormone release. Others (e.g. prostanoids) however may act locally at the site of the inflammatory lesion to stimulate the primary nociceptive afferents and thereby activate central pathways which precipitate CRH/AVP release. In addition, many of the mediators provoke widespread pathological effects in the body (e.g. hypotension, hypoglycaemia) which are perceived as stressful by the organism and may therefore activate the HPA axis by other means. A further potential mechanism for communication between the immune and HPA systems lies in the propensity of the two systems to produce and use common chemical mediators and receptors in conditions such as infection and inflammation. For example, in rodents a peripheral endotoxin challenge stimulates the synthesis of cytokines such as IL-1 and IL-6 in the hypothalamus and other areas of the CNS, possibly via mechanisms dependent on the generation of prostanoids at the level of the blood–brain barrier or on the integrity of vagal afferents. Furthermore, activated immune or inflammatory cells produce ACTH, β-endorphin and other POMC products together with CRH- and AVP-like peptides. Teleological arguments favour a local regulatory role (autocrine, paracrine or intracrine) for these agents, a view supported by the wealth of evidence that IL-1 and IL-6 are potent activators of the HPA axis at the level of the hypothalamus and that ACTH, β-endorphin, CRH and AVP each exhibit significant immunoregulatory properties. However, since migratory cells of immunological lineage are found in abundance in both the anterior pituitary gland and the adrenal cortex, it is possible that the peptides they release target the endocrine cells directly and thereby provoke the release of ACTH and the glucocorticoids. The activation of the HPA axis by immune insults is thus a complex event potentially requiring the integration of a broad spectrum of stimuli, the complement of which will reflect the nature and intensity of the insult.

1.3.3   Negative Feedback Control of the HPA Axis

The adrenocortical responses to incoming stimuli (i.e. stress and circadian factors) are effectively contained within appropriate limits by a complex series of mechanisms through which the glucocorticoids negatively regulate their own secretion—see (20–22) for detailed review. Thus, the reductions in circulating corticosteroids (evident, for example, in Addison's disease or following adrenalectomy) are accompanied by a sustained hypersecretion of ACTH and an exaggeration of the pituitary adrenocorticotrophic responses to stress, both of which are readily corrected by replacement therapy with glucocorticoids. Conversely, increases in steroid levels, brought about for example by adrenocortical tumours or administration of exogenous glucocorticoids, effectively suppress the resting and stress-induced ACTH release. Perhaps not surprisingly, the HPA responses to immune insults are particularly sensitive to alterations in glucocorticoid status. This is due in part to the powerful ability of the steroids to suppress the release and/or pathophysiological actions of various cytokines and other inflammatory mediators (e.g. eicosanoids) which normally trigger the HPA response (see also Chapter 8). However, there is also evidence that the stimulatory actions of various immunokines within the HPA axis are subject to glucocorticoid regulation—see also Chapter 13 and (19, 20).

The feedback actions of steroids are highly complex, as they are exerted at multiple sites within the brain and pituitary gland and they utilise at least three distinct mechanisms which are effective over different time domains. These are termed: (a) rapid or fast feedback, (b) early delayed feedback, and (c) late delayed feedback (21, 22).

Phases of Glucocorticoid Feedback

Rapid feedback develops within seconds of an increase in glucocorticoid levels; it is of short duration (< 10 min) and is followed by a "silent period" during which the stress response is intact, even though the plasma steroid level may remain elevated. Rapid feedback is sensitive to the rate of change rather than the absolute concentration of steroid in the blood and may therefore provide an important means whereby the stress response can be blunted if the corticoid level is already rising in response to a previous stimulus.

The second or "early delayed" phase of feedback develops approximately 1–2 h after the initial elevation of plasma steroid levels; it is normally maximal within 2–4 h and, depending on the intensity of the stimulus, may persist for up to 24 h. Both the circadian and the stress-induced excursions in ACTH secretion are suppressed with an intensity that is directly proportional to the concentration of steroid previously reached in the blood.

Late delayed feedback, which has a latency of about 24 h, develops only after a very substantial rise in steroid levels and is frequently the consequence of repeated or continuous administration of high doses of corticosteroids. It may persist for days or weeks after the steroid treatment is withdrawn and is thus largely responsible for the potentially life-threatening suppression of the HPA axis associated with the abrupt cessation of long term treatment with high doses of steroids in, for example, patients with rheumatoid arthritis.

Mechanisms of Glucocorticoid Feedback

The rapid feedback actions of the glucocorticoids are exerted primarily at the hypothalamic level; weaker actions also occur at the pituitary level but the contribution, if any, of extrahypothalamic sites in the CNS is ill-defined. The underlying molecular mechanisms are poorly understood. Although there are some reports to the contrary, the majority of data suggests that these effects are non-genomic (and hence do not involve MR or GR) and that they may be mediated by receptors that are located close to or within cell membranes and which, when activated, inhibit exocytosis, possibly by blocking Ca^{2+} influx (see Section 1.3.1).

The early and late delayed phases of feedback inhibition, by contrast, are mediated by classical intracellular corticosteroid receptors located primarily in the anterior pituitary gland, the hypothalamus and the hippocampus, but also elsewhere in the brain. Both the high affinity MRs and the lower affinity GRs (see Section 1.3.1) are involved. Current evidence suggests that MRs (located predominantly in the hippocampus) may maintain the tonic inhibitory influence of steroids on HPA function in non-stress conditions as these receptors, which are not "protected" by 11β-hydroxysteroid dehydrogenase, are normally almost fully occupied by glucocorticoids even at the nadir of the circadian rhythm. GRs on the other hand (found in particular abundance in the anterior pituitary gland and hypothalamus) are extensively occupied only when the glucocorticoid level is raised, for example by stress, disease or administration of exogenous steroids. Thus, unlike MR, these receptors detect phasic changes in steroid levels and serve to restore glucocorticoid release to the basal (i.e. non-stress) level (23).

Several lines of evidence suggest that early delayed feedback is dependent on the de novo generation of protein second messengers, which inhibit the release rather than the synthesis of ACTH and its hypothalamic releasing factors. The nature of the second messenger proteins is unclear but recent studies in our laboratory suggest that lipocortin 1 (LC1) (a Ca^{2+} and phospholipid binding protein strongly implicated in anti-inflammatory and anti-proliferative actions of the steroids) may be important in this regard—see Chapter 8 and (20).

Unlike the early delayed phase, late delayed feedback is characterised by inhibition of the synthesis and the release of CRH/AVP and ACTH in the hypothalamus and anterior pituitary gland respectively (20). The inhibition of synthesis is in effect an exaggeration of the tonic, GR-mediated inhibitory influence of the endogenous glucocorticoids on the genes encoding each of the three peptides. The concomitant inhibition of peptide release cannot be explained in this way as peptide stores are rarely fully depleted. Reductions in the pools available for release may be important in this regard but the underlying molecular mechanisms await explanation.

Short Loop and Ultra-short Loop Feedback Mechanisms

In addition to the corticosteroids, other hormones of the HPA axis participate in the feedback regulation of ACTH secretion (22). Of particular importance are the POMC derived peptides, ACTH and β-endorphin, both of which have been shown to exert powerful inhibitory actions on the secretion of CRH/AVP by the hypothalamus. Since neither peptide readily penetrates the blood–brain barrier, their "short loop" feedback actions are probably exerted at the level of the median eminence, which lies outside the blood–brain barrier. Ultra-short loop feedback actions have been attributed to both CRH and AVP but the physiological significance of such responses is unclear.

1.3.4   HPA Responses to Repeated or Sustained Stress

The bulk of studies on stress and HPA function have focused on acute stresses and relatively little is known of either the characteristics or the mechanisms controlling the HPA responses to repeated or sustained stress—for detailed review see (24). Such conditions are of course inherent to our lifestyle and environment and a deeper understanding of their influence on neuroendocrine function is thus highly desirable. However, for both ethical and practical reasons it is difficult to develop appropriate animal models and, as described below, the data available suggest that the profile of the HPA responses observed may vary considerably according to the nature of the stress.

In some cases, the HPA responses to repeated (successive or intermittent) or sustained (chronic) stressful stimuli are attenuated. For example, "tolerance" develops to stresses such as cold, handling, saline injection or water deprivation (induced by replacement of drinking water with physiological saline). Some degree of "cross tolerance" may occur between stresses that invoke similar pathways or mechanisms to increase CRH/AVP release. Thus, for example, repeated handling reduces the subsequent adrenocortical response to a saline injection; however, rats tolerant to the C-fibre dependent stress of exposure to a cold environment respond to a novel psychological stress (e.g. immobilisation) with a normal or even exaggerated rise in serum corticosterone. In other situations however, the HPA responses to intermittent stress (e.g. electric foot shock, insulin-induced hypoglycaemia) or chronic stress (e.g. septicaemia) are maintained or even enhanced; i.e. tolerance does not develop. The mechanisms whereby this "adaptation" occurs are poorly understood. It has been suggested that the continued release of CRH/AVP in repetitive restraint stress is facilitated by an increase in the neuronal drive to the PVN which effectively overcomes the increased negative feedback drive exerted by the elevated levels of glucocorticoids. Others however have described marked reductions in the expression of MRs in the hippocampus and GRs in the PVN in conditions of chronic stress and suggested that the negative feedback mechanism itself may be disrupted. A further hypothesis has emerged from studies in rats subjected to repeated stresses such as immobilisation or insulin-induced hypoglycaemia, namely the sustained hypersecretion of ACTH is driven primarily by AVP which is synthesised in and released from the parvocellular neurones in the PVN in preference to CRH (24). To our knowledge the factors driving AVP synthesis in this condition are not known, although impaired glucocorticoid feedback is a likely candidate. Interestingly the expression of AVP but not CRH in the parvocellular division of the PVN is also increased in rats subjected to the sustained stress of experimentally induced arthritis (see Chapter 9). Moreover, AVP has recently been implicated in the aetiology of the hypercortisolaemia evident in depression. More studies are now required to distinguish between different types of stress in terms of the anatomical pathways and the corticotrophin releasing factors they employ.

1.3.5 Age and Gender Related Changes in HPA Function

The functional development of the HPA axis begins in fetal life and in the later stages of gestation the fetus secretes substantial quantities of cortisol/corticosterone. It also responds to stress with increases in adrenocortical activity which are driven by the hypothalamo–pituitary axis and which are sensitive to the negative feedback actions of the glucocorticoids. Paradoxically, in the rat and several other species HPA function regresses postnatally and a period ensues during which the neonate fails to release adequate amounts of glucocorticoids in response to traumatic stimuli (e.g. endotoxaemia). Interestingly, this potentially hazardous phase of adrenocortical insufficiency, termed the stress hyporesponsive phase (SHRP), coincides with an important phase of immunological development and may be significant in this respect. Its aetiology is ill-defined although it has been attributed to immaturity of the hypothalamic CRH/AVP neurones, which fail to respond to neurochemical and humoral stimuli, and to a "supersensitivity" of the axis to the feedback actions of the steroids (25). Increasing evidence suggests that disturbances in the programming of the HPA axis in fetal and early neonatal life may predispose the individual to hypertension and other disease states in adult life. In the same vein, exposure to emotional trauma during this critical period has been shown to have important long term consequences for HPA function. For example removal of neonatal rats from their mothers for one day results in adrenal hypertrophy and raised serum corticosterone concentrations in adulthood; moreover, the adrenocortical response to stress is prolonged and immune function is compromised. By contrast, regular but brief separation of neonatal rats from their mothers is not associated with overt changes in HPA function in the adult and, indeed, animals reared in this way are particularly well equipped to cope with stress throughout their adult life (see also Chapter 2).

In adults, distinct sexually dimorphic patterns of glucocorticoid secretion emerge. Serum glucocorticoid concentrations are consistently higher in the female than the male with further increases occurring towards the middle of the menstrual or oestrous cycle just prior to ovulation and in the late stages of pregnancy. These changes are due partly to the positive effects of oestrogen on the expression of the corticosteroid binding globulin (transcortin). In addition, oestrogen exerts significant effects at the hypothalamic level increasing the synthesis and the release of CRH, a phenomenon which may be implicated in the aetiology of the relatively high incidence of emotional disorders (e.g. depression, anxiety) in the female which are characterised by enhanced CRH secretion (26). Further modulation may be brought about by progesterone which, when present in large amounts (e.g. in the pre-menstrual phase or pregnancy), binds readily to, but is only weakly active at, mineralocorticoid receptors in the hippocampus.

In both sexes, the serum glucocorticoid concentrations tend to increase in ageing individuals, particularly in disease states (19). The reasons for this are unknown but several lines of evidence suggest that this phenomenon may be an important contributory factor to the age-related decline in immunocompetence.

1.4 OTHER NEUROENDOCRINE RESPONSES TO STRESS

1.4.1 Prolactin

PRL is frequently described as a "stress hormone". This nomenclature originated from reports that various acute stressors elicit the release of PRL both in experimental animals and in man. However, serum PRL levels are not always raised by stress and increasing evidence suggests that the profile of the PRL response depends on the nature and duration of the stimulus and on the endocrine status of the individual—for detailed review see (27).

There is now general agreement that stresses such as ether anaesthesia, surgery, restraint, insulin-induced hypoglycaemia and cold normally precipitate a prompt, short lasting hypersecretion of PRL. The literature concerning PRL responses to acute immunological insults is, however, less consistent and, while some data suggest that exposure to endotoxin, IL-1 or IL-6 may increase PRL release, others show that PRL secretion is either unchanged or inhibited by these stimuli (28, 29). Several lines of evidence suggest that the capacity of an individual to release PRL in acute stress is influenced markedly by the pre-existing serum PRL concentration. Thus, stresses such as ether anaesthesia and restraint readily stimulate PRL release when the serum PRL is low; however, if applied at a time when the circulating levels of the pituitary hormone are raised (e.g. on the afternoon of pro-oestrus or during lactation), these stimuli para-doxically produce a prompt inhibition of PRL release (27). The stress induced secretion of PRL is also sensitive to alterations in glucocorticoid tone (29). Exogenous glucocorticoids thus attenuate the hypersecretion of PRL provoked by psychological trauma and by physical stresses such as foot shock, hypogly-caemia, ether anaesthesia and restraint. Conversely, adrenalectomy, whether surgical or pharmacological (by administration of a GR antagonist) produces a glucocorticoid-reversible augmentation of the PRL responses to a variety of stressors. The inhibitory actions of the steroids have been attributed to actions in the CNS, in particular the hypothalamus, and in the pituitary gland where both the synthesis and the release of PRL are blocked.

The mechanisms by which acute stress increases PRL secretion are unknown. Limited evidence suggests that the responses reflect increased secretion of prolactin releasing factors (notably VIP) by the hypothalamus rather than suppression of the release of dopamine (the major PRL release inhibiting factor), and that central histaminergic and 5-hydroxytryptaminergic pathways are in-volved in driving the responses. In addition, the neurohypophysial hormones, in particular AVP, may play a significant role. Interestingly, there are reports which suggest that certain stressors augment the activity of the hypothalamic dopami-nergic neurones (27). Such an action is unlikely to temper the stress-induced hypersecretion of PRL observed when pre-existing levels of PRL are low, as the dopaminergic tone to the lactotrophs is already maximal or near maximal. It could, however, contribute significantly to the stress-induced depression of PRL release observed when PRL levels are high as, in these circumstances, the tonic dopaminergic drive to the lactotrophs is minimal.

The significance of alterations in PRL secretion observed in stress is obscure and studies in the rat suggest that the physiological consequences are minimal and, in particular, that reproductive function is near normal (27). PRL has significant immune enhancing properties (see Chapter 16 for further details) and it is therefore possible that the prompt changes in serum PRL observed in stress serve to fine tune immune status and thus to modulate the immunosuppressive actions of the corticosteroids that are released subsequently.

1.4.2   Growth Hormone

Many stresses influence the secretion of GH but the profile of the observed response depends upon the species. Thus, in man and other primates stresses such as insulin-induced hypoglycaemia, exercise, sudden perturbations in environment, painful stimuli, haemorrhage, administration of histamine or adrenaline, emotional stress, pyrogen injection, major surgery, restraint, high intensity sound and ether anaesthesia all evoke overt increases in GH release. In contrast, these and other stimuli (e.g. electric shock, cold, handling and hypertonic glucose) produce marked decreases in plasma GH in rats. Endotoxin also inhibits GH secretion in rats, although a rebound increase in GH secretion may occur on the following day (30). When administered repeatedly, stresses such as immobilisation, noise or exposure to ether continue to depress the secretion of GH in the rat with little, if any, sign of adaptation. Moreover, rats exposed to a repetitive stress respond to a novel acute stress with a reduction in GH secretion which is quantitatively similar to or more marked than that observed in control rats (31, 32). Little is known about the effects of repeated or sustained stress on GH secretion in man although long term stress prior to puberty is associated with stunted growth and development.

Although there are data to the contrary, increasing evidence suggests that the inhibition of GH release provoked in the rat by many stresses is due primarily to increased secretion of the hypothalamic neuropeptide, SRIH. For example, passive immunisation of rats against SRIH prevents the decrease in serum GH induced by endotoxin and other stresses (30). In the same vein, studies using push–pull cannulae have shown that immobilisation stress, applied acutely or repetitively, increases the release of SRIH in the median eminence whilst acute exposure to ether is associated with an increase in SRIH in the anterior pituitary gland (33–35). Other workers, however, have failed to demonstrate an increase in hypothalamic SRIH release in rats exposed to endotoxin, raising the possibility that the inhibition of GH release provoked by the stress is due, at least in part, to inhibition of GHRH secretion (36). This concept is supported by findings that IL-1, which appears to be an important mediator of the GH response to endotoxin, inhibits GHRH release *in vitro* (37).

Little is known about the neural pathways which converge upon the hypothalamus to effect the stress-induced inhibition of GH secretion. Several lines of evidence suggest that the GH responses to acute exposure to ether are temporarily correlated with increases in noradrenaline metabolism in several hypothalamic nuclei including the PVN, the dorsomedial nuclei and the arcuate nucleus. In addition, dopamine metabolism is selectively augmented in the rostral division of the arcuate nucleus while 5-HT metabolism is differentially affected by stresses such as ether, with decreases occurring in the PVN and SON and increases in the suprachiasmatic nucleus (38). Observations that CRH inhibits GH release and that the inhibition of GH secretion produced by electric shock is abolished by central administration of a CRH antagonist favour a role for CRH in the GH response to stress (39). Since the responses to CRH *in vivo* are blocked by antisera against SRIH (40) and CRH stimulates SRIH release from cultured fetal hypothalamic cells (41), it seems likely that the actions of this neuropeptide are mediated by an increase in SRIH release.

Although long-term therapy with glucocorticoids is well known to depress the secretion of GH and to impair growth, the extent to which endogenous adrenal steroids modulate the GH response to stress is unclear. It seems unlikely that the glucocorticoids released in response to an acute stress contribute to the decrease in GH secretion provoked by the stimulus as the GH response occurs too rapidly. However, glucocorticoids may modulate the GH responses to repetitive stress. Their actions may be explained, in part, by inhibition of the release of SRIH from the hypothalamus, as immunoneutralisation of SRIH enhances the GH response to GHRH in dexamethasone treated rats (42). Furthermore, administration of dexamethasone *in vivo* increases hypothalamic SRIH mRNA and immunoreactivity, while decreasing the hypothalamic content of immunoreactive GHRH (43). In addition, the steroids may exert significant actions at the pituitary level.

1.4.3   The Hypothalamo–Pituitary–Gonadal Axis

It is well known that the activity of the hypothalamo–pituitary–gonadal (HPG) axis is sensitive to stress. The nature of the response depends on several factors including the species, the duration of the stress, the age and sex of the animals and the gonadal steroid milieu. Chronic stress results invariably in a decrease in plasma LH concentration and consequent disruption of reproductive function. In contrast, the LH responses to acute stress are more variable and, dependent on the conditions, LH secretion may be inhibited, stimulated or unchanged. Alternatively, a biphasic response may emerge, in which an initial rise in serum LH is followed by a phase of impaired LH secretion. The divergent effects of acute stress on LH release have been attributed, at least in part, to differences in oestrogen levels for, while acute stress increases LH secretion in oestrogen primed female rats, when applied to ovariectomised rats not receiving oestrogen replacement it inhibits the secretion of the pituitary hormone. The stimulatory effects of acute stress on LH secretion are mimicked by acute injections of ACTH or corticosteroids, with the responses to the former being dependent upon the release of adrenal steroids. On the other hand, when given chronically, ACTH and corticosteroids depress reproductive function and thus mimic the effects of long-term stress.

Much remains to be learnt about the mechanisms by which the corticosteroids exert their stimulatory and inhibitory effects on LH secretion but the data available suggest that, in both instances, the anterior pituitary gland and the hypothalamus are important targets (44). Corticosteroid receptor immunoreactivity has been detected in catecholaminergic neurones of rat brain and, since catecholamines are important regulators of GnRH secretion, it has been proposed that the inhibitory effects of corticosteroids and stress on LH secretion are exerted in part via actions on catecholaminergic pathways. This concept is supported by findings that the stress induced inhibition of LH is blocked by an inhibitor of noradrenaline synthesis and by the α-adrenoceptor antagonist, phenoxybenzamine (44). Intrahypothalamic opioidergic pathways also play a key role in effecting the stress-induced suppression of GnRH secretion, acting via μ or ϵ and κ but not δ opioid receptors (45). Reports that opioid receptor antagonists reverse the suppressive effects of corticosteroids and ACTH on LH secretion raise the possibility that the steroid-induced inhibition of gonadotrophin secretion may also involve modulation of opioidergic transmission (44).

Substantial evidence suggests that CRH and AVP participate in the inhibition of HPG activity induced in the rat by physical but not immunological stresses. For example, *in vivo* i.c.v. administration of the CRH receptor antagonist, α-helical CRH_{9-41} prevents the decrease in plasma LH concentration caused by mild electric shocks or fasting although not by IL-1. Moreover, the LH response to acute stress is attenuated in rats congenitally lacking hypothalamic AVP (Brattleboro strain) and both CRH and AVP depress the release of GnRH from the rat hypothalamus *in vitro*. In primates by contrast, CRH is also implicated in the LH responses to IL-1 and thus peripheral administration of α-helical CRH_{9-41} prevents IL-1α-induced inhibition of LH release in ovariectomised monkeys (46). Emerging data suggest that the population of CRH neurones concerned with the regulation of HPG function is distinct from that controlling ACTH secretion and it is now apparent, for example, that the inhibition of LH release provoked by foot shock stress in unaffected by electrolytic lesioning of the PVN (46), although whether this holds true for other stresses is not known. It is also unclear whether CRH or AVP act directly on the GnRH neurones or whether their actions involve intermediary pathways. Reports that the CRH-induced inhibition of LH secretion is blocked by the opioid receptor antagonist, naloxone, argue for an intermediary role for endogenous opioid peptides (47). On the other hand, immunocytochemical studies have revealed direct synaptic connections between CRH and GnRH containing neurones in the medial preoptic area (i.e. the locus of the GnRH perikarya) and infusion of CRH into the medial preoptic area inhibits the release *in vivo* of GnRH in the median eminence. Other data show that CRH also inhibits GnRH release from fragments of medial basal hypothalamus (which exclude the medial preoptic area), suggesting that CRH may also depress GnRH secretion via an action on the nerve terminals (46).

1.4.4   The Hypothalamo–Pituitary–Thyroid Axis

The hypothalamo–pituitary–thyroid (HPT) axis is unaffected by mild stresses but generally responds to more severe acute stresses (such as ether exposure, restraint, orbital sinus puncture under light anaesthesia, forced exercise, infection and immobilisation) with a rapid decrease in serum TSH. However, some stresses produce marked increases in TSH secretion in the rat and man, for example acute noise, forced swimming and exposure to cold. Furthermore, the suppression of TSH secretion induced by endotoxin in rats is followed by a rebound increase in TSH release (30). Repetitive stress (e.g. immobilisation and noise) either fails to influence or decreases serum TSH levels. Cross tolerance between stresses has not been reported and the evidence available suggests that animals subjected to repeated stress respond to a novel acute stress with alterations in TSH release which are typical of those mounted to the acute stimulus (31, 32).

Little is known about the mechanisms whereby TSH release is inhibited by certain stresses. Repetitive immobilisation stress does not affect the TSH response to exogenous TRH, suggesting that the pituitary response to the releasing factor is intact (31). A decrease in the release of hypothalamic TRH appears more likely since the inhibitory effects of IL-1 and IL-6 on TSH secretion are associated with a decrease in hypothalamic TRH. In addition, IL-1α decreases hypothalamic proTRH mRNA (31).

More information is available on the TSH response to cold stress, probably because cold is an important physiological stimulus to the HPT axis and the consequent release of the thyroid hormones serves to raise the basal metabolic rate and, hence, to increase core temperature. Studies in experimental animals have shown repeatedly that acute exposure to cold results in increased TSH secretion, raised blood levels of T_3 and variable changes in serum T_4, with the rises in TSH and T_3 levels emerging within 15–30 min and 1–2 h respectively. However, there are conflicting reports on the HPT responses to chronic cold exposure and, although several workers have shown that plasma levels of TSH and T_3 are significantly raised, others have claimed that the plasma TSH concentration remains unchanged (48–50). These discrepancies may reflect differences in experimental technique, such as intensity and duration of the stimulus, sampling times and procedures. It is generally accepted that hyper-secretion of TSH provoked by acute cold stress is due to increased release of TRH from the hypothalamus. Evidence to support this concept includes findings that the TSH responses are diminished by administration of TRH antiserum or by destruction of PVN, a procedure which reduces hypothalamic TRH. Further-more, cold exposure raises the TRH content of the median eminence and anterior hypothalamus–preoptic area and causes an increase in TRH release in vivo in both the mediobasal hypothalamus and the median eminence (51, 52). The TRH responses have, in turn, been attributed primarily to activation of central noradrenergic systems since drugs which block α-adrenoceptors (phentolamine or prazosin) reduce the release of TRH into the median eminence induced by cold (51) while phenoxybenzamine (another α-adrenoceptor antagonist) blocks the associated rise in serum TSH as also do inhibitors of dopamine-β-hydro-xylase (53). The role of other central neurotransmitters in the TSH responses to cold is less clear; some studies suggest that 5-hydroxytryptaminergic and cholinergic pathways may be involved but other data do not support this view (54, 55). Other studies which demonstrate a failure of naloxone to modulate the TRH response argue against a role for the endogenous opioid peptides (56).

1.4.5   Neurohypophysial Responses to Stress

The release of both AVP and oxytocin from the neural lobe of the pituitary gland into the general circulation is influenced by various stresses. As already mentioned in Section 1.2.5, increases in plasma AVP levels are produced by stresses involving changes in plasma osmolality, blood volume and blood pressure (for example, water deprivation and haemorrhage). In man, non-osmotic stresses such as nausea, surgery, exercise, insulin-induced hypoglycaemia and psychological stress also increase vasopressin secretion. There are reports that hypoglycaemia, foot shock and ether also raise serum AVP levels in the rat but the majority of data available suggest that, in this species, AVP secretion is normally unaffected by these and other non-osmotic stresses, such as cold, restraint, noise and novel environment. Stress-induced increases in plasma AVP levels are not always associated with changes in AVP mRNA in magnocellular neurones. Thus, although AVP mRNA is increased during salt loading and prolonged dehydration, it is unaffected by acute osmotic stress. Exposure to stress also increases AVP mRNA in parvocellular neurones which are involved in the control of ACTH secretion—for review see (57).

In contrast to vasopressin, oxytocin release in rats is increased both by osmotic stimuli (e.g. administration of hypertonic saline) and by non-osmotic stresses such as immobilisation, swimming, ether and hypoglycaemia. Insulin-induced hypoglycaemia and other stimuli also increase plasma oxytocin levels in humans but behavioural stresses decrease oxytocin secretion in other primates. Changes in magnocellular oxytocin mRNA levels have not been demonstrated in the acute response to stress. There is evidence, however, that oxytocin released in response to immobilisation stress originates from the parvocellular division of the PVN. The physiological role of oxytocin released during stress is not clear but a hypophysiotrophic action on the corticotrophs seems likely, since oxytocin and CRH are co-localised in parvocellular and magnocellular neurones. In addition, oxytocin may contribute to the metabolic and immune responses to stress—for review see (57).

1.5   CONCLUSION

The activity of the neuroendocrine system is altered markedly in conditions of acute or chronic stress. The profile of the hormonal responses observed is tailored to the stimulus and thus depends on the nature of the stress, its intensity and its duration and may be further modified according to the individual and its state of health. Invariably, the most overt response is the activation of the HPA axis which confers resistance to stress and is thus critical to the survival of the host. The physiological significance of the alterations in other aspects of pituitary function provoked by stress is less clear, although the reductions in the secretion of TSH and GH evident in many situations may be regarded as energy conserving, particularly in the case of intermittent or sustained chronic stress. Similarly, the concomitant impairment of HPG function may be regarded as protective.

The stress-protective properties of the corticosteroids have been attributed, at least in part, to their modulatory actions on the immune system and, hence, on the body's defence system (15). In normal circumstances, glucocorticoids exert a tonic inhibitory action on immune and inflammatory cells but they are not present in sufficient quantities to prevent the host mounting an effective response to an immune insult. The hypersecretion of glucocorticoids evoked by such insults is largely dependent on and thus occurs after the activation of immune and inflammatory cells. This sequence precludes any possibility that steroids released in response to the immune insult modulate important events that occur in the early stages of the immune or inflammatory response (e.g. clonal proliferation of lymphocytes); however, it provides ample opportunity for the steroids to contain events at a later stage and thus to prevent the response proceeding to a point where it threatens the host (15). Nevertheless, there are some circumstances in which such a hypersecretion of glucocorticoids may not be advantageous to the host, for example, the immunosuppression consequent on steroid release in response to a viral challenge is well known to render the host susceptible to opportunist bacterial or fungal infections. Similarly, numerous studies suggest that the persistent elevation of glucocorticoids caused by chronic stress may increase susceptibility to infection (58). For example, repeated restraint stress reduces the ability of mice to combat infections such as influenza virus or mycobacterium. Inevitably, the data from human studies are more difficult to interpret but, nonetheless, the positive correlation between psychological stress (e.g. bereavement, unemployment) and the prevalence of diseases such as infections cannot be denied.

While excessive glucocorticoid secretion leads to immunosuppression, further evidence from studies on experimental animals suggests that adrenocortical insufficiency may be an important contributory factor in the pathogenesis of autoimmune and inflammatory disorders—see also Chapters 8 and 9 and (58). Again, hard clinical data are difficult to obtain but evidence is beginning to emerge that the HPA axis is disturbed in at least some patients with autoimmune disease and that peripheral glucocorticoid resistance may be a further factor in the aetiology of inflammatory disease. For example, reductions in the basal a.m. serum cortisol levels and in the cortisol responses to surgery have been described in patients with rheumatoid- but not osteo-arthritis. Small reductions in adrenal function have also been reported in cohorts of patients with multiple sclerosis and fibromyalgia while, interestingly, patients with systemic lupus erythematosus are frequently glucocorticoid resistant, possibly because the glucocorticoid receptor is expressed in an aberrant form or the associated signal transduction mechanisms are defective (see also Chapter 8). These important findings have rekindled research into the physiology and pathology of the HPA axis and its complex relationship with the immune system; many new avenues await investigation and it is predicted that the data accrued from both basic and clinical studies will enhance our understanding of the pathogenesis of immune and inflammatory disease and may ultimately lead to the identification of novel targets for therapeutic intervention.

REFERENCES

1. Harris G. W. *Neural Control of the Pituitary.* London, Edward Arnold, 1955.
2. Ju G., Liu S.-J. and Ma D. Calcitonin gene-related peptide and substance P-like immunoreactive innervation of the anterior pituitary in the rat. *Neuroscience*, 1993, **54**: 981–9.
3. Houben E. and Denef C. Bioactive peptides in anterior pituitary cells. *Peptides*, 1994, **15**: 547–82.
4. Horvath E. and Kovacs K. Fine structural cytology of the adenohypophysis in the rat and man. *J Electron Microscop Tech*, 1988, **8**: 401–32.
5. Yoshimura F., Haremiya K., Yachi H., Soji T. and Yokoyama M. Degranulated acidophils as a possible source of "thyroidectomy cells" in the rat hypophysis. *Endocrinol Jpn*, 1973, **20**: 181–9.
6. Allaerts W., Carmeliet P. and Denef C. New perspectives in the function of pituitary folliculo-stellate cells. *Mol Cell Endocrinol*, 1990, **71**: 73–81.
7. Allaerts W., Fluitsma E. C. M., Hoefsit P. H. M., Jeucken H., Morreau F. T., Bosman F. T. and Drexhage H. A. Immunohistochemical, morphological and ultrastructural resemblance between dendritic cells and folliculo-stellate cells in normal human and rat anterior pituitaries. *J Neuroendocrinology*, 1996, **8**: 17–30.
8. Buckingham J. C. and Gillies G. E. Hypothalamus and pituitary gland – xenobiotic induced toxicity and models for its investigation. In C. K. Atterwill and J. D. Flack (eds) *Endocrine Toxicology*. Cambridge University Press, Cambridge, 1992, pp 83–114.
9. Marshall L. A., Monroe S. E. and Jaffe R. B. Physiologic and therapeutic aspects of GnRH and its analogues. *Frontiers in Neuroendocrinology*, 1988, **10**: 239–78.
10. Frohman L. A., Downs T. R. and Chomczynski P. Regulation of growth hormone secretion. *Frontiers in Neuroendocrinology*, 1992, **13**: 344–405.
11. Gillies G. E., Linton E. A. and Lowry P. J. Corticotrophin releasing activity of the new CRF is potentiated several times by vasopressin. *Nature*, 1982, **299**: 355–7.
12. Page R. B. The anatomy of the hypothalamo–pituitary complex. In E. Knobil and J. D. Neill (eds) *The Physiology of Reproduction*. New York, Raven Press, 1994, pp 1527–619.
13. Brodal P. Central Autonomic System: The Hypothalamus. In *The Central Nervous*

System: Structure and Function. New York, Oxford University Press Inc, 1992, pp 368–82.

14. Baylis P. H. The posterior pituitary. In G. M. Besser and M. O. Thorner (eds) *Clinical Endocrinology*. London, Mosby-Wolfe, 1995, pp 5.1–14.

15. Munck A., Guyre P. and Holbrook N. J. Physiological function of glucocorticoids in stress and their relation to pharmacological actions. *Endocrine Reviews*, 1984, **5**: 25–44.

16. Buckingham J. C., Christian H. C., Gillies G. E., Philip J. G. and Taylor A. D. The hypothalamo–pituitary adrenal immune axis. In J. A. Marsh and M. D. Kendall (eds) *The Physiology of Immunity*, New York, CRC Press, 1996, pp 331–54.

17. Bamberger C. M., Bamberger A. M., de Castro M. and Chrousos G.P. Glucocorticoid receptor beta, a potential endogenous inhibitor of glucocorticoid action in humans. *J Clin Invest*, 1995, **95**: 2435–41.

18. Owens M. J. and Nemeroff C. B. Physiology and pharmacology of corticotrophin releasing factor. *Pharmacological Reviews*, 1991, **43**: 425–73.

19. Buckingham J. C., Loxley H. D., Christian H. C. and Philip J. G. Activation of the HPA axis by immune insults: roles and interactions of cytokines, eicosanoids and glucocorticoids. *Pharmacology, Biochemistry and Behaviour*, 1996, **51**: 285–96.

20. Buckingham J. C. Stress and the neuroendocrine immune axis: the pivotal role of glucocorticoids and lipocortin 1. *Br J Pharmacol*, 1996, **118**: 1–19.

21. Kellerwood M. E. and Dallman M. F. Corticosteroid inhibition of ACTH secretion. *Endocrine Reviews*, 1984, **5**: 1–25.

22. Buckingham J. C., Smith T. and Loxley H. D. The control of ACTH secretion. In V. H. T. James (ed.) *The Adrenal Cortex*, New York, Raven Press, 1992, pp 131–58.

23. de Kloet E. R. Brain corticosteroid receptor and homeostatic control. *Frontiers in Neuroendocrinology*, 1991, **62**: 543–644.

24. Aguilera G. Regulation of pituitary ACTH release during chronic stress. *Frontiers in Neuroendocrinology*, 1994, **15**: 321–50.

25. Rosenfeld P., Suchecki A. J. and Levine S. Multifactorial regulation of the hypothalamic–pituitary–adrenal axis during development. *Neurosci Behav Rev*, 1992, **129**: 384–8.

26. Vamvakopoulos N.C. and Chrousos G.P. Hormonal regulation of human corticotrophin releasing hormone gene expression: implications for the sexual dimorphism of the stress response and immune/inflammatory reaction. *Endocrine Reviews*, 1994, **15**: 409–20.

27. Gala R. R. The physiology and mechanisms of the stress-induced changes in prolactin secretion in the rat. *Life Sci*, 1990, **46**: 1407–20.

28. Yirmiya R., Shavit Y., Ben-Eliyahu S., Gale R. P., Liebeskind J. C., Taylor A. N. and Weiner H. Modulation of immunity and neoplasia by neuropeptides released by stressors. In M. A. McCubbin, P. G. Kausmann and C. B. Nemeroff (eds) *Stress, Neuropeptides and Systemic Disease*. New York, Academic Press Inc., 1991, pp 261–86.

29. Taylor A. D., Cowell A. M., Flower R. J. and Buckingham J. C. Dexamethasone inhibits the release of prolactin from the rat anterior pituitary gland by lipocortin 1 dependent and independent mechanisms. *Neuroendocrinology*, 1995, **62**: 530–42.

30. Kasting N. W. and Martin J.B. Altered release of growth hormone and thyrotropin induced by endotoxin in the rat. *Am J Physiol*, 1982, **243**: E332–7.

31. Armario A., Lopez-Calderon A., Jolin T. and Balasch J. Response of anterior pituitary hormones to chronic stress. The specificity of adaptation. *Neurosci Behav Rev*, 1986, **10**: 245–50.

32. Armario A., Marti O, Gavalda A., Giralt M. and Jolin T. Effects of chronic

immobilization stress on GH and TSH secretion in the rat: response to hypothalamic regulatory factors. *Psychoneuroendocrinology*, 1993, **18**: 405–13.

33. Aguila M. C., Pickle R. L., Yu W. H. and McCann S. M. Roles of somatostatin and growth hormone-releasing factor in ether stress inhibition of growth hormone release. *Neuroendocrinology*, 1991, **54**: 521–5.

34. Benyassi A., Roussel J.-P., Rougeot C., Gavalda A., Astier H. and Arancibia S. Chronic stress affects in vivo hypothalamic somatostatin release but not in vitro GH responsiveness to somatostatin in rats. *Neurosci Lett*, 1993, **159**: 166–70.

35. Benyassi A., Gavalda A., Armario A. and Arancibia S. Role of somatostatin in the acute immobilization stress-induced GH decrease in rat. *Life Sci*, 1993, **52**: 361–70.

36. Fukata J., Kasting N. W. and Martin J. B. Somatostatin release from the median eminence of unanaesthetized rats: lack of correlation with pharmacologically suppressed growth hormone secretion. *Neuroendocrinology*, 1985, **40**: 193–200.

37. Peisen J. N., McDonnell K. J., Mulroney S. E. and Lumpkin M. D. Endotoxin-induced suppression of the somatotropic axis is mediated by interleukin-1β and corticotropin-releasing factor in the juvenile rat. *Endocrinology*, 1995, **136**: 3378–90.

38. Johnston C. A., Spinedi E. J. and Negro-Vilar A. Effect of acute ether stress on monoamine metabolism in median eminence and discrete hypothalamic nuclei of the rat brain and on anterior pituitary hormone secretion. *Neuroendocrinology*, 1985, **41**: 83–8.

39. Rivier C. and Vale W. Involvement of corticotropin-releasing factor and somatostatin in stress-induced inhibition of growth hormone secretion in the rat. *Endocrinology*, 1985, **117**: 2478–82.

40. Rivier C. and Vale W. Corticotropin-releasing factor CRF acts centrally to inhibit growth hormone secretion in the rat. *Endocrinology*, 1984, **114**: 2409–11.

41. Peterfreund R. A. and Vale W. W. Ovine corticotropin-releasing factor stimulates somatostatin secretion from cultured brain cells. *Endocrinology*, 1983, **112**: 1275–8.

42. Wehrenberg W. B., Janowski B. A., Piering A. W., Culler F. and Jones K.L. Glucocorticoids: potent inhibitors and stimulators of growth hormone secretion. *Endocrinology*, 1990, **126**: 3200–3.

43. Nakagawa K., Ishizuka T., Shimizu C., Ito Y. and Wakabayashi I. Increased hypothalamic somatostatin mRNA following dexamethasone administration in rats. *Acta Endocrinol*, 1990, **127**: 416–9.

44. Brann D. W. and Mahesh V. B. Role of corticosteroids in female reproduction. *FASEB J*, 1991, **5**: 2691–8.

45. Petraglia F., Vale W. and Rivier C. Opioids act centrally to modulate stress-induced decrease in luteinizing hormone in the rat. *Endocrinology*, 1986, **119**: 2445–50.

46. Rivest S. and Rivier C. The role of corticotropin-releasing factor and interleukin-1 in the regulation of neurons controlling reproductive functions. *Endocrine Reviews*, 1995, **16**: 177–99.

47. Petraglia F, Sutton S., Vale W. and Plotsky P. Corticotropin-releasing factor decreases plasma luteinizing hormone levels in female rats by inhibiting gonadotropin-releasing hormone release into hypophysial-portal circulation. *Endocrinology*, 1987, **120**: 1083–8.

48. van Haasteren G. A. C., van der Meer M. J. M., Hermus A. R. M. M., Linkels E., Klootwijk W., Kapstein E. *et al.* Different effects of continuous infusion of interleukin-1 and interleukin-6 on the hypothalamic-hypophysial-thyroid axis. *Endocrinology*, 1994, **135**: 1336–45.

49. Fukuhara K., Kvetnansky R., Cizza G., Pacak K., Ohara H., Goldstein D. S. and Kopin I. J. Interrelationships between sympathoadrenal system and hypothalamo–pituitary–

adrenocortical/thyroid systems in rats exposed to cold stress. *J Neuroendocrinology*, 1996, **8**: 533–41.

50. Hauger R. L. and Aguilera G. Regulation of corticotropin-releasing hormone receptors and hypothalamic pituitary adrenal axis during cold stress. *J Neuroendocrinology*, 1992, **4**: 617–24.

51. Arancibia S., Tapia-Arancibia L., Astier H. and Assenmacher I. Physiological evidence for α1-adrenergic facilitatory control of the cold-induced TRH release in the rat, obtained by push–pull cannulation of the median eminence. *Neurosci Lett*, 1989, **100**: 169–74.

52. Rondeel J. M. M., de Greef W. J., Hop W. C. J., Rowland D.L. and Visser T.J. Effect of cold exposure on the hypothalamic release of thyrotropin-releasing hormone and catecholamines. *Neuroendocrinology*, 1991, **54**: 477–81.

53. Mattila J., Mannisto P.T. and Tuominen J. Studies on the mechanism of the enhanced cold-induced TSH secretion in spontaneously hypertensive rats. *Experientia*, 1983, **39**: 423–4.

54. Kotani M., Onaya T. and Yamada T. Acute increases of thyroid hormone secretion in response to cold and its inhibition by drugs which act on the autonomic or central nervous system. *Endocrinology*, 1973, **92**: 288–94.

55. Tuomisto J., Ranta T., Mannist P., Saarinen A. and Leppaluoto J. Neurotransmitter control of thyrotropin secretion in the rat. *Eur J Pharmacol*, 1975, **30**: 221–9.

56. Arancibia S., Tapia-Arancibia L., Roussel J. P., Assenmacher I. and Astier H. Effects of morphine on cold-induced TRH release from the median eminence of unanaesthetized rats. *Life Sci*, 1985, **38**: 55–66.

57. Jezova D., Skultetyova I., Tokarev D. I., Bakos P. and Vigas M. Vasopressin and oxytocin in stress. *Ann N Y Acad Sci*, 1995, **771**: 192–203.

58. Derjik R. and Sternberg E. M. Corticosteroid action and neuroendocrine–immune interactions. *Ann NY Acad Sci*, 1994, **746**: 33–41.

59. Reichlin S. Neuroendocrine control of pituitary function. In G. M. Besser and M. O. Thorner (eds) *Clinical Endocrinology*, London, Mosby-Wolfe, 1994, 1.3.

Chapter 2

The Autonomic and Behavioural Responses to Stress

Sandra V. Vellucci

The Babraham Institute, Cambridge, UK

2.1 INTRODUCTION

Exposure to stress results in a co-ordinated series of responses which enable an organism to anticipate and react rapidly to threats to its survival or well-being and thus preserve its internal milieu. Characteristically, the activity of the sympathetic division of the autonomic nervous system (ANS) and hypothalamo–pituitary–adrenocortical (HPA) axis is increased (see Chapter 1); in addition, profound changes in behaviour ensue. Cessation or removal of the stress usually terminates the response and the organism reverts to its "normal" state. However, if the stress is prolonged or severe, adaptive responses may occur which lead to a new

Stress, Stress Hormones and the Immune System. Edited by J. C. Buckingham, G. E. Gillies and A.-M. Cowell
© 1997 John Wiley & Sons, Ltd.

equilibrium. In some instances these may be beneficial, for example, regular exercise can improve cardiovascular function. In others, however, the effects are detrimental. Inappropriate or excessive compensatory mechanisms (which counter the stress responses) lead to a failure of homeostasis and consequently to the development of physical and psychological disorders. In man these typically include cardiovascular or gastrointestinal disease, compromised immune function, suppression of growth and reproductive function and development of psychological or psychiatric disorders such as anxiety or depression.

The aims of this chapter are to describe the major autonomic and behavioural responses which occur when an organism is exposed to stress and to show how they are mediated by the central nervous system (CNS). Particular emphasis is placed on the proposed role of the 41-amino acid corticotrophin releasing hormone (CRH) as a neurotransmitter or neuromodulator essential for the central integration of the stress response (see also Chapter 1). As not all individuals respond to a given stress in a similar manner (particularly if the stress is chronic), consideration is also given to factors which may underlie these differences. In addition, details of studies carried out on experimental animals living in social groups (e.g. non-human primates) are included as these permit investigations of the effects of more complex variables or constraints on behaviour. Such studies are of particular relevance when considering the possible involvement of stress in the aetiology of psychiatric disorders in man. As psychological factors and alterations in autonomic function exert a significant influence on immune function, this chapter will also provide a basis for the information detailed in Chapters 15, 18 and 19.

2.2 THE AUTONOMIC NERVOUS SYSTEM—BASIC PRINCIPLES

2.2.1 Organisation

The autonomic nervous system (ANS) innervates the heart, blood vessels, visceral organs, smooth muscle, exocrine glands, lymphoid tissues and some endocrine glands. It thus plays a vital role in the regulation of those functions over which there is no conscious control, namely cardiovascular function, respiration, digestion, excretion, body temperature, metabolism, sweating and other exocrine secretions and aspects of immune and endocrine function. The efferent pathways of the ANS comprise two main divisions, termed the parasympathetic (cranio-sacral) and sympathetic (thoraco-lumbar) nervous systems respectively. Most target tissues are innervated by neurones from both divisions, which exert mutually antagonistic effects; the levels of cellular activity thus reflect the integration of stimuli from both components. Nonetheless, in many instances one system exerts a functional dominance. For example, the sympathetic system has the major role in controlling blood pressure while in the gut the parasympathetic system is dominant. See (1) for detailed review.

Both branches of the ANS are organised in such a way that neurones leaving the spinal cord reach their effector organ via synapses at a ganglion or ganglia. In the parasympathetic system the ganglia are located close to or within the effector organ, with few (if any) connections between them. The organisation of the sympathetic system is more complex because the ganglia, the majority of which are located close to the spinal column in the sympathetic (paravertebral) chain, are closely interconnected. Thus, a pre-ganglionic sympathetic fibre may pass through several ganglia before synapsing with a post-ganglionic neurone; moreover its terminals may make contact with several post-ganglionic fibres. Furthermore, the sympathetic system includes a neuroendocrine component, the adrenal medulla, which has been likened to a specialised ganglion and which releases its products directly into the systemic circulation. The differential organisation of the parasympathetic and sympathetic nervous systems (Fig. 2.1) is critical to their respective functions. The lack of connections between ganglia in the parasympathetic system enables nerves arising in the spinal cord to exert discrete influences on each of their respective target tissues, varying their tone specifically according to physiological demand. The sympathetic system also has the capacity to vary its tone specifically to individual organs as required. However, the complex neuronal network between ganglia gives this system the additional ability to discharge as a single unit. This synchronous event is particularly important in conditions of stress where the simultaneous stimulation of the sympathetically innervated structures in the body is critical to host defence as it prepares the organism for "fight or flight".

Autonomic outflow is tightly regulated by specific centres in the central nervous system (CNS). These centres receive inputs from a variety of ascending and descending central nervous pathways which, in turn, may be influenced by a wide range of physical, emotional and environmental stimuli as well as by alterations in the physiological milieu. The main controlling and integrating centre is the hypothalamus which sends impulses to autonomic efferent neurones through the dorsal longitudinal fasciculus and mammillotegmental tract, with relays in the reticular formation. The hypothalamus thus influences autonomic function by a mechanism distinct from that which it uses to control pituitary function (see Chapter 1). The autonomic centres in the hypothalamus receive impulses from several sources. These include afferents from:

(a) the viscera via the ascending fibres in the brain-stem,
(b) the olfactory cortex and limbic system via the medial forebrain bundle,
(c) the medial and anterior thalamic nuclei, amygdala and hippocampus, and
(d) the neocortex via fibres originating mainly in the orbital cortex of the frontal lobe.

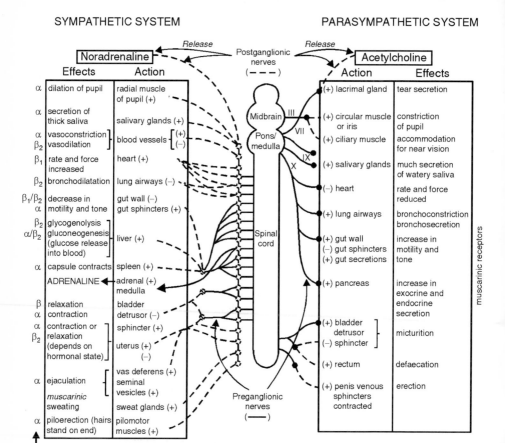

Figure 2.1 Schematic diagram showing the basic organisation of the autonomic nervous system. (+), excitation; (−), inhibition. In the sympathetic system (+) and (−) generally correspond to responses mediated by α- and β-adrenoceptors respectively. Reproduced by permission from M. J. Neal, *Medical Pharmacology at a Glance*, 1989, p. 20, Oxford, Blackwell Scientific Publications

In addition, the hypothalamic neurones are sensitive to changes in body temperature and to the osmolarity and concentrations of specific chemicals in the circulation (e.g. glucose). The second major centre integrating autonomic outflow comprises the visceral afferent nuclei and visceral centres in the brain-stem reticular formation. These centres relay impulses to the intermediolateral cell column of the spinal cord and the sacral parasympathetic nucleus via reticulo-spinal connections (descending autonomic fibres). Like the hypothalamus, autonomic brain-stem nuclei receive inputs from a variety of sources. These include:

(a) the viscera via the vagus nerve which relays impulses centrally to autonomic preganglionic neurones through the nucleus of the solitary tract and the reticular formation, and
(b) the olfactory and limbic systems through the olfacto-tegmental component of the medial forebrain bundle and via a complex pathway which includes the habenular nucleus, midbrain nuclei and dorsal longitudinal fasciculus.

2.2.2 Neurotransmitters and Receptors

The preganglionic fibres of both the sympathetic and the parasympathetic systems use acetylcholine as a transmitter, which acts via nicotinic cholinoceptors to stimulate the post-ganglionic fibres. In the parasympathetic system the post-ganglionic fibres are also cholinergic, but the cholinoceptors on the effector organs they innervate are muscarinic, and dependent on the target tissue, may belong to one of three main subclasses (M_1, M_2 or M_3, see Table 2.1). By contrast, the vast majority of post-ganglionic sympathetic fibres are noradrenergic although in a few instances they too may use acetylcholine and muscarinic receptors (e.g. fibres supplying the sweat glands). The primary product of the adrenal medulla is adrenaline although smaller amounts (20%) of noradrenaline are also released into the systemic circulation. The actions of noradrenaline and adrenaline on their target tissues are effected by specific adrenoceptors of which five major sub-classes (α_1, α_2, β_1, β_2 and β_3) have been identified, which differ in their ligand specificity, distribution and signal transduction systems (see Table 2.2).

While acetylcholine, noradrenaline and adrenaline are the major transmitter substances used by the ANS, other agents undoubtedly modulate or contribute to

Table 2.1 Muscarinic cholinoceptors: classification, ligand selectivity and signal transduction systems. *NB Acetylcholine also stimulates nicotinic cholinoceptors; oxotremorine is selective for muscarinic receptors. No selective agonists of the muscarinic sub-types are yet available. HHSD, hexahydrosiladifenidol; IP_3, inositol trisphosphate; DAG, diacylglycerol; cAMP, cyclic adenosine monophosphate; G, guanine nucleotide binding protein (class in subscript)—for further details see Chapter 4 and (3)

Muscarinic cholinoceptor subtype	M_1	M_2	M_3
Agonists*	Acetylcholine Oxotremorine	Acetylcholine Oxotremorine	Acetylcholine Oxotremorine
Antagonists	Atropine Pirenzepine	Atropine Gallamine	Atropine HHSD
Signal transduction	$G_{q/11}$ ↑ IP_3/DAG ↑ K^+ channel	$G_{i/o}$ ↓ cAMP ↓ Ca^{++} channel	$G_{q/11}$ ↑ IP_3/DAG

Table 2.2 Adrenoceptors: classification, ligand selectivity and signal transduction systems. IP_3, inositol trisphosphate; DAG, diacylglycerol; cAMP, cyclic adenosine monophosphate. G, guanine nucleotide binding proteins (class in subscript)—for further details see Chapter 4 and (3)

Adrenoceptor Subclass	α_1	α_2	β_1	β_2	β_3
Endogenous agonist potency	Noradrenaline ≫ adrenaline	Adrenaline ≥ noradrenaline	Noradrenaline ≥ adrenaline	Adrenaline ≫ noradrenaline	Noradrenaline > adrenaline
Selective agonists	Phenylephrine	Clonidine	Isoprenaline Dobutamine Xamoterol	Isoprenaline Salbutamol Procaterol	Isoprenaline BRL37344
Selective antagonists	Phentolamine Prazosin Indoramine	Phentolamine Yohimbine	Propranolol Atenolol	Propranolol Butoxamine	Propranolol Bupranolol
Signal transduction	$G_{q/11}$ ↑ IP_3/DAG	$G_{i/o}$ ↓ cAMP ↑ K^+ channel ↓ Ca^{2+} channel	G_s ↑ cAMP	G_s ↑ cAMP	G_s ↑ cAMP

the responses. Many substances have been implicated in the non-adrenergic, non-cholinergic (NANC) control of autonomic function; not all fulfil the criteria of neurotransmitters or neuromodulators but included in the list are purines (adenosine triphosphate and adenosine), nitric oxide, prostanoids, peptides, amino acids and other biogenic amines.

2.3 THE EFFECTS OF STRESS ON THE ACTIVITY OF THE AUTONOMIC NERVOUS SYSTEM

Perception of a stressful stimulus causes immediate activation of the sympathetic nervous system with the consequent release of noradrenaline and adrenaline from sympathetic nerve endings and the adrenal medulla respectively. Acetyl-choline release from the few existing post-ganglionic sympathetic cholinergic fibres (e.g. those innervating the sweat glands) is also enhanced. In contrast, the parasympathetic drive to autonomically innervated tissues is generally reduced, although in some instances (e.g. lower gastrointestinal tract) it too may be increased (see Section 2.3.3). The magnitude of the sympathetic response depends on both the nature of the stress and the species concerned. For example in man, adrenaline output normally is provoked more readily by emotional trauma (e.g. anxiety and difficulty in coping) than by physical stressors. By contrast, rodents are more sensitive to physical stressors e.g. cold. The release of catecholamines is viewed as an integrated adaptive response designed to preserve life, preparing the organism for "fight or flight" and thus for increased physical (particularly locomotor) and mental activity (see Table 2.3). The most overt of the responses are the dilated pupils (α_1-adrenoceptor-mediated contraction of the radial muscle of the iris), increased sweating (stimulation of muscarinic cholino-ceptors), piloerection (α_1-adrenoceptor-mediated) and tremor (β_2-mediated in-creased contractility of skeletal muscle). Importantly, the blood flow to skeletal

Table 2.3 Responses to sympathoadrenal activation

Tachycardia	Sweating
Vasoconstriction in:	Piloerection
gastrointestinal tract	
kidney	Hyperglycaemia
spleen	
skin	Hyperlipidaemia
Vasodilation in skeletal muscle	Pupil dilation
Inhibition of gastrointestinal motility and secretions	Activation of renin–angiotensin– aldosterone system
Hyperventilation	Platelet activation
Bronchodilation	

muscle is selectively increased, thereby facilitating the delivery of nutrients and removal of metabolites. In addition, availability of oxygen and nutrients (glucose and fatty acids) is increased to support the increased energy demand. In many instances anticipatory autonomic responses precede and prepare the individual for stress, a phenomenon first described by Canon (1929). On the other hand, in conditions of chronic intermittent stress adaptation (i.e. a reduced autonomic response) may occur, although subsequent exposure to an acute (novel) stress will still result in a normal or enhanced autonomic response.

2.3.1   Cardiovascular and Respiratory Effects

Activation of the sympathetic nervous system in stress causes an increase in the rate and force of contraction of the heart, leading to an increase in cardiac output, together with a significant increase in mean arterial pressure (MAP). A substantial redistribution of the blood also occurs, with flow to the skeletal muscle beds being increased at the expense of the splanchnic region and skin, while perfusion of the heart, lungs and brain is maintained or even enhanced. These responses are essential to ensure adequate delivery of oxygen and nutrients to and removal of metabolites from these organs and thus to equip the individual with the physical and mental energy for "fight or flight".

The cardiac responses are due primarily to the actions of noradrenaline and adrenaline on β_1-adrenoceptors in the myocardium and are reduced substantially in subjects taking β-adrenoceptor blocking drugs. However, in cases in which vagal tone is apparent (e.g. young subjects) a complementary reduction in parasympathetic tone may also be important. The concomitant rise in blood pressure is attributable partly to the increase in cardiac output and partly to an increase in total peripheral resistance effected by α_1-adrenoceptor-mediated constriction of the resistance vessels. In addition, a β_2-adrenoceptor-mediated increase in renin release which triggers the formation of angiotensin II (a potent pressor agent) and aldosterone (which increases blood volume) may contribute to the response, although surprisingly angiotensin-converting enzyme inhibitors (e.g. captopril) have little effect on the response. The redistribution of blood which accompanies the pressor response is explained largely by the differential distribution of α_1- and β_2-adrenoceptors within the vascular system and their opposing influence on vascular tone and resistance (α_1, constriction; β_2, dilatation). The vessels supplying skeletal muscles are particularly rich in β_2-adrenoceptors and thus dilate when exposed to adrenaline thereby facilitating increased flow. By contrast, vessels in the splanchnic regions and skin possess a preponderance of α_1-adrenoceptors and therefore constrict when challenged with either noradrenaline or adrenaline.

In normal circumstances, increases in MAP are associated with a decrease in heart rate brought about by activation of the baroreceptor reflex. The stress response is thus unusual as the baroreceptor reflex is overcome and increases in arterial blood pressure and heart rate occur simultaneously. Reports that central administration of CRH produces changes in MAP, heart rate, regional blood flow and baroreceptor reflexes similar to those seen in many conditions of physical and emotional stress favour a role for the neuropeptide in orchestrating this unusual series of cardiovascular responses. This is supported by evidence that the effects of CRH are attenuated by ganglion blockade or intracerebroventricular (i.c.v.) administration of the CRH antagonist, α-helical CRH_{9-41}. Interestingly, however, peripheral administration of CRH causes hypotension due largely to a direct vasodilator action. Situations where peripheral CRH or CRH-like peptides may be elevated are discussed elsewhere (Chapters 10 and 11) and may have particular significance in conditions in which the immune system is activated.

The cardiovascular responses to stress are accompanied by significant changes in respiratory activity. Gaseous exchange in the lung is greatly facilitated by bronchodilation, which results from the activation by adrenaline of the β_2-adrenoceptors located on bronchial smooth muscle and from a complementary reduction in parasympathetic tone. In addition, the oxygen carrying capacity of the blood is increased as the spleen contracts (an α_1-adrenoceptor-mediated effect) and large numbers of red cells are released into the circulation. Hyperventilation with associated disturbances in acid–base balance is also a common occurrence.

Chronic stress is frequently associated with pathological changes in cardiovascular function. For example, the sustained vasoconstriction in peripheral vascular beds which results from prolonged sympathetic stimulation may give rise to arteriosclerosis as well as hypertension. This has been reported in a range of animals, including rodents, chickens, pigs and primates, in which the responses may be exacerbated by chronic high levels of glucocorticoids which increase serum lipids. Other cardiovascular abnormalities resulting from sustained overactivity of the sympathetic nervous system include myocardial necrosis and fibrosis both of which have been described in a variety of species including pigs and primates.

2.3.2 Metabolic and Thermoregulatory Responses

Activation of the sympathetic nervous system in acute stress results in mobilisation of energy stores. Blood glucose levels rise due to the stimulation of hepatic β_2-adrenoceptors, which increase glycogenolysis or gluconeogenesis or both; plasma glucagon is also raised but insulin levels normally remain unchanged. In addition, the stimulation of β_1/β_3-adrenoceptors in adipose tissue promotes lipolysis. The metabolic responses to stress are accompanied by an increase in thermogenesis which is determined by both autonomic and behavioural influences (see Chapter 16). Core temperature thus rises due to increased sympathetic activity, which drives brown adipose tissue (BAT) non-shivering thermogenesis, and to associated bouts of physical activity. Other factors undoubtedly also contribute to the response for human subjects undergoing anxiety-associated psychological stress (e.g. examinations) show an increase in body temperature which is not accompanied by increased physical activity and which, unlike the concomitant tachycardia, is insensitive to peripheral β-adrenoceptor blockade.

CRH is strongly implicated in the central initiation and co-ordination of the metabolic and thermogenic responses to stress and, when injected centrally in experimental animals, it mimics many of the effects normally induced by stress (typically producing increases in blood glucose, free fatty acids and BAT thermogenesis) while the CRH antagonist, α-helical CRH_{9-41} and anti-CRH antisera oppose these responses. For example, in rodents transfer from one cage to another, which constitutes a psychological stress, gives rise to an increase in body temperature which is mimicked by central injection of CRH and blocked by α-helical CRH_{9-41}. The anxiolytic benzodiazepines also attenuate this type of stress response, possibly by enhancing the γ-amino butyric acid$_A$ ($GABA_A$)-receptor-mediated inhibitory tone on CRH secretion (see Chapter 1).

2.3.3 The Gastrointestinal and Urinary Tracts

Acute physical or psychological stress has profound effects on gastrointestinal and urinary tract function. Characteristically, both gastric emptying and small intestine transit time are reduced whereas colonic transit is increased markedly, leading to increased defecation; gastric acid and pepsin release are also increased as are pancreatic secretions. An increase in urinary frequency is also normally apparent. Chronic stress is associated both with the development of gastric lesions and ulcers and with the manifestation of the irritable bowel syndrome. The peripheral nervous mechanisms underlying these events are far from fully understood and cannot be simply explained by an increase in sympathetic drive or a decrease in parasympathetic tone since each would be expected to impair defecation and reduce urinary frequency. Recent studies have emphasised a central role for CRH in generating some, but not all, of the gastrointestinal responses to stress and, from these, some insight of the peripheral mechanisms is beginning to emerge.

When given centrally, CRH mimics and α-helical CRH_{9-41} antagonises the effects of restraint stress and other experimental stress paradigms on gastric emptying and intestinal and colonic transit time. The inhibition of gastric emptying is pronounced and appears to depend on the central activation of both opioidergic and sympathetic-noradrenergic pathways; it is thus overcome by the opioid receptor antagonist naloxone, by the ganglion blocker chlorisondamine and by the noradrenergic neurone blocking drug bretylium but not by truncal vagotomy. The locus of action of naloxone is unclear although it has been suggested that it acts centrally to depress sympathetic outflow to the stomach. Alternatively, it may antagonise the inhibitory actions of locally produced opioid peptides on gastric emptying. The inhibitory effects of CRH on small intestinal transit, although relatively modest, are also dependent on opioidergic and autonomic mechanisms and thus are reversed readily by naloxone and by ganglion blocking drugs. However, these responses, unlike those of the stomach, are readily abolished by truncal vagotomy but not by bretylium, suggesting the involvement of a different autonomic pathway, namely an inhibitory vagal efferent. The stimulation of large bowel transit by CRH (given i.c.v.) has been attributed exclusively to activation of the parasympathetic system. Thus, the pronounced contractile responses elicited by the peptide are mimicked by stimulation of the dorsal vagal complex, blocked by ganglion blockade or surgical vagotomy but unaffected by administration of bretylium or naloxone. From these studies it appears that the changes in gastrointestinal motility associated with stress are due, at least in part, to the central activation by CRH of three distinct autonomic pathways which innervate the stomach, the small intestine and the large bowel respectively.

Considerable attention has focused on the pathogenesis of stress-induced gastric ulceration. Paradoxically, central injections of CRH exert a protective effect on the gastric mucosa in that they attenuate the ulcerogenic responses to stress. The responses to the peptide, which are readily blocked by the CRH antagonist α-helical CRH_{9-41}, are complex and involve not only inhibition of gastric acid release but also enhanced bicarbonate production, increased mesenteric blood flow and, as discussed above, reduced gastric motility. The mechanisms responsible are ill-defined although neuroanatomical and electrophysiological studies have indicated that the noradrenergic system arising in the locus coeruleus is important in this regard. On the other hand, the increased secretion of bicarbonate appears to be secondary to the activation of the HPA axis for it is abolished by hypophysectomy, antagonised by naloxone and mimicked by systemic injections of β-endorphin, a polypeptide which is co-released with corticotrophin (ACTH) from the anterior pituitary gland in conditions of stress (see Chapter 1). Several other peptides also protect the gut from stress-induced ulceration when given centrally (e.g. bombesin, opioids, calcitonin, neurotensin). By contrast, others, e.g. thyrotrophin releasing hormone (TRH), vasoactive intestinal polypeptide (VIP), pancreatic polypeptide and neuropeptide Y (NPY) have powerful ulcerogenic actions which are associated with increased gastric acid and pepsin secretion and enhanced gastric contractility and emptying. Particular attention has focused on TRH which is now strongly implicated in the pathogenesis of stress-induced gastric ulceration. In support of this concept, TRH-positive nerve fibres and receptors are found in abundance in brain structures such as the hypothalamus, amygdala and dorsal motor nucleus which are concerned with gastric function and the manifestation of gastric ulcers. Furthermore, the increases in gastric secretion and ulceration provoked by cold stress (an important activator of the hypothalamo–pituitary–thyroid axis) are associated with increased release of TRH within the CNS and are abolished by central administration of anti-TRH antisera. The ulcerogenic responses to TRH, which are mimicked by several stable TRH analogues, are dependent on increased vagal (i.e. parasympathetic) drive to the stomach and are therefore blocked readily by the muscarinic cholinoceptor antagonist, atropine, but not by antagonists of adrenoceptors or dopamine receptors.

Several lines of evidence suggest that the ulcerogenic responses to stress may depend both on the nature of the stress and on the individual's prior stress experience. The majority of studies in experimental animals have been based on stresses such as handling, tail or foot shock, restraint and forced activity (e.g. forced swimming). In rodents, prenatal stress and early weaning have been shown consistently to be potent risk factors which predispose individuals to stress ulcers in adult life; for example, restraint-induced ulceration is exacerbated in the adult offspring of rats subjected to handling stress during pregnancy. On the other hand, post-natal exposure to handling stress prior to weaning exerts a protective effect against subsequent ulcerogenic stresses. The picture with other types of stresses, e.g. electric foot shock, is not always so clear and there are inconsistencies in terms of the direction of the effects. What does emerge from the circumstances of the first stress is the degree of controllability which the individual can exert over a subsequent stress, i.e. whether it is avoidable (controllable) or unavoidable (uncontrollable). This aspect is discussed in more detail in Section 2.4.5.

2.3.4 Immunological Responses

Increasing anatomical and pharmacological evidence suggests that the lymphoid organs (e.g. thymus and spleen) and circulating immune and inflammatory cells (lymphocytes and leukocytes) are important targets for the ANS. The physiological role of the ANS in the regulation of immune function is unclear but data from a number of laboratories now suggest that activation of the sympathetic system and consequent release of catecholamines (either locally from nerve terminals or into the systemic circulation from the adrenal medulla) may be an important factor in the pathogenesis of stress-induced immunosuppression. This phenomenon will be discussed in detail in Chapter 15.

2.4 THE EFFECTS OF STRESS ON BEHAVIOUR

Stress elicits a broad spectrum of behavioural responses, the profile of which depends on the type, severity and duration of the stress, the species, the individual's prior experience and whether or not it is able to cope appropriately with the challenge. Generally, the responses are adaptive and include, for example, activation of neural pathways that mediate arousal, attention and avoidance behaviours and inhibition of pathways involved in the regulation of growth, reproduction and feeding. Not surprisingly, many of the behaviours are indicative of fearfulness or anxiety. Thus animals frequently exhibit reductions in exploratory activity, social interaction and conditioned emotional responses, whilst behaviours such as shock-induced freezing, shock-induced fighting and acoustic startle responses are generally increased. Brief descriptive accounts of some of the characteristic responses are presented below.

2.4.1 Fear and Anxiogenesis

When presented with an acute, fear-provoking stimulus, an animal typically adopts a vigilant or "orienting" posture. In some instances it may "freeze" or become immobile. This is particularly common in species which are preyed upon (e.g. rodents and rabbits) and has the advantage of making the animal less liable to detection by a predator. Freezing, which may be triggered in rodents by the sight or smell of a predator, a loud noise or an electric shock, is characterised by the adoption of a crouched or sitting posture with rigid muscular tone; there is no discernible movement, heart rate is reduced (resulting, paradoxically, from increased *parasympathetic* drive to the myocardium) while respiration is rapid and shallow. In other instances, fear may cause an animal to attempt to escape (the "flight" response), particularly to avoid environments or situations associated with a previous unpleasant experience (e.g. an electric shock). Further fear-induced behaviours include frequent urination and defecation and the manifestation of inappropriate behaviours (termed "displacement activities", see Section 2.4.3) such as excessive self-grooming. In addition, locomotor, exploratory and feeding behaviours are normally reduced as too are social interactions. Many of these responses can be readily observed by placing an animal (usually a rat) in a novel environment (e.g. a large open arena) where, typically, it will remain close to the outer walls of the arena and exhibit reduced locomotor and rearing activity, increased defecation and self-grooming and exaggerated startle responses to acoustic stimuli. Some species, notably rodents, also signal their distress to their conspecifics by ultrasound vocalisation, using frequencies which depend on the nature of the aversive stimulus to warn of impending dangers.

Anxiety is a more generalised and long-lasting emotion than fear and occurs when an animal is anticipating an unpleasant or painful stimulus. For example, an animal may become anxious when it is placed in a situation which it associates with danger (such as a brightly lit arena) and exhibit behaviours which may include increased vigilance, jumpiness and frequent urination and defecation. These behaviours are exploited in experimental models of anxiety (see

Chapter 6). Other behaviours influenced by fear and anxiety include sexual activity (see Section 2.4.5), feeding, motivation, learning and memory.

Food intake is reduced considerably in conditions of stress. For example, hungry rats eat less when exposed to a novel environment. Similarly, after a one hour period of restraint rats eat less than controls when presented with food. As with many other aspects of the behavioural responses to stress (see Section 2.5), the neuropeptide CRH has been strongly implicated in this response. In support of this concept, central administration of CRH mimics the reduction in food intake provoked by stress while the CRH receptor antagonist, α-helical CRH_{9-41}, opposes the response. CRH also reduces food intake triggered by stimuli such as muscimol, dynorphin, noradrenaline and insulin although, paradoxically, in low doses it increases feeding in animals which have been food deprived for 24 h. Furthermore, tolerance may develop to the inhibitory effects on feeding of higher doses of CRH.

The effects of stress on learning and memory are well documented and, indeed, many behavioural tests of anxiety are based on the premise that anxiogenic drugs (e.g. β-carbolines, CRH) enhance motivation and learning capacity in rats exposed to aversive stimuli while, conversely, anxiolytics (e.g. benzodiazepines) disrupt learning and memory (see Chapter 6). For example, exogenous CRH exerts effects which resemble those provoked by an aversive stress and in a learning paradigm it acts as an "aversive reinforcer". On the other hand, benzodiazepines have been known for some years to have the capacity to produce anterograde amnesia in human subjects. These cognitive effects are not surprising as there is a high degree of interplay between the brain areas involved in mediating the stress responses (notably the limbic structures) and those concerned with information processing and action initiation as well as emotional outlook.

2.4.2 Anti-nociceptive Responses

Studies in rodents have shown that, in many instances, physical or emotional stresses increase nociceptive thresholds and thus induce a state of "stress-induced analgesia". The mechanisms underlying this phenomenon are unclear but several investigators have been able to distinguish between effects which are dependent upon opioidergic and non-opioidergic pain inhibitory systems. The former are naloxone-reversible and include responses elicited in experimental animals by stressors such as tail pinch, prolonged intermittent foot shock, immobilisation, food deprivation and intraperitoneal (i.p.) injection of 2-deoxy-glucose in animals, as well as the anticipation of foot shock in humans. Non-opioid dependent analgesia has been evoked in laboratory animals by foot shock, centrifugal rotation, cold water swimming and i.p. injection of hypertonic saline. Interestingly, humans receiving CRH following dental surgery have reported less post-operative pain than those given placebo. Furthermore, in the rat, intravenous administration of CRH can elicit an anti-nociceptive effect in the hotplate test, similar to that of morphine. The mechanism responsible is unclear but may involve β-endorphin since this peptide is released from the anterior pituitary gland in response to CRH infusions and the anti-nociceptive effects of CRH are reversed by hypophysectomy.

2.4.3   Inappropriate Behavioural Responses to Stress

In some cases the behavioural responses to stress appear to be inappropriate for the particular circumstances and may be regarded as displacement activities. For example, rats exposed to a novel environment display an increase in self-grooming which ceases as the animal becomes habituated to the environment. Other inappropriate behavioural patterns may occur as a result of frustration or if animals are kept in an inadequate environment. These include stereotypies (repeated patterns of movement with little or no variation and no obvious function, e.g. circling and pacing) which occur in situations where the environment is restricted (e.g. when an animal is held in captivity) or if there is conflict or lack of control of the stressful situation (see Section 2.6). It has been suggested that stereotypies represent a form of coping strategy, since in some cases they have been associated with a reduction in plasma glucocorticoid concentrations.

2.4.4   Social Stress

Some mammalian species exhibit social behaviour only at certain times of the year (e.g. in the breeding season), whereas others, e.g. most primates, live permanently in social groups adhering to a well-defined dominance hierarchy (4). This can generate stress between group members (e.g. as far as access to food, mates and preferred positions are concerned), but can also prove to be useful in dealing satisfactorily with external stressors (e.g. predators). The most important property of a social group is that it has a well-defined structure; that is, the relationships which exist between the different members are not merely random or equal. The relationships formed can be divided into various classes, each of which has specific behavioural features (e.g. mother–infant relationships, interjuvenile interactions or sexual consortships). Interactions within and be-tween classes occur frequently; the former are often aggressive but the response, for example of an adult male to a juvenile, is likely to differ from that to a fellow adult male. These interactions determine not only the response of individual members of the group to one another but also their access to favoured objects and their reaction to a common stressor from within or outside the group. Early social experiences, especially peer interactions, are essential for normal emotional and behavioural development and greatly influence the way in which an animal relates to other members of its social group in its adult life. Studies in primates have shown that infants are influenced either directly or indirectly (via their mother or their peers) by any event which influences the group as a whole even though at that stage the infant can understand and is concerned with only a very small part of its social group. For example, monkeys show little play and no sexual behaviour in adulthood when raised with their mother only while those deprived of both maternal and peer–peer interactions exhibit severe behavioural abnormalities in adult life, with mating behaviour being absent and social interaction being greatly reduced in the presence of behaviourally "normal" adults. On the other hand, infants raised with their peers but without their mothers develop "normal" adult behaviours.

It is important to recognise that not all members of a social group are affected in the same way by a particular stress. For example, chronic social stress and overcrowding have a marked influence on subordinate animals whereas dominant animals are more sensitive to the trauma of a novel environment or the introduction of a strange (potentially threatening) male into the group. Social stress in both experimental animals and in man is frequently derived from, or expressed through, aggressive interactions. Indeed, non-human primates living in social groups form hierarchies where dominance is defined in terms of the outcome of aggressive interactions. Thus, if animal A attacks animal B and B fails either to retaliate or to initiate aggression towards A, then A is said to be dominant over B. If animal B attacks C and C attacks D, a linear hierarchy is said to exist in which A is the dominant animal. However, it does not necessarily follow that A is the most aggressive animal in the group, as dominance is defined on the basis of the line of aggression (i.e. A to B etc.) and not by the total amount of aggression shown by an individual. This is well illustrated in established social groups of monkeys where instances of overt aggression are rare and the dominant male may deal with any conflict or potential conflict within the group by a change in posture or facial expression. Thus, in a social group, the ultimate impact of stress on an animal will depend not only on the severity, duration and type of stress but also on the rank that the animal holds within the group and on the coping strategies it has developed.

2.4.5 Adaptation to Stress

Repeated exposure to a given stress frequently results in adaptation or habituation. This response is critical to the well-being of the organism as it enables it to cope more successfully with the insult. The rapidity with which adaptation occurs depends on the severity, duration and type of stress and appears to be consequent on facilitation of adaptive neural pathways and reciprocal inhibition of non-adaptive mechanisms. The behaviours affected are wide-ranging and include altered cognitive and sensory thresholds, increased alertness, selective memory enhancement and suppression of feeding and reproduction.

The effects of stress on reproduction are complex and involve both sexual behaviour and reproductive function. For example, in the female rat stress inhibits lordosis, i.e. the receptive posture (immobile with back arched concavely and tail deviated laterally) necessary for mounting and penile intromission. In addition, stress may cause delayed puberty, failure of ovulation or embryo implantation, spontaneous abortion and increased infant mortality. The effects of stress in the male are essentially complementary and typically include inhibition of testosterone production, spermatogenesis, sexual behaviour and libido. These complex behavioural and physiological events involve several hormones, including CRH which has been shown to inhibit gonadotrophin release (see Section 2.5 and Chapter 1).

Behavioural habituation to chronic or repeated stress is coupled with a series of peripheral adaptive events which provide the energy required. These involve a shift of energy substrates from storage sites to the blood stream and complementary increase in cardiovascular and pulmonary function (see Section 2.3). In addition, anabolic processes such as digestion, growth and immune function are suppressed. Adaptive responses are partly genetically determined. Other important epigenetic factors (i.e. factors "of the earth") which enable an effective coping strategy to be developed are early life experiences (which may determine the predictability of the stress and whether any degree of control can be exercised over it) and social buffering (see Section 2.6).

2.5   THE PUTATIVE ROLE OF CRH IN THE CENTRAL INTEGRATION OF THE STRESS RESPONSE

Many neural pathways and neurotransmitter substances have been implicated in the complex central mechanisms which effect the body's integrated responses to acute and chronic stress. A discussion of our current state of knowledge is beyond the scope of this chapter and the reader is referred to the reviews detailed in the reading list (4–7). However, it is pertinent to consider briefly the apparently critical role of CRH in this regard. This peptide, together with vasopressin, is essential for the activation of the pituitary–adrenal system; it also contributes at the hypothalamic level to the stress-induced suppression of the growth and reproductive axes (see Chapter 1 for further details). Early evidence that CRH may fulfil a wider brief in the central integration of the stress response emerged from reports that central injections of the peptide mimic many of the effects of stress on autonomic function and behaviour in both rodents and primates; many of these actions are still evident after hypophysectomy, adrenalectomy or systemic administration of antibodies to ACTH and are thus independent of the pituitary–adrenal axis. Furthermore, many of the autonomic and behavioural responses evoked by stress are attenuated by pretreatment with anti-CRH antisera or the CRH antagonist α-helical CRH$_{9-41}$ (5, 6). Some examples of this work have already been discussed (see Sections 2.3.1, 2.3.2, 2.4.1, 2.4.3 and 2.4.5).

Within the CNS, CRH has a widespread but specific distribution. Importantly, apart from being expressed in the hypothalamus (see Chapter 1), it is also found in abundance in the cerebral cortex and other regions associated with sensory information processing, the limbic system (e.g. amygdala and bed nucleus stria terminalis) and brain-stem autonomic nuclei (e.g. nucleus of the solitary tract and the dorsal and ventral parabrachial nuclei); particularly high levels occur in the amygdala, lateral hypothalamus, central grey region, dorsal tegmentum, locus coeruleus, parabrachial nuclei, dorsal vagal complex and inferior olive. Specific, high affinity, saturable CRH receptors are also abundant in the CNS. These receptors, which are positively coupled to adenylyl cyclase, exist in multiple subtypes (CRH-R1, CRH-R2α and CRH-R2β) which are each expressed in discrete, non overlapping areas and may therefore subserve distinct functional roles. The CRH-R1 receptor, which may exist in two alternatively spliced forms (see Chapters 1 and 11), is expressed mainly in the anterior pituitary gland, the cerebellum, the cerebral cortex and the olfactory bulb. The CRH-R2α form is located neuronally and shows a significant correlation with the distribution of CRH mRNA, being prevalent in the hypothalamus, cerebral cortex, limbic system, cerebellum and spinal cord. In contrast, the CRH-R2β receptors are non-neuronal and are found in the choroid plexus arterioles and in peripheral tissues such as the lung, cardiac muscle and skeletal muscle.

Many functional studies have aimed to identify the sites within the CNS at which CRH exerts its various actions on autonomic function and behaviour; for reviews see (5–7). The literature is complex but the bulk of evidence accords with the neuroanatomical data and thus points to the hypothalamus, the limbic structures (notably the amygdala), the cortex, the pons, the locus coeruleus, the dorsal vagal complex and other brain-stem areas as major sites of action. In addition, the basal ganglia may contribute to the effects of CRH on locomotion.

2.6 STRESS AND ANIMAL MODELS OF PSYCHIATRIC DISORDERS

Chronic stress may give rise to a broad spectrum of pathophysiological and behavioural disturbances, particularly if the glucocorticoid concentration is raised. To cope effectively with such conditions animals must develop an effective mechanism whereby they can either regulate or modulate any potentially severe disturbances in HPA activity. The most important is the ability to exert an element of control over a potentially stressful situation by making active responses. Such responses may allow the animal to avoid or escape from the stimulus, or to replace that stimulus with another. For example, rats with the ability to terminate unpredictable electric shocks by pressing a lever show less severe disturbances in glucocorticoid secretion than corresponding controls which lack these skills. Similarly, the plasma cortisol concentrations of rhesus monkeys trained to terminate an aversive noise by pressing a lever are similar to those of unstressed controls. In contrast, monkeys which lack the skills to actively regulate the noise have greatly elevated cortisol concentrations. In male baboons in the wild, low plasma cortisol concentrations are not indicators of social dominance *per se* but they are associated with a specific type of dominance which involves a degree of controllability. Thus, the basal cortisol concentrations are lower in males which exhibit any of the following behaviours: a marked ability to distinguish between threatening and neutral interactions with rivals, a propensity to initiate a fight in a threatening situation, skills at distinguishing between winning and losing a fight and, on losing, an ability to displace the aggression onto a third animal. Overall these behaviours indicate a high degree of skilfulness, control and predictability over social contingencies, all of which are recognised as psychological features which minimise the pathophysiological impact of stress. Dominant baboons which lack these behavioural strategies have plasma cortisol concentrations which are similar to those of subordinate animals.

Exposure of naive animals to unpredictable and uncontrolled (i.e. inescapable) aversive stimuli leads to subsequent deficits in their ability to learn the skills required to terminate aversive stimuli, even if they are escapable. This gives rise to a condition known as "learned helplessness", suggesting that the inability to control or terminate a stress results from the initial learning of inescapability. Experimentally-induced behavioural deficits of this type are used as animal models of depression (see Chapter 6) and are considered analogous to some of the mood or cognitive disturbances noted in patients with this disorder. Evidence suggests that a fundamental biochemical change underlying these behavioural defects is the depletion of noradrenaline or a decrease in tyrosine hydroxylase activity in the locus coeruleus or both. This view is supported by evidence that direct effects of CRH on locus coeruleus noradrenergic neurones are very similar to those provoked by stress. However, stress also affects other parts of the CNS which play an important role in information processing, action initiation and emotional outlook. For example, the mesocortical dopaminergic system, which innervates the prefrontal cortex and is linked closely to the nucleus accumbens, is implicated in motivational and reinforcement-reward phenomena. This system is activated by the locus coeruleus noradrenergic system during stress as also is the amygdalo-hippocampal complex.

In the context of animal models relevant to psychiatric disorders in man, observations on groups of rhesus monkeys have shown that early experience of controllability may have long term consequences on social behaviour and social status. In one study, groups of rhesus monkeys were raised under conditions differing in the degree of control or "mastery" over appetitive stimuli in the first year of life. Those having the ability to control access to the stimulus by pressing a lever (the so-called "learned mastery" animals) were paired with "yoked" controls which received identical appetitive stimuli, but only at times chosen by the "learned mastery" group. Significant behavioural differences emerged at 7 to 10 months of age, with the "learned mastery" group demonstrating minimal fearful behaviour and enhanced exploratory activity when challenged by environmental stressors (e.g. novel environment). Furthermore, although in their own surroundings there was little difference between the behaviours of the two groups, the "yoked" group exhibited raised plasma cortisol concentrations. When, at the age of approximately two years, the animals were treated with an anxiogenic compound (β-carboline), the "learned mastery" group responded with aggression whereas the "yoked" group became fearful. Interestingly, when the animals were placed in new social groups, the "learned mastery" animals became the dominant members of the group whereas the "yoked" animals became the subordinates. Thus, early experience of controllability has important long-term consequences on social behaviour and social status. This may have relevance to humans in that individuals reared in an environment where they always lack controllability may be more likely to develop psychiatric disorders such as anxiety or depression.

Mother–infant or peer–peer separation also has important long-term behavioural consequences which may be relevant to depression. For example, separation of young rhesus monkeys from their mothers or peers results in a severe behavioural syndrome described as "despair" which may lead ultimately to the development of life-threatening illness which is characterised by failure to maintain adequate food and water intake, lethargy, withdrawal and lack of responsiveness to external stimuli. Similar behavioural effects have been reported when human infants are separated from their mothers. In species in which the young animals exhibit a high degree of interaction but the mother–infant relationship is less didactic (e.g. certain monkeys) a similar type of despair response is seen when a young animal is separated from its peers. Thus the autonomic, behavioural and neuroendocrine responses to a stressful situation will depend not only on the severity, duration and type of stress but also on past experience of the individual and the available options for coping with the stress, including the presence of conspecifics (i.e. the degree of social support).

It is now widely accepted that stress is a significant factor in the aetiology of certain psychiatric disorders in humans, for example major depression, panic attacks and anxiety and anorexia nervosa. A critical factor underlying these disorders is believed to be a disturbance of the mechanisms regulating CRH function in the brain. Thus, a large proportion of patients suffering from

Table 2.4 Summary of some of the behavioural effects evoked by stress

---

Fear and anxiogenesis
Reduced ingestive behaviour
Locomotor activity (in rodents)
    reduced in novel environment, accompanied by freezing and increased defecation and
    self-grooming; increased in familiar environment
Increased nociceptive threshold
Inhibition of normal reproductive behaviour
Manifestation of inappropriate behaviours and displacement activity

---

endogenous depression have elevated plasma cortisol concentrations which cannot be suppressed by dexamethasone treatment. In addition, they exhibit a blunted ACTH response following CRH stimulation, which is believed to be due to a decrease in pituitary responsiveness to the releasing hormone. The concentrations of CRH in the cerebrospinal fluid of untreated patients with endogenous depression or suicide victims are higher than those of either healthy age-matched controls or patients with other psychiatric disorders such as schizophrenia or dementia. They are also higher in females than males as is the incidence of depression and anxiety. Recently studies have shown that i.c.v. injections of CRH can produce kindling (i.e. repeated exposure results in increasing responses); this may be an important factor in panic disorders where the symptoms increase in frequency and intensity with time. Some of the effects of stress on behaviour are summarised in Table 2.4.

2.7 CONCLUSIONS

Exposure to stress gives rise to a variety of autonomic and behavioural effects that, depending on their exact nature, may ultimately be either beneficial or detrimental to an animal's well-being. Thus a variety of pathological and mental disorders may occur following stress exposure, particularly if it is chronic, severe or uncontrollable. CRH is found in those areas of the brain that are involved in the regulation of autonomic function and behaviour and there is strong evidence to suggest that it plays an important role in the initiation and integration of these responses. The possible role of stress, and of CRH, in the aetiology of human psychiatric disorders is also considered.

REFERENCES

1. Lefkowitz R. J., Hoffman B. B., Taylor P. Neurotransmission. The autonomic nervous and somatic nervous systems. In G. H. Hardman, L. E. Limbard, P. B. Molinoff, R. W.

Raymond and A. Gilman (eds) *Goodman and Gilman's The Pharmacological Basis of Therapeutics*. New York, McGraw-Hill, 1995, pp 105 –39.

2. Neal M. J. *Medical Pharmacology at a Glance*. Oxford, Blackwell Science Ltd., 1989, p 20.

3. Watson S., Girdlestone D. Receptor and ion channel nomenclature supplement. *TIPS*, 1996, **18** (suppl): 5–13.

4. Vellucci S. V. Primate social behaviour: anxiety or depression. In S. E. File (ed) *Psychopharmacology of Anxiolytics and Antidepressants*. New York, Pergamon Press, 1991, pp 83–105.

5. De Souza E. B. Corticotropin-releasing factor receptors: physiology, pharmacology, biochemistry and role in central nervous system and immune disorders. *Psychoneuroendocrinology*, 1995, **20**: 789–819.

6. Dunn A. J., Berridge C. W. Physiological and behavioral responses to corticotropin-releasing factor administration: is CRF a mediator of anxiety or stress responses? *Brain Research Reviews*, 1990, **15**: 71–100.

7. Owens M. J., Nemeroff C. B. Physiology and pharmacology of corticotropin-releasing factor. *Pharmacological Reviews*, 1991, **43**: 425–473.

Chapter 3

The Immune System

Richard Aspinall

Imperial College School of Medicine, London, UK

3.1 INTRODUCTION

There are few safe natural environments and indeed, unless free from all predators and competitors, all environments are potentially hazardous. Survival is thus an active process that involves competition for finite resources not only with fellow members of the species but also with all other species. The prize for the winners of this competition is the long-term maintenance of their DNA, both in the present population and in future generations. The continuance of DNA within the gene pool requires both its successful replication and the survival of that replicated DNA in the next generation for further replication and, hence, transmission to offspring. For humans, this demands a survival period of approximately 40 years, i.e. from birth until the attainment of sexual maturity of offspring. Throughout this period humans have to face the onslaught of bacteria, viruses, fungi and other parasites, whose sole aim is to ensure that their DNA is established in the next generation for which humans provide the resources.

Stress, Stress Hormones and the Immune System. Edited by J. C. Buckingham, G. E. Gillies and A.-M. Cowell
© 1997 John Wiley & Sons, Ltd.

Humans have probably been subject to major epidemics periodically for the last 5000 years. Such epidemics have coincided largely with the time required for the population to reach a critical density and for individuals to migrate between groups to establish the conditions for the spread of infectious pathogens. Survival of the human species has thus become dependent on the ability to cope with infectious agents both from local sources and from afar. Similar arguments apply to other mammalian species and indeed to lower vertebrates and other organisms. The life cycles of the invading organisms are, however, much shorter than that of their hosts and thus the genetic mutations that occur naturally allow the organisms to take advantage of weaknesses in the host's defence mechanisms. This has placed a major selective pressure on genes that enable individuals to resist infection and survive. As a result, a powerful defence mechanism has evolved to counteract this onslaught and protect the host; this is termed the immune system.

The mammalian immune system, which has reached a particularly high level of sophistication in man, has two major components; one is non-specific and capable of acting against a wide variety of agents while the other is highly specific and discriminates between different invading organisms. This chapter describes the basic mechanisms of non-specific and specific immunity and aims to present an overview of the wide array of complex mechanisms that are brought into play when a foreign substance enters the body. The cells involved in mediating the immune-inflammatory response are summarised in Table 3.1a and b.

Table 3.1a Cells involved in immune/inflammatory responses

Present within the tissue	Vascular endothelial cells
	Mast cells
	Tissue mononuclear phagocytes/macrophages
Enter from the blood	Platelets (contain no nucleus, therefore, not strictly a cell)
	Leukocytes/white blood cells (actively mobile)

Table 3.1b Classification of leukocytes (white blood cells)

		Proportion of leukocyte population (%)
Polymorphonuclear cells/granulocytes	Neutrophils	55
	Eosinophils	3
	Basophils	0.5
Mononuclear cells	Lymphocytes	35
	Monocytes	6.5

3.2 NON-SPECIFIC IMMUNITY

Non-specific immunity, also termed natural, native or innate immunity, encompasses defence mechanisms which are present in the body prior to exposure to foreign antigen.

Factors which play important roles in non-specific immunity include physicochemical barriers, circulating molecules (e.g. complement and acute phase proteins) and phagocytic cells.

3.2.1 Physical and Chemical Barriers

The environment which bathes our cells, providing them with nutritional support and removing waste products, also provides an ideal environment for the support of potential invading organisms. Physical barriers exist between the external environment and this nutritionally rich internal environment to prevent the influx of such organisms. Many of the barriers are not just physical walls to the entry of organisms but contain various chemical protective elements. These include, for example, the acid of the stomach which produces an environment of low pH, the antibacterial peptides produced by the intestinal cells and enzymes such as lysozyme in the saliva, sweat and tears or pepsin produced by the cells of the gut. Any organism able to breach these barriers and lodge itself within the body tissues will be counteracted initially by a blanket form of defence. This innate or non-specific form of defence is immediate and ever present in healthy, nutritionally normal individuals and is able to discriminate in a limited way between self and non-self components. The speed of response is crucial because, for example, a bacterium which can replicate in 20 min will produce 4.7×10^{21} progeny within 24 h of invasion. The innate system, therefore, provides a crucial first line of defence, playing a fundamental role in preventing more tissue damage, in isolating and destroying the infectious agent and in activating the repair processes.

3.2.2 Complement

The factors that initiate a non-specific immune response are usually products of the invasive organism itself. The complement system, a collection of soluble serum proteins that acts in a cascade fashion to enhance the inflammatory response in various ways, is of primary importance in destroying such organisms. The C3 component is central to the complement pathway and is normally present in serum, largely in the inactive form, at a concentration of approximately 1300 μg/ml. Activation of this component may occur in a non-specific manner via the "alternative" pathway, which is described below, or in an antibody-dependent manner via the "classical" pathway of specific immunity (see Section 3.3.1). (No relative importance of the pathways should be inferred from this nomenclature. These pathways were so named because the classical pathway was the first to be discovered).

Activation of C3 occurs constantly, albeit at a very slow rate, due to a natural hydrolysis reaction and results in the formation of an activated form termed C3b which possesses an unstable bond. This molecule can react avidly with the proteins and carbohydrates present on the surfaces of all cells. In the normal situation any C3b in the circulation is rapidly inactivated and normal cells possess co-factors that cause the break down of any C3b which binds to their plasma membrane. Host tissue is thus protected from damage by complement. However, these protective co-factors are not present on bacteria and thus the C3b remains bound on their surface and will subsequently bind the three other components essential to this alternative pathway, namely Factor B, Factor D and properdin. The ensuing combination of these components forms the all important C3 convertase enzyme which converts more C3 into its activated form, and hence potentially greatly amplifies this critical component in the complement pathway. One report estimates that a single molecule of C3b deposited on an organism can become 4×10^6 molecules in about 4 min. Thus large amounts of activated C3 convertase build up on the bacterial cell surface. This complex then binds C3b which changes the C3 convertase to C5 convertase, thus permitting the cleavage of the C5 component into C5a and C5b. In the classical complement pathway analogous C3 and C5 convertases are formed and from this point onwards the two pathways converge, resulting in the formation of the cytocidal "membrane attack complex" (MAC). This requires, firstly, the binding of C5b to the membrane complex and subsequently binding of the C6, C7, C8 and C9 complement components. C9 is a monomer of 79 kDa and it has been suggested that between 12 and 15 C9 molecules bind to the C5b–C8 complex. This greatly enhances the ability of the complex to enter the lipid bilayer and to form pores in the plasma membrane that are large enough to allow free diffusion of small molecules (water, ions) but too small to permit the passage of large molecules (e.g. proteins). This results in an influx of water and cell death by osmotic lysis.

In addition to cell death, activation of complement results in the recruitment of other immune mechanisms to eliminate foreign macromolecules from host tissues. The products released by the breakdown of C3 and C5, that is C3a and C5a, act as chemotactic factors for neutrophils (see Section 3.2.3.) which are consequently drawn from the vasculature to the point of the injury. C3a and C5a also cause smooth muscle contraction and degranulation of mast cells and basophils with consequent release of histamine and other vasoactive substances which induce capillary leakage. Clearly these are powerful molecules and, not surprisingly, their life span is limited; inactivation is effected by serum carboxy-peptidases which cleave the terminal arginine from the peptides and thereby reduce biological activity.

3.2.3 Macrophages, Neutrophils and Inflammatory Mediators

Macrophages and neutrophils have been termed the "professional phagocytes" of the body as they engulf and effectively remove exogenous pathogens and cell debris. Macrophages originate in the bone marrow as promonocytes and mature macrophages are distributed throughout the tissues and serous cavities of the body. In general they are long-lived cells which depend upon mitochondria for the generation of their metabolic energy. At sites where physical or chemical barriers are breached by invading pathogens, local macrophages are activated by a number of factors including microbial products such as lipopolysaccharide (LPS) and also complement components (C5a) and certain cytokines (tumour necrosis factor, TNFα; interferon-γ, IFN-γ; interleukin-4, IL-4). The activated macrophages generate active oxygen species which promote phagocytosis and bacterial cell killing. Macrophage activation also promotes local inflammation directly, via the production of inflammatory mediators including platelet activating factor (PAF), prostaglandins and leukotrienes (see also Chapter 8). An indirect route may also be brought into play via the initiation of the plasma clotting cascade and hence thrombin production which, in turn, stimulates neutrophils and endothelial cells to synthesise PAF.

Activated macrophages also release a broad spectrum of cytokines including IL-1 and TNF which act both locally and systemically on stromal cells such as fibroblasts and epithelial cells, leading to a secondary wave of cytokine release. Although some of these cytokines may also have been released earlier by the activated monocytes, this secondary wave is important because it plays a major role in initiating the acute phase response (see below).

Products both of macrophages and complement activation assist in the mass migration of neutrophils to the site of the injury. For example, IL-1 and TNF induce changes in the local vasculature that increase permeability and stimulate the expression of adhesion molecules by the endothelial cells. As a result, neutrophils attach to the local endothelial cells and pass from the vasculature into the tissues. In addition, factors such as IL-8 and monocyte chemoattractant factor are produced within the local lesion and serve as potent chemoattractants to neutrophils and mononuclear cells respectively.

Neutrophils are non-dividing, short-lived cells which are terminally differentiated. They are produced in the bone marrow from their precursors and are programmed to die within a matter of two to three days. Since they constitute from 50–66% of all of the white cells in the circulation and have such a short life span they are produced in great numbers. In the marrow about 60% of all haemopoietic activity is directed towards neutrophil production compared with 20–30% devoted to producing erythrocytes. Neutrophils are devoid of mitochondria and depend on their abundant cytoplasmic glycogen stores for energy. This cytoplasmic glycogen pool enables the cells to be active and metabolise in anaerobic conditions. Along with macrophages, neutrophils are the main cell types seen in early inflammatory responses and their function is to engulf any bacterial cell debris or foreign particular matter. Particles that have been taken in by the neutrophil are contained within membrane-bound vesicles called phagosomes; storage granules from the cytoplasm of the neutrophil fuse with these phagosomes and fill them with compounds which are able to kill and degrade bacteria.

As will become clear later, macrophages and neutrophils also play important roles in all phases of the specific immune response. In addition, they contribute to the processes of wound cleaning and the elimination from the body of the antigens that initiate the specific immune response by the host cells and tissues.

3.2.4   Acute Phase Reactants

Thus far, invasion of the host by a foreign body has evoked complement activation and a storm of cytokines which, in turn, lead to changes in the local vasculature and the insurgence of neutrophils. In addition, cytokines produced at the site of the lesion may also induce systemic changes, which include the induction of the acute phase response. The acute phase response is characterised by fever, more generalised changes in vascular permeability and changes in the biosynthetic, metabolic and catabolic profiles of many organs. It depends to a large extent on a cytokine-driven increase in the hepatic production of a range of plasma proteins including complement C-reactive protein and mannose binding protein. Both C-reactive protein and mannose binding protein have the ability to bind to bacterial cell surfaces to promote complement activation and bacterial cell lysis. They may also act as opsonins to enhance bacterial phagocytosis.

The immediate, innate response described above is often followed by a lymphoid cell-mediated response which shows a greater degree of specificity in terms of coping with invaders. The specificity of the lymphoid cell-mediated response derives from the recognition of a foreign antigen by specific receptors located on the surface of the lymphocytes.

3.3   SPECIFIC IMMUNITY

Specific immune reactions, also termed adaptive or acquired immune reactions, are carried out by the lymphocytes which are the only cells in the body capable of recognising foreign antigens. There are of the order of 1×10^{12} lymphocytes in the adult human. Complex processes early in development ensure that each lymphocyte expresses an unique protein on its cell surface which recognises foreign, but not host or "self", molecules and therefore functions as an "antigen receptor". The first phase of a specific immune response, often called the "cognitive" phase, is the binding of antigen to its specific receptor. This leads to the "activation" phase which involves cell proliferation (clonal expansion), differentiation and migration and, subsequently, to the "effector" phase in which the activated cohort of lymphocytes destroys and eliminates the foreign substance. The mechanisms of the effector phase vary greatly and may extend to recruitment of components of the natural immune system. The specific immune system may thus confer some specificity to the non-specific immune response.

There are two major classes of lymphocytes, termed B cells and T cells. B cells secrete antibodies. These recognise and bind to specific antigens which are then destroyed; this process is called *humoral immunity* and is the principal defence mechanism against extracellular microbes and their secreted toxins. By contrast, T lymphocytes serve to eliminate invading pathogens by recognising and binding directly (via cell surface receptors) to antigens on the surface of cells termed "antigen presenting cells". This process, which is called *cell mediated immunity*, is directed towards intracellular microbes such as viruses and certain bacteria which proliferate inside host cells. In addition, T cells may recognise potential tumour antigens as non-self. Despite clear differences in their function, T and B cells are similar morphologically. They are typically 8–10 mm in diameter with a large nucleus surrounded by a thin rim of cytoplasm. Natural killer (NK) cells may also be categorised as lymphocytes but, unlike T and B cells, they are usually large and granular.

3.3.1   B Cell Lymphocytes

B Cell Receptors, Immunoglobulin Structure and Diversity

B lymphocytes, which are the only cells in the body capable of producing antibodies, are key players in the processes of humoral immunity. They recognise their respective antigens via cell-specific receptors located on their surfaces. These receptors are membrane-bound antibodies and, in any given cell, they are identical in structure to the antibody eventually secreted by that cell into the blood stream, with the exception of a short amino acid sequence which allows their insertion into the cell membrane.

Antibodies, or immunoglobulins (gamma globulins with immune properties) as they are also called, all have the same basic structure and physico-chemical features (Fig. 3.1). They are constructed of two identical proteins, each of which is comprised of a heavy chain and a light chain. The heavy and light elements refer to the length of the polypeptide chains, with the light chain being approximately half the length of the heavy chain. There are two types of light chain, termed κ or λ. Greek letters are also used to denote the different types of heavy chain; in man there are five, termed γ, α, μ, δ and ϵ. The classes or isotypes of antibodies are named according to the heavy chain, but using English

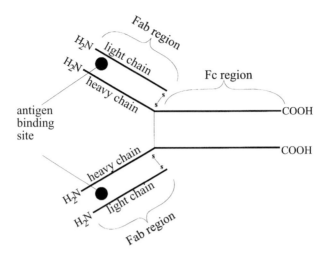

Figure 3.1   Diagrammatic representation of an immunoglobulin molecule

capital letters to denote the subclass, i.e. IgG, IgA, IgM, IgD, or IgE. Each class is characterised by extensive regions of homology within the heavy chain although further subdivisions of IgG and IgA have been described on the basis of sequence homologies.

Despite overall structural similarity, there are an estimated 1×10^{7}–1×10^{9} different antibody molecules in every individual, each with an unique amino acid sequence in its antigen binding domain. If each antibody were encoded by a single gene, approximately half the genome would be required to produce the full spectrum of antibody molecules present in a given individual. Complex genetic mechanisms have thus developed which enable B cells to produce an enormous number of molecules from a limited number of immunoglobulin genes. The diversity in the antibody repertoire depends on three short regions (each approximately 10 amino acids long) in the N-terminus of the heavy and long chains, termed the hypervariable regions or complementarity determining regions, which are generated by complex genetic mechanisms. Alignment of the hypervariable regions of each heavy chain with the light chain produces a three-dimensional shape with a unique ability to recognise the complementary three-dimensional shape of a specific antigen; this forms the antigen binding site.

B Cell Maturation and Activation

All lymphocytes are generated from stem cells, which are first formed in the yolk sac blood islands during embryogenesis. As development of the embryo proceeds, the site of stem cell production moves to the liver and subsequently to the bone marrow which is the major site of production in the adult. Precursors of mature B cells pass through distinct developmental stages. These include pro-B cells, which do not express immunoglobulin products and pre-B cells, which express the heavy chain of IgM in their cytoplasm only and thus cannot respond to antigen. This is followed by production of a light chain and assembly of an IgM with a distinct antigen specificity on the cell surface. The immature B cell goes on to express surface IgD and then migrates from the bone marrow to the peripheral lymphoid tissues and circulates in blood and lymph.

Virgin B lymphocytes which fail to encounter their antigen die within days. Interaction of the B cell with antigen, however, results in cross-linking of the membrane-bound immunoglobulin and hence to B cell activation, proliferation and antibody secretion. Some of the daughter cells will express the γ, α or ϵ heavy chains in addition to the μ and δ heavy chains expressed previously, while preserving the antigen specificity. This process is called "isotype switching" and, as the heavy chain isotype influences the effector mechanisms whereby antibodies eliminate foreign molecules (see below), it will expand the effectiveness of the response. This pattern of immunoglobulin expression may be useful in determining the stages of B cell maturation. Some activated lymphocytes are not secretory but retain their immunoglobulin which remains associated with the membrane. Such cells are termed memory cells and, although because of isotype switching they may produce antibodies of any class, they retain their original antigen specificity. Memory B cells survive for weeks, months or even years and serve to mount the secondary antibody response which will normally produce antibodies of higher affinity, but constant specificity (affinity maturation).

The antigens recognised by B cells are foreign proteins, glycoproteins, polysaccharides or lipids. Responses to some molecules in the latter two classes can be made by B cells without T cell help and so have gained the name "thymus-independent antigens". B cell responses to other antigens (thymus-dependent antigens), such as foreign proteins, however, require not only the stimulus provided by the antigen binding to the membrane immunoglobulin but also a second stimulus provided by a subpopulation of T lymphocytes, often called helper T cells. Although thymus-independent antigens induce antibody responses, the generation of memory cells, isotype switching and affinity maturation occur only when the humoral immune response is activated by thymus-dependent antigens, suggesting that the helper T cells play a prime role in the generation of these phenomena.

A critical step in B cell activation by protein antigens involves the generation of intracellular second messengers which stimulate resting B cells to move from the G_0 to the G_1 stage of the cell cycle, a process which takes approximately 12–24 hours. In addition, protein antigens are internalised, processed and presented on the B cell surface in combination with class II molecules of the major histocompatibility complex (MHC) which enables them to be recognised by specific antigen receptors on helper T cells. (Further explanation of MHC-restricted lymphocyte reactions can be found on page 84). The B cell thus becomes an "antigen presenting cell". In certain circumstances, other cells such as macrophages and dendritic cells may also internalise, process and present antigens on their cell surface and perform the function of an antigen presenting cell.

The role of the helper T cells in activating the B cells relies on an ill-defined physical contact as well as on the production and secretion of cytokines, which are the principal molecules of communication between immune and inflammatory cells and are increasingly being recognised as important communicators between the immune, nervous and endocrine systems. Different cytokines appear to be active at different stages during B cell growth and differentiation and the precise characteristics of the humoral response may be influenced by the relative amounts of the various cytokines secreted. The principal cytokines involved in the humoral response are listed in Table 3.2. Much of this information has been obtained from *in vitro* studies on clonal cell lines and it remains to be determined whether there are any significant differences *in vivo*.

B Cell Effector Mechanisms

There are two major regions within the immunoglobulin molecule, namely the Fab region and the Fc portion (see Fig. 3.1), which are associated with different functions. The Fab region contains the antigen binding domain which is clearly important. It may act as an anti-toxin to deactivate the soluble toxic products of bacteria, or as opsonin to change the surface characteristics of a bacterium to make phagocytosis easier. Alternatively, the antibodies that bind to antigens on the surface of invading pathogens may act to neutralise and prevent the entry of viruses into cells (thus reducing their chances of survival) or act as anti-adhesins which, for example, prevent the attachment of bacteria to mucosal surfaces.

Other effector functions consequent upon antibody–antigen interactions depend on the Fc portions once the antibodies are complexed with the antigen. The relevant sites lie in the constant regions of the heavy chain in the Fc portion. Thus all antibodies belonging to a particular class will activate the same effector pathways, irrespective of their antigen specificity. These isotype-specific functions involve the activation of natural immunity and inflammatory mechanisms via several different pathways.

(a) When complexed with their antigens, IgG and IgM bind the first serum protein in the complement cascade (C1q). This results in the activation of complement via the "classical" pathway with the consequent activation of C3 and the generation of the membrane attack complex followed by lysis of the invading organisms. Complement activation also allows opsonisation (see below) and consequently enhanced phagocytosis as well as the local recruitment of inflammatory cells (e.g. mast cells and granulocytes; see pages 74–6).

(b) The Fc portion of the immunoglobulin molecule also has a directional role in opsonisation. Mononuclear phagocytes and neutrophils have receptors for the Fc region of IgG and through these they can be directed towards a coated bacterium whose membrane properties will have changed because of the binding of the antibody molecule. Opsonisation therefore leads to enhanced phagocytosis. Alternatively, C3b generated by complement activation can act as an opsonin to enhance phagocytosis via C3b receptors on leukocytes.

(c) Although cells can be lysed by complement this is a less efficient means of cell lysis than antibody-dependent cell-mediated cytotoxicity (ADCC). Here, the Fc portion of an antibody bound to its antigen on the surface of a cell is recognised by leukocytes such as macrophages or NK cells which bear Fc receptors on their cell surfaces. Lysis of the antibody-bearing target cell then proceeds. ADCC is distinct from the cell mediated reactions mounted by cytolytic T lymphocytes, as will be described later (pages 86–8).

(d) Mast cells and basophils possess specific high affinity receptors for IgE which bind their immunoglobulin, even in the absence of antigen. Addition of antigen causes cross linkage of the bound immunoglobulin molecules leading to degranulation within these cells which release their stored potent inflammatory and vasoactive mediators (e.g. histamine) and synthesise *de novo* lipid-derived mediators (leukotrienes, prostaglandins, PAF) which they subsequently release.

(e) At mucosal surfaces, such as the epithelial cells in the gut, a specific transport system exists for the transfer of IgA molecules from the blood to the mucosa where it may neutralise antigens in mucosal secretions.

B Cell Subsets

Although different B cells produce immunoglobulins belonging to different classes, until recently B cells were not thought of as a heterogeneous population and were subdivided only according to their developmental stage, as discussed on page 79 above. However, subdivisions have now been defined on the basis of the molecules expressed on the cell surface; the molecules are termed complementarity determining or cluster differentiation (CD) molecules and there is evidence to suggest an association between phenotype and function. Most attention has been given to the CD5$^+$ B cells which represent approximately 5% of the B cell population and arise early in development. In contrast to the majority of B cells, these cells are not replenished from stem cells in the bone marrow but have an inherent capacity for self-renewal. They appear to be involved in the humoral immune response to carbohydrates but not the response to protein antigens. Also of considerable interest are the CD40$^+$ B cells which interact with a "receptor" (CD40L) on T helper cells and appear to play a key role in the development of a memory pool of B cells. The biochemical and functional characterisation of B cell subsets is a rapidly growing area of research

Table 3.2 A brief guide to the cytokines

		Family: Haematopoietins
IL-2	Alternative name	T cell growth factor (TCGF)
	Production	T cells
	Function	T cell growth, B cell growth and differentiation, NK cell activation
IL-4	Alternative name	B cell growth factor 1, B cell stimulating factor, mast cell growth factor 2
	Production	Mainly T_H2 cells and mast cells
	Function	B cell activation, T cell growth, B cell production of IgE, mast cell growth
IL-5	Alternative name	T cell replacing factor, B cell stimulating factor, B cell, growth factor II, eosinophil differentiation factor
	Production	Mainly by T_H2 cells and mast cells
	Function	Growth and differentiation of eosinophils, B cell proliferation and IgA production
IL-6	Alternative name	Include B cell stimulating factor 2, interferon-$\beta2$, hepatocyte stimulating factor, plasmocyte growth factor
	Production	Mainly monocytes, T cells, fibroblasts and endothelial cells
	Function	T and B cell growth, B cell differentiation and IgG production, synthesis of acute phase proteins from the liver
		Family: Interferons
IFNα	Alternative name	Type-1 interferon, leukocyte interferon
	Production	Leukocytes
	Function	Anti-viral activity, increased MHC class I expression, increases NK function
IFNβ	Alternative name	Type-1 interferon, fibroblast interferon
	Production	Fibroblasts
	Function	Anti-viral activity, increased MHC class I expression, increases NK function
IFNγ	Alternative name	Type-II interferon, immune interferon
	Production	T_H-1 cells, NK cells
	Function	Macrophage activation, improves MHC class I and II expression on many cells, anti-viral activity, inhibits proliferation of T_H-2 cells

		Family: Tumour Necrosis Factor
TNFα	Alternative name	Cachetin
	Production	Mainly macrophages, T cells and B cells
	Function	Induces cachexia (weight loss), mediates local inflammatory responses, activates endothelium, activates macrophages and neutrophils, tumour cytoxicity
TNFβ	Alternative name	Lymphotoxin
	Production	T cells
	Function	Tumour cytoxicity, endothelial activation
		Family: Chemokines
IL-8	Alternative name	Monocyte derived neutrophil chemotactic factor, neutrophil activating factor, monocyte derived neutrophil activating peptide
	Production	Mainly by monocytes, endothelial cells and fibroblasts
	Function	Neutrophil chemotaxis, T cell chemotaxis at high doses
MCP-1	Alternative name	Monocyte chemo attractant factor (MCAF)
	Production	Macrophages and other cells
	Function	Chemotactic for monocytes
		Unassigned Family
IL-10	Alternative name	Cytokine synthesis inhibitor factor
	Production	Mainly by T_H2 cells and monocytes
	Function	Inhibition of antigen presentation to T_H1 cells, inhibition of IFNγ production, inhibition of IL-1, TNFα, IL-6 and IL-8 by macrophages, stimulation of mast cells, induction of class II MHC on B cells
IL-1	Alternative name	Lymphocyte activating factor (LAF), thymocyte proliferation factor, endogenous pyrogen, T cell replacing factor, B cell replacing factor, osteoclast activating factor (OAF), procoagulant inducing factor and muscle proteolysis inducing factor
	Production	Cells which produce IL-1 include macrophages, epithelial cells, endothelial cells, dendritic cells, Langerhans cells, B cells, some T cells and astrocytes
	Function	Role in T and B cell activation and macrophage activation, initiating phases of the acute phase response, and in promoting the fever response

and includes an understanding of ways in which B cells trigger death in tumour cells and mechanisms that underlie the generation of autoimmune conditions.

3.3.2   T Lymphocytes

T Cell Receptors, Subtypes and MHC-restricted Recognition of Antigen

Like B cells, T cells recognise their antigen by cell surface receptor, termed T cell receptors. The enormous diversity in the specificity, and hence structure, of the T cell receptor also arises from complex genetic mechanisms that involve somatic rearrangement during T cell development. The T cell receptor is a complex of at least seven polypeptide chains. In normal human venous blood the majority (>90%) of T cell receptors consist of one α and one β polypeptide chain, which are the antigen recognition elements, associated with a group of at least five proteins, the CD3 complex, which is essential for the function of all T cell receptors. The remaining T cell population expresses receptors composed of γ and δ chains along with the CD3 complex. The functional significance of the two subtypes of receptor is unclear but T cells bearing receptors with the $\gamma\delta$ configuration are located mainly in surface epithelial tissue. A normal peripheral blood T cell may have 20–30 000 $\alpha\beta^+$ receptor complexes on its surface. The chains which constitute the antigen recognition elements reveal similarities to immunoglobulin molecules, in that they also contain constant and variable regions. Between the constant and variable regions the β chain has portions termed the J (joining) region and the D (diversity region), whereas the α chain has only the J region. Recognition of specific antigens is determined by the V, D and J regions of the β chain and the V and J regions of the α chain. Further variability within the antigen binding domain, and hence specificity, may be introduced by the addition of extra nucleotides at the segments between these regions. There are approximately 130 genomic segments coding for the variable region of the $\alpha\beta^+$ T cell receptor (30 for the β chain and 100 for the α chain), about 62 genomic segments coding for the J region (50 for the α chain and 12 for the β chain) and 2 D regions for the β chain. Taking all possible combinations into account it has been suggested that the T cell receptor may express somewhere in the order of 10^{16} antigen binding specificities.

T cells detect only short peptide sequences in protein antigens which must be presented on the surfaces of other cells (antigen presenting cells) in association with the molecules of the MHC before they are recognised by their specific T cell receptors. The recognition is thus MHC restricted. MHC molecules are encoded by genes within a highly polymorphic region of the genome. Of importance in T cell receptor engagement are the MHC class I molecules and MHC class II molecules (see below). MHC molecules also play an important role in shaping the repertoire of mature T cells, i.e. in determining which cells survive and in ensuring that cells of the immune system can discriminate between self and non-self.

MHC class I. This is an ubiquitous molecule expressed on the surface of almost every nucleated cell in the body. It is composed of two protein chains of specific structure and an associated peptide of variable structure which may be a "self" molecule or a foreign antigen. The longer α chain is encoded by a gene within the MHC and has a cytoplasmic, a transmembrane and an extracellular portion. The second shorter chain is termed $\beta2$ microglobulin and the peptide fragment associated with these two chains is derived from the cytosol. Cytoplasmic proteins produced normally by the cell have a very short half-life; they are degraded and the products are transported to the lumen of the endoplasmic reticulum. There they associate with the α chain and the $\beta2$ microglobulin chain to form the final class I molecule which is transported to and expressed at the cell surface. This process is continuous and can be envisaged as the class I molecule sampling the cytoplasmic proteins at intervals and displaying peptides from the cytoplasmic contents at the cell surface. The majority of peptides expressed at the surface would not normally excite attention from the immune system because they are "self" peptides, and there should be no self reactive T cells in the peripheral tissues. However, if a cell becomes infected with virus its internal machinery may be switched to making viral particles which, like any other protein produced in the cytoplasm, would be degraded to short peptide fragments. These foreign peptides would then be displayed as part of the class I molecule at the cell surface. T cells with receptors specific for that MHC class I-associated peptide would then become alerted to the fact that the cell was making a non-self peptide. The MHC class I molecules are therefore presenting antigenic peptides from *endogenous* sources at the cell surface. The T cells which recognise class I restricted antigens represent a distinct subset which express CD8 molecules on the cell surface that bind to the non-polymorphic region of the class I molecule.

MHC class II. Unlike MHC class I, the MHC class II molecules have a restricted distribution. Cells that express MHC class II constitutively are usually cells that are moving about the body. MHC class II molecules are composed of two chains, termed α and β, both of which are encoded by genes within the MHC. Newly synthesised class II molecules are present in vesicles which are produced from the endoplasmic reticulum and are directed to the Golgi apparatus, which acts as a form of traffic policeman and directs these vesicles to the endosomal pathway. The cell utilizes this endosomal pathway to internalise resources from outside the cell which are then contained in vesicles or coated pits. Equally, invading organisms may take advantage of this mechanism for entering the cell. Eventually the proteases within the endosomal vesicle are activated to degrade the proteins to peptide fragments. Vesicles containing the

MHC class II molecule then meet and fuse with the vesicle containing these degraded peptide fragments which associate with the class II molecules. The now complete class II molecule is then expressed at the cell surface. Clearly the MHC class II molecule is constantly analysing the pathway by which substances enter the cell, including antigenic peptides derived from exogenous sources which are then expressed at the cell surface. The T cells which recognise class II MHC-restricted antigens express CD4 molecules on their cell surface, which bind to the non-polymorphic region of the MHC class II molecule.

T cells may also be classified on the basis of their effector functions as discussed in the following section.

T Cell Activation and Effector Mechanisms

T cell activation requires that the T cell receptor–CD3 complex on the T cell surface recognises and binds the processed peptide antigen fragment that is expressed on the surface of the antigen-presenting cell in association with the relevant MHC molecule. Additional molecules on the T cell surface, termed accessory molecules, may also be necessary for full activation to proceed. For example, as well as aiding in the ability of a T cell to recognise its antigen, CD4 and CD8 molecules participate in the activation and response of a T cell. For $CD4^+$ cells, which are MHC II restricted, the expression of co-stimulatory molecules may also be required on the antigen-presenting cells. (Principally macrophages, B cells and dendritic cells express MHC II). For example, B7 interacts with CD28 on T cells. The need for the simultaneous delivery of signals from an antigen presenting cell and a responding MHC-restricted T cell is a fail-safe mechanism used by the immune system to combat any self-reactive T cells present in the somatic tissues and thus prevent their clonal expansion. For example, $CD4^+$ T cells recognising peptide presented by MHC class II molecules on somatic cells in the absence of a co-stimulatory molecule will not invoke the clonal expansion of those T cells, but will lead instead to the induction of a state of anergy (a state of non-responsiveness) in those T cells.

Once the interaction between the T cell and the presenting antigen has occurred, a number of early membrane or intracellular signals are induced within the T cell; these include inositol phospholipid hydrolysis, increased Ca^{2+} levels, protein phosphorylation and ion fluxes. These then trigger transcriptional activation and expression of T cell genes which, in turn, causes cell proliferation, differentiation and stimulation of effector functions. Over 70 T cell genes are thought to be involved in these processes, including cellular proto-oncogenes (e.g. *c-myc* and *c-fos*) which are induced in minutes, cytokine genes which are stimulated within minutes or hours and, finally, cytokine receptor genes which enable the T cell itself to mount a proliferative response to its own cytokine growth factors.

$CD4^+$ cells appear to be central to many T cell-mediated responses since activation of these cells results in the generation of cytokine-producing cells which, in turn, provide the necessary extra signals to stimulate B and T cell effector functions. This observation led to the concept of "immunological help" and the idea that the CD4$^+$ population contained the T helper cell population. Similarly, experiments on defining the phenotype of cytotoxic cells revealed that they were CD8$^+$. The idea that all cytotoxic cells are CD8$^+$ and that all CD4$^+$ cells are helper cells is somewhat of a generalisation and does not prove to be the case every time.

CD4$^+$ effector mechanisms. The cytokines secreted by the helper CD4$^+$ T lymphocytes serve to recruit and activate leukocytes involved in the inflammatory process (typically the components involved in non-specific immunity) and to enhance proliferation and differentiation in T and B lymphocytes as well as other cell types, including macrophages and venular endothelial cells. These events will thus greatly amplify both humoral and cell-mediated immune responses as well as recruiting and directing non-specific immune reactions towards a defined stimulus.

Early *in vitro* investigations on cloned CD4$^+$ cell lines suggested a subdivision of CD4$^+$ T cells into T$_H$1 and T$_H$2 populations based on the spectrum of cytokines which they produced when activated. T$_H$1 cells are characterised by the production of IL-2, TNF-β and IFN-γ which can drive the activation of macrophages, thus leading some to consider them as inflammatory T cells. T$_H$2 cells are characterised by the production of IL-4 and IL-5 which activate B cells. Consequently, some use the term "helper cells" for this subset alone. Both T$_H$1 and T$_H$2 cells are produced from a precursor designated T$_H$0. The exact mechanism which influences a CD4$^+$ cell to become a T$_H$1 or T$_H$2 cell is not known. Differentiation down a specific pathway may be influenced by the spectrum of cytokines produced by an immune stimulus which may vary depending on the nature and intensity of that stimulus. The major activities of cytokines involved in the immune response are summarised in Table 3.2. It must be remembered, however, that cytokines have overlapping functions and this, coupled with the stimulus-dependent cytokine cocktail which will prevail, will influence the precise course of the response and hence the consequent effector mechanisms recruited to eliminate a foreign antigen.

CD8$^+$ effector mechanisms. Cytotoxic lymphocytes are generally CD8$^+$ MHC class-I restricted but on rare occasions they may be CD4$^+$ MHC class-II restricted. They leave the thymus and circulate as "pre-cytolytic" cells which express T cell receptors with antigen specificity but they have no inherent cytolytic activity. They require activation which may be achieved by interaction of the CD8$^+$ cell with a dendritic cell expressing high levels of the co-stimulating molecules in addition to the specific antigen appropriately displayed on MHC molecules. The presence of these signals activates the CD8$^+$ cell to produce

IL-2, driving its own proliferation. Alternatively, CD8$^+$ cells can be activated with the help of CD4$^+$ T cells which may be needed because co-stimulatory molecules on the dendritic cells did not reach levels adequate to induce self-activation of the CD8$^+$ cell. Once activated, the cytolytic cell kills its target by one of two independent mechanisms, depending on the cytokine environment. One method is analogous to the osmotic lysis caused by complement activation (see Section 3.2.2) and involves the granular synthesis of pore-forming molecules, called perforin or cytolysin, which are inserted into the membrane of the target cell but which have no effect on the T cell. The second method involves the induction of apoptosis in the target cell, which involves DNA cleavage, nuclear disruption and cell death.

Activated CD8$^+$ cells also secrete IFN-γ which has antiviral activity and induces the expression of MHC class I molecules in infected cells, thus increasing their chances of becoming target cells for cytotoxic CD8$^+$ T cells. Both of these features assist in the removal of intracelluar viral particles, one of the prime physiological functions of cytolytic T lymphocytes.

At one time, a category of CD8$^+$ cells which were dependent on CD4$^+$ T cell help, were classified as suppressor T lymphocytes. These cells were thought to secrete suppressor factors which limit the cell mediated response by interacting with T cell receptors to inhibit the interactions of the T cells with their antigen-presenting cells. More recently the significance and even existence of such cells has been questioned.

T Cell Development

Throughout life pre-T cells originate in the bone marrow stem cells and migrate to the thymus, which is the major site for T cell development in mammals. The thymus is a bilobed organ located, after birth, at the base of the great vessels overlying the heart. It is formed from tissues derived from disparate sites during gestation, including tissues from the third pharyngeal pouch and cleft and the neural crest, together with stem cells, macrophages and dendritic cells from haemopoietic centres. The thymus is relatively large at birth (typically 10–15 g in humans) and continues to grow until puberty (30–40 g in humans) after which it involutes (10–15 g at 60 years of age). There is little evidence for extra-thymic sites for T cell differentiation but, despite the thymic involution, T cell maturation continues throughout life.

Each lobe of the thymus consists of lobules divided into an outer, cell-dense area which is called the cortex and contains the immature thymocytes, and an inner region or medulla where T cells at later stages of development are found. The main pathway of development of $\alpha\beta$ T cells in the thymus is well characterised and the cell may be readily phenotyped at the different stages of development (see also Chapter 17). Separation on the basis of expression of the CD4 and CD8 molecules reveals four distinct populations. The CD4$^-$/CD8$^-$

(double negative cells), the $CD4^+/CD8^+$ (double positive cells) and the $CD4^+/CD8^-$ and $CD4^-/CD8^+$ cells (both termed single positive). The double negative thymocyte population represents the T cell precursors, which then proliferate and differentiate to produce the double positive population. Both of these populations are found in the cortex where complex processes of random somatic rearrangement of different gene segments occurs to generate functional T cell receptor genes. At this stage the T cell receptor–CD3 complex and accessory molecules are detectable in the cortex. Selection processes based on the specificity of the receptor expressed by the double positive cells then occur in the cortex and only those cells with the ability to recognise MHC molecules presenting foreign peptides are allowed to differentiate further into the single positive thymocytes, which are located in the medulla. This involves a process of positive selection (only thymocytes with receptors recognising self MHC molecules survive) followed by negative selection (elimination of potentially auto-reactive T cell clones). The cells which exit from the thymus represent only a small proportion of the total number of cells in the thymus and the majority of thymocytes will never leave the thymus but die there by a process of pro-grammed cell death.

T cells released from the thymus are antigenically naive and migrate around the secondary lymphoid tissue for a limited period only. (Experiments in mice suggest this may be a period of months). If they do not meet and interact with their respective antigens, they are functionally lost from the peripheral T cell pool. Interaction of the cell with antigen leads to activation, clonal expansion and the production of effectors which serve both to remove the antigen (by destroying the pathogen carrying that antigen) and to produce memory cells. Memory T cells respond more rapidly and with a greater magnitude of reaction to the antigen, should it reappear. Recent phenotyping studies have centred on the expression of the CD45 molecule, a glycoprotein that is expressed in various forms on all haemopoietic cells with the exception of erythrocytes. Memory T cells in humans express the CD45RO variant of the CD45 molecule whereas naive cells express the CD45RA variant. Both the $CD4^+$ and $CD8^+$ subsets are reported to contain functional naive and memory cells that express these CD45 variants.

3.3.3 Natural Killer Cells

Natural killer (NK) cells are large, granular lymphocytes that have the ability to kill some tumour cells and some virally infected cells as well as some normal cells. They are derived from the bone marrow and do not undergo thymic maturation. These cells do not have cell surface receptors that would allow for the type of MHC restricted antigen recognition found on T cells and, unlike T cells, they do not require priming before they kill their target. They are present in the blood of normal, healthy individuals and their numbers may vary with age. The exact mechanism by which they distinguish virally infected from normal cells is still not formally demonstrated. However, the fact that NK cells can kill targets expressing low levels of MHC molecules has led to the suggestion that in virally infected cells there is some alteration in either the levels of expression of MHC class I or its conformation which is recognised by the NK cell and leads to the induction of NK cell mediated killing.

3.4   LYMPHOID TISSUE

3.4.1   Primary Lymphoid Tissue

Primary lymphoid tissues are concerned with generating and maintaining a pool of lymphocytes. Events in the primary lymphoid tissue (i.e. the bone marrow and thymus) which are concerned with B and T cell development are described above (pages 78–9 and 88–9).

3.4.2   Secondary Lymphoid Tissue

The lymphocytes produced by and released from the primary lymphoid organs have such a diversity of receptor specificity that the possibility of one antigen meeting one specific B or T cell with the appropriate receptor would be remote, were it not for the organisation of the secondary lymphoid tissues.

Lymph Nodes

The capillary channels that make up the lymphatics are most numerous beneath the skin and the mucosa of the gastrointestinal, respiratory and genitourinary tracts, but are not found in the central nervous system, or the globe of the eye. The network of capillaries in a given region converges into vessels that empty into lymph nodes, forming the afferent lymphatics. Lymph nodes are encapsulated, bean-shaped organs which vary in size according to their level of activity. The afferent lymphatic channels enter the sub-capsular region of the lymph node bringing, amongst other things, antigen from the tissues that the lymph node serves. Lymphocytes released from primary lymphoid tissues which have not been stimulated by antigen enter lymph nodes from the blood via specialised venular epithelial cells (high endothelial venules). The lymph node thus provides an environment for the components of a potential immune response to meet and react together.

Spleen

The spleen is a highly vascularised organ lying between the fundus of the stomach and the diaphragm and is the largest aggregation of lymphoid tissue in the body. The lymphoid tissue is concentrated in the areas within the spleen, defined histologically as the white pulp, which contain distinct regions of B and T cells. The red pulp acts as a generalised filter removing particles and damaged erythrocytes from the blood. The spleen also contains large numbers of phagocytic cells, many of which are in the marginal zone of the white pulp. The splenic phagocytes remove cell debris and the products of effete erythrocytes, leukocytes and platelets as well as micro-organisms from the blood. This large concentration of phagocytes and lymphoid tissue thus allows the spleen to play a major role in the initiation of the immune response to circulating antigens.

Gut Tissue

The mucosal lymphoid tissue of the gastro-intestinal tract is subdivided into organised tissue (Peyer's patches), where antigen enters the system to induce an immune response, and diffuse tissue (the lamina propria containing lymphocytes and the intra-epithelial lymphocytes), where antigen interacts with effector lymphocytes.

3.5 STRESS AND ITS EFFECTS ON THE IMMUNE SYSTEM

Understanding the endogenous factors that regulate immune function has long been a challenge to the immunologist. Recognition of the interactions between the neuroendocrine, autonomic and immune systems has been an exciting development and is likely to bring research scientists and clinicians from these disciplines closer together. In particular, there has been a growing interest in how stress, with its accompanying influences on autonomic, endocrine and psychological and behavioural responses, may affect the functioning of the immune system, with wide-ranging implications for the pathophysiology and treatment of disease. Glucocorticoids are by far the best studied of the stress hormones that influence immune function and the underlying mechanisms are covered in detail in Chapter 8. Further aspects of stress–immune system interactions may be found in Chapters 9–19.

There are many studies, supported by anecdotal evidence, about the linkage between increased stress and an increased susceptibility to infectious disease. Retrospective studies have revealed that stressful life events increase the risk of contracting upper respiratory tract infections and studies on the reactivation of latent herpes virus infection suggest that disease episodes follow emotional distress. Similar results have been obtained in studies with bacterial infections and the effect of stress has also been extended to wound healing. In support of this, there are reports that peripheral leukocytes taken from women responsible for the care of elderly demented relatives produce significantly lower levels of IL-1β following stimulation with LPS when compared with leukocytes from control subjects. In addition, punch biopsy wounds in these female carers took significantly longer to heal than wounds from controls.

The critical step for the generation of an adequate response to an infectious organism is the bringing together of the antigen, the professional antigen presenting cell and the lymphocyte with the correct receptor specificity, in an environment which is conducive to supporting clonal expansion of the lymphocyte. The structure of the secondary lymphoid organs and the movement around the body of both naive lymphocytes and antigen presenting cells are intended to optimise the surveillance of the host's tissues and, most importantly, to improve the chances of encounter between a lymphocyte bearing a specific receptor and the antigen for which it is specific. Assuming an average of 2500 lymphocytes per μlitres of blood (2.5×10^9 lymphocytes per litre) and an average of 4 litres of blood per individual, a normal healthy individual may expect to have about 10^{10} lymphocytes in their blood. Some estimates suggest that approximately 2% of the lymphocytes in the body are present in the blood at any one time, making the total number of mature lymphocytes in the body approximately 5×10^{11}. Of these lymphocytes, about 3.5×10^{11} may be T cells and approximately 1.2×10^{11} B cells with the rest being NK cells. As mentioned earlier, the T cell receptor may be able to produce approximately 10^{16} antigen specificities but with only 3.5×10^{11} T cells in the peripheral pool, only a proportion of the potential repertoire can be represented at any one time. Any condition which reduces the chances of an antigen meeting a lymphocyte with the appropriate receptor specificity will reduce the efficiency of the immune response. Stress has this effect: it alters the migration characteristics of leukocytes, changes their cytokine production and also may alter the repertoire of receptors present in the T cell pool by virtue of the effect that stress has on T cell development. Each of these effects will be a factor in reducing the chances of the T cell with the correct receptor specificity coming into contact with the antigen presenting cell displaying the specific antigen. Any equation used to calculate the chances of an antigen meeting a lymphocyte receptor of the appropriate specificity should, therefore, take into consideration the degree of stress which will reduce the chances of this encounter.

FURTHER READING

Abbas A. K., Lichtman A. H., Pober J. S. *Cellular and Molecular Immunology*, Philadelphia, W. B. Saunders, 1991.

Ader R., Cohen N., Fetern D. Psychoneuroimmunology: Interactions between the nervous system and the immune system. *Lancet*, 1995, **345**: 99–103.

Baumann H., Gauldie J. The acute phase response. *Immunology Today*, 1994, **15**: 74–80.

Black P. Central nervous system–immune system interactions: Psychoneuro-endocrinology of stress and its immune consequences. *Anti-microbial Agents and Chemotherapy*, 1994, **38**: 1–6.

Black P. Immune system–central nervous system interactions: Effect and immunomodulatory consequences of immune system mediators on the brain. *Anti-microbial Agents and Chemotherapy*, 1994, **38**: 7–12.

Hanner I. *et al.* Lymphocyte populations as a function of age. *Immunology Today*, 1992, **13** 215–9.

Howard M. C., Miyajima A., Coffman R. T cell derived cytokines and their receptors. In W. E. Paul (ed) *Fundamental Immunology*. New York, Raven Press, 1993, pp 763–793.

Janeway C. A. Jr, Travers P. *Immunobiology: The Immune System in Health and Disease.* Oxford, Blackwell Scientific Publications, 1994.

Kiecolt-Glaser J. K., Marucha P. T., Malarkey W. B., Mercado A. M., Glaser R. Slowing of wound healing by psychological stress. *Lancet*, 1995, **346**: 1194–6.

Lentner C. (ed) *Geigy Scientific Tables 3*. Basle, CIBA Geigy, 1984, pp 65–6.

Ottaway C. A., Husband A. J. The influence of neuroendocrine pathways on lymphocyte migration. *Immunology Today*, 1994, **15**: 511–17.

Shreiber R. D., Chaplin D. D. Cytokines, inflammation and innate immunity. In M. M. Frank, K. F. Austen, H. N. Claman, E. R. Unanue (eds) *Samter's Immunological Disease*, 5th edition. Boston, MA, Little Brown and Co., 1995.

Steel D. M., Whitehead A. S. The major acute phase reactants: C-reactive protein, serum amyloid P component and serum amyloid A protein. *Immunology Today*, 1994, **15**: 80–7.

Stites D. P., Terr A. I., Parslow T. G. *Basic and Clinical Immunology*, 8th Edition. Connecticut, Appleton Lange, 1994.

Wilder R. Neuroendocrine–immune system interactions and autoimmunity. *Ann Rev Immunol*, 1995, **13**: 307–38.

Chapter 4

Hormone Receptors and Signal Transduction

G. P. Vinson

Queen Mary and Westfield College, London, UK

4.1   INTRODUCTION

The ability of cells to respond to chemical transmitter substances, whether they be hormones, immunokines or neurotransmitter substances, depends on the presence in the target cell of highly specific, saturable, high affinity binding proteins which are termed receptors; these may be located within the cell membrane (termed cell surface or membrane-bound receptors) or within the cell (intracellular receptors). The binding of a transmitter substance to its receptor causes the receptor to undergo a transformational change which triggers a sequence of events within the cell. These culminate in a specific physiological response, for example increased glucose uptake (insulin), synthesis and release of thyroid hormones (thyrotrophin), increased heart rate (adrenaline and nora-drenaline), increased or decreased synthesis of specific target proteins (steroids). The speed with which the physiological response occurs depends on the mechanisms of signalling downstream of the receptor and may vary from milliseconds to minutes, hours or even days. This chapter will review briefly the major families of receptors and the signal transduction mechanisms they use, with

Stress, Stress Hormones and the Immune System. Edited by J. C. Buckingham, G. E. Gillies and A.-M. Cowell
© 1997 John Wiley & Sons, Ltd.

particular reference to the endocrine system. For further details of this complex and rapidly advancing area the reader is referred to the reading list. A list of commonly used abbreviations is appended.

4.2   HORMONES, RECEPTORS AND THEIR INTERACTIONS: BASIC CONCEPTS

The binding of a transmitter substance (also called an "agonist" or "ligand") to its receptor and the subsequent initiation of a cellular event is often likened to unlocking and opening a door. The binding of the substance (the insertion of the key) is the rate limiting step which permits a conformational change in the receptor (the turning of the lock) and thereby triggers the cellular response (the opening of the door) via intracellular components which mediate the responses downstream of the receptor. Many factors can influence the efficiency with which this sequence of events is effected. These include:

(a) *The concentration of the agonist at the receptor.* The cellular responses to an agonist are normally concentration-dependent with a sigmoidal relationship between the logarithm of the concentration of agonist at the receptor and the magnitude of the response.

(b) *The binding characteristics of the agonist.* The affinity of the agonist for the receptor determines the potency or sensitivity of the response (Fig. 4.1). Affinity is usually measured by the dissociation constant (K_d) which in practical terms is the concentration of free ligand which gives half-maximal saturation of the receptor complement. Thus, a lower value for K_d implies a greater affinity. As the affinity increases (and K_d decreases), the propensity for forming ligand–receptor complexes is increased and the curve for agonist concentration vs. response is shifted to the left. The potency of an agonist in initiating a biological response may be measured in different ways but most commonly, following pharmacological practice, it is given as the ED-50 which is the concentration that gives half maximal response. In a single cell *in vitro* system (i.e. where the accessibility of the ligand to its receptors is not limited by pharmacokinetic factors) the ED-50 may be expected in principle to be numerically similar to the K_d; in actuality however, it is sometimes considerably lower than the predicted value because only a small percentage of the receptors needs to be occupied to elicit a maximal cellular response, the remaining receptors being termed "spare receptors". An alternative measure of ligand potency is the lowest concentration of hormone to give a response which is statistically different from zero. This value cannot be predicted from the K_d, and therefore increases the knowledge about the ligand–receptor interaction.

(c) *The efficacy of the ligand.* Some substances are termed full agonists as they will trigger a maximal (100%) cellular response and thus have "high efficacy" or "high intrinsic activity"; others, termed partial agonists, produce a maximal response which is substantially lower than that elicited by a full agonist even though they may bind to the receptor with high affinity. Receptor antagonists also bind with high affinity but they fail to elicit the conformational change in the receptor required to elicit a response, i.e. they have no efficacy. Thus, by virtue of occupying the receptor, they limit the access of agonist. Antagonists which bind reversibly to the receptor and thus compete with agonists for occupancy are called "competitive antagonists"; they cause a parallel shift to the right of the concentration response curve for a given agonist. Antagonists which bind irreversibly to the receptor reduce the magnitude of the maximum response to agonist and produce a non-parallel shift of the agonist dose response curve to the right.

(d) *The number and affinity state of the receptors.* An alteration in receptor number or affinity state will have a profound influence on the biological response, particularly for those receptor populations which require full occupancy to elicit a maximal cellular response. In the long term receptor concentration is regulated to a high degree by the ligand concentration, with chronic stimulation frequently resulting in a reduction in receptor density (termed "down-regulation"); conversely understimulation leads to receptor "upregulation". Such regulation does not normally occur in the acute stimulatory period which characterises many physiological responses. None-theless, since receptors are saturable, vigorous stimulation, even in the acute period, will result in fewer free receptors being available. Moreover, in the case of membrane bound receptors the ligand–receptor complex may be internalised (see Section 4.3) or, alternatively, the receptor may be trans-formed to a low affinity state.

(e) *The cellular factors required to transduce the response.* Although these factors are invariably present in the target cells, they do not exist in a steady state but are subject constantly to tight regulation. Alterations in their status may be expected to have a significant impact on the final cellular response and, indeed, they provide an important target for novel therapeutic interventions.

4.3 MEMBRANE-BOUND RECEPTORS

Neurotransmitter substances, cytokines and many hormones—typically amino acid derivatives such as adrenaline (but not thyroid hormones), peptides, proteins and glycoproteins—bind to receptors that are embedded in the cell membrane and it is here that the receptor conformational change triggers the intracellular signalling cascade. Receptor activation may also lead to internalisation of the ligand–receptor complex; however, this process is not associated with the

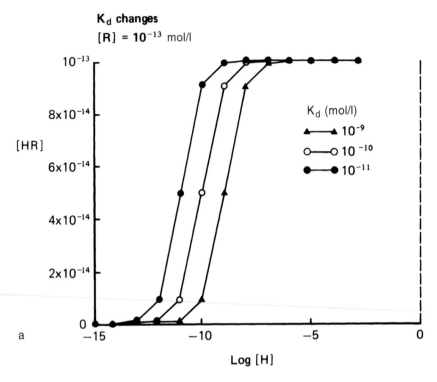

Figure 4.1a The effect of changing the dissociation constant (K_d) on the formation of the hormone receptor (HR) complex at different hormone concentrations. These computer generated curves illustrate responses in a system in which the receptor concentration is 10^{-13} mol/l, and the K_d is 10^{-9}, 10^{-10} or 10^{-11} mol/l

manifestation of the cellular response, although in some instances it may aid the delivery of the ligand to an intracellular target (see Chapter 1). In general however, the internalisation process is associated with receptor regulation and leads either to hormone–receptor degradation or to recycling of the functional receptor back to the membrane after an indeterminate refractory period. Membrane-bound receptors are classified on the basis of their structure and the signal transduction sequences they use; broadly they fall into four main classes:

(a) ion channel linked receptors,
(b) guanine binding protein (G-protein) coupled receptors,
(c) tyrosine kinase receptors, and
(d) cytokine receptors.

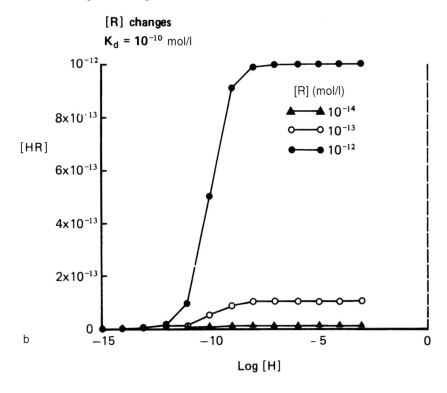

Figure 4.1b The effect of changing receptor concentration on the formation of the hormone receptor (HR) complex. In these curves, the K_d is constant at 10^{-10} mol/l, while receptor concentration varies between 10^{-12} and 10^{-14} mol/l. In both **a** and **b** data are presented as semilog plots, the conventional form for dose response data. This seemingly exaggerates the effect of receptor concentration compared with K_d. However, a corollary is that, in general, the amplitude of response is often easier to evaluate precisely than is the sensitivity, that is, the minimum effective dose. The biological response does not necessarily precisely reflect the formation of HR since full responses may often be achieved when only a proportion of the total receptor population available is occupied; equally, a biological response may occur only after a large proportion of the receptors is occupied. (Both figures from Vinson G. P., Whitehouse B., Hinson J. P. (1992), *The Adrenal Cortex* p 143. Reprinted by permission of Prentice Hall, Upper Saddle River, New Jersey)

4.3.1   Ion Channel Linked Receptors

These receptors mediate very rapid events, with the manifestation of the cellular event taking only milliseconds from the binding of ligand to receptor. They are found predominantly, although not exclusively, in the central and peripheral nervous systems and skeletal muscle (i.e. in excitable tissues) where they mediate fast synaptic transmission. Important examples include the nicotinic acetylcholine receptor, the type A γ-amino butyric acid (GABA$_A$) receptor, the type 3 5-hydroxytryptamine (5-HT$_3$) receptor and the N-methyl, D-aspartate (NMDA) glutamate receptor. Structurally these receptors are composed of five oligomeric protein subunits arranged in the lipid membrane around an aqueous ion channel; each subunit includes four sequences of some 20–25 hydrophobic amino acids which form α-helices and span the cell membrane (the "transmembrane domain"). The most extensively studied of these receptors is the nicotinic receptor which comprises four different subunit proteins (α, β, γ and δ) arranged in a pentameric structure (α_2, β, γ, δ); each receptor has two acetylcholine binding sites, both of which must be occupied for receptor activation. Binding of ligand causes a conformational change which opens the channel and thus permits a rapid influx of Na$^+$ which, in turn, depolarises the cell membrane. Molecular studies have demonstrated tissue-specific variants in subunit sequences which provide opportunity for a high degree of receptor heterogeneity; thus, distinct subpopulations of nicotinic receptors occur in different regions of the brain and these differ again from those found in skeletal muscle.

Molecular heterogeneity is also a feature of other ion channel linked receptors. Its functional significance is unclear but pharmacological studies indicate that it may provide opportunity for selective allosteric modulation by drugs and possibly by endogenous factors. For example, the main subunits which form the GABA$_A$ receptor (α, β, γ and δ) each exist in several isoforms; the α-subunit is essential for the enhancement of GABA binding by benzodiazepines, an important class of drug used in the treatment of anxiety, insomnia, epilepsy and muscle spasm (see Chapters 2 and 6). One α-subunit variant (α_6) lacks a benzodiazepine binding site and those GABA$_A$ receptors which contain this subunit are thus insensitive to benzodiazepines. Other variants in this subunit give rise to two distinct classes of benzodiazepine receptor which differ in their pharmacological specificity and distribution in the brain. The γ-subunit is also required for benzodiazepine action and variants in this protein may also affect the selectivity for different ligands.

4.3.2 G-protein Coupled Receptors

The G-protein coupled family of receptors is very large and includes receptors for many peptides (e.g. the hypothalamic hypophysiotrophic peptides), glycoproteins (e.g. the gonadotrophins) and classical neurotransmitters (e.g. adrenaline and noradrenaline). Structurally, these receptors comprise a single protein with seven hydrophobic segments with distinctive sequence patterns which are predicted to form α-helices spanning the membrane (Fig. 4.2). The N-terminal region forms a presumptive extracellular strand of varying length, but the three proposed external and three internal loops are generally shorter, thus the transmembrane domains are close to each other. In general, the seven transmembrane domains are thought to be clustered together to form a barrel-shaped configuration, the outer part of which may contain the region to which the hormone binds. In the case of many peptide hormones, the extracellular N-terminal domain does not play a part in hormone recognition, but for glycoproteins, a large N-terminal domain may be involved. Activation of the receptors is detected by a membrane-bound protein, the G-protein, possibly via interactions with the intracellular loops and the C-terminus of the receptor. The G-protein in turn acts as a transducer and thereby triggers a sequence of events within the cell which culminates in the cellular response. The effector systems employed by G-proteins fall broadly into two categories:

(a) enzymes that regulate the levels of intracellular second messengers, and
(b) ion channels (e.g. Ca^{2+} and K^+ channels) that alter the excitability of the cell membrane.

Attention has focused primarily on the activities of two target enzymes, adenylyl cyclase and phospholipase C (PLC) and their respective second messengers, $3'5'$-cyclic adenosine monophosphate (cAMP) and inositol trisphosphate/diacylglycerol (IP_3/DAG), which directly or indirectly activate protein kinases and thereby regulate specific cell functions (see below for further details). However, it is important to recognise that G-proteins may also modulate the activity of other effector enzymes, notably phospholipase A_2 which causes the release of arachidonic acid and hence the eicosanoids (see Chapter 8). Perhaps not surprisingly, events mediated by G-protein-coupled receptors occur over a variable time period and, dependent on the response, may emerge within seconds (e.g. vasopressin-induced contraction of vascular smooth muscle), minutes (corticotrophin (ACTH) induced glucocorticoid secretion) or hours (e.g. corticotrophin releasing hormone (CRH)-induced synthesis of ACTH).

G-proteins

These membrane proteins are heterotrimeric in structure with three subunits termed α (~40 kDa), β (37 kDa) and γ (8 kDa). The α-subunit has a high affinity

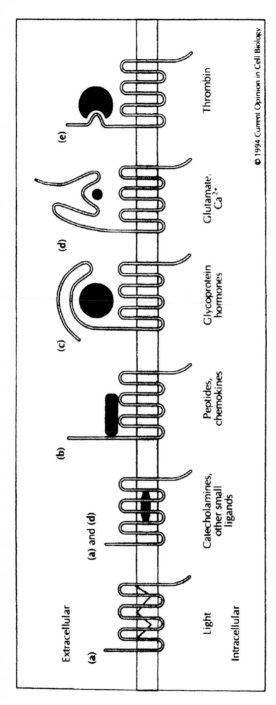

Figure 4.2 Diverse strategies for ligand detection by G-protein coupled receptors. (**a**) Ligands bind via the transmembrane domains to members of the rhodopsin and adrenergic receptor subfamily. (**b**) Peptide receptors appear to utilise the receptors' exofacial surfaces. (**c**) High-affinity binding of glycoprotein hormones is mediated by their receptors' long amino-terminal exodomain; whether this domain serves only to bind and orient the hormone or plays a more active role in forming the agonist for the seven transmembrane segment is not clear. (**d**) Receptors for glutamate and Ca^{2+} appear to use a mechanism very different from that used by the adrenergic receptors for detecting small ligands. Glutamate or Ca^{2+} bind to a domain in their receptors' amino-terminal exodomain, which resembles the binding proteins that capture amino acids and other small nutrients in the bacterial periplasmic space. Liganding of these binding proteins is known to cause a large pincer-like conformational change. In the receptor, the analogous conformational change in the amino-terminal exodomain presumably creates a "tethered ligand" (see below), which then binds to the seven transmembrane segment to effect receptor activation. Such a mechanism is better known for the thrombin receptor. (**e**) The protease thrombin recognises and cleaves its receptor's amino-terminal exodomain. This cleavage event unmasks a new amino terminus, which then serves as a tethered peptide ligand, binding intramolecularly to the seven transmembrane segment to effect receptor activation. A synthetic peptide mimicking the first five amino acids after the cleavage site is a full agonist for thrombin receptor activation. (Reproduced from Coughlin S.R. *Current Opinion in Cell Biology*, 1994, **6**: 191–197, by permission of Current Biology Ltd)

binding site for guanine nucleotides and possesses intrinsic GTPase (guanine triphosphatase) activity. In the resting state the G-protein exists as a free trimer (α, β, γ) with GDP (guanine diphosphate) bound to the α-subunit. When the receptor is activated by binding of an agonist, a conformational change occurs which causes the receptor to bind to the trimeric G-protein. This in turn triggers a conformational change in the α-subunit which causes GDP to dissociate and to be replaced with GTP (guanine triphosphate). At the same time the α-subunit dissociates from both the receptor and from the $\beta\gamma$ moiety. The α-subunit, with its associated GTP, is the active form of the G-protein, which translocates within the membrane in order to bring about the cellular response by associating with target enzymes or ion channels. The process is halted by hydrolysis of GTP which is effected by the GTPase activity of the α-subunit. The inactivated GDP-bound α-subunit then reassociates with the $\beta\gamma$ moiety to complete the cycle. The complex in its fully associated condition is located in the cell membrane through myristoylation of the α- or prenylation of the γ-subunit or both (Fig. 4.3).

Many G-protein subtypes have now been characterised and cloned. These include more than 20 α-subtypes (distinguished by simple subscript numbers) which are widely expressed with most individual cell types expressing several variants. In addition, there are five known mammalian β-subunits, which have a high degree of sequence homology (53–90%), and six γ-subunits which have less homology and hence vary in their capacity to bind to the different β-subunits. Despite their molecular heterogeneity, the $\beta\gamma$ complexes appear to be relatively promiscuous and may bind to different α-subunits.

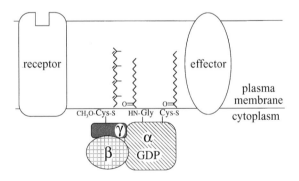

Figure 4.3 The three types of lipid modifications found on guanine binding proteins (G-proteins). A "typical" heterotrimeric G-protein situated at the inner face of the plasma membrane is shown. The γ-subunit contains both a myristoyl group linked through an amide bond to the amino terminus as well as a thioester-linked palmitoyl group. The α-subunit contains a thioether-linked geranylgeranyl isoprenoid as well as a methylated carboxyl terminus. All three lipids are shown inserted into the membrane bilayer, although there may be additional membrane proteins involved in this interaction. (Reproduced from Casey P. J. *Current Opinion in Cell Biology,* 1994, **6**: 219–225; by permission of Current Biology Ltd)

The α-subunits are divided into four families which form the basis for the classification of the G-protein complexes as a whole. These families are designated as G_s, G_i/G_o, G_q/G_{11} and G_{12}, a classification that partly reflects their actions and partly their homology and the history of their isolation. The subscripts "s" and "i" reflect the respective stimulatory and inhibitory actions of the protein on adenylyl cyclase. These actions were identified originally on the basis of interactions with cholera toxin and pertussis toxin which interact directly with the α-subunits causing ADP ribosylation of an arginine residue in G_s and a cysteine residue in G_i. Cholera toxin thus enhances the α-subunit stimulation of adenylyl cyclase activity directly, while pertussis toxin blocks the suppression of adenylyl cyclase brought about by some effectors (e.g. somatostatin). From this it emerged that those receptors which function through activation of adenylyl cyclase are linked to members of the G_s family while others may inhibit adenylyl cyclase activity via interactions with G_i. More recent evidence which has shown that G_i is more heterogeneous in structure and function than G_s has complicated this simple interpretation. It now appears that G_i may also regulate Ca^{2+} and K^+ channels as too does G_o which may also depress adenylyl cyclase. The G-protein dependent activation of PLC is also complex and may involve G_q or G_{11} while G_{12} is associated with regulation of Na^+/K^+ exchange. Further data advocate a role for the $\beta\gamma$ complex in effecting cellular responses and thus refute the dogma that only the α-subunits trigger responses.

Adenylyl Cyclase

Adenylyl cyclase is the enzyme responsible for the conversion of adenosine triphosphate to cAMP. Eight subtypes of the enzyme have been identified to date, each with a characteristic tissue distribution and a molecular weight of approximately 120 kDa. All isoforms conform to a unique structure, consisting of two groups of six transmembrane helices separated by a large (40 kDa) cytoplasmic domain (C1), with a short cytoplasmic N-terminus and a long cytoplasmic C-terminus (C2, see Fig. 4.4). Two large highly conserved sections of the intracellular loop (C1a) and the cytoplasmic C-terminus (C2a) are thought to represent the catalytic subunits which are targetted and regulated by GTP-bound $G_{\alpha s/i}$-subunits. Type I adenylyl cyclase is also inhibited by $G\beta\gamma$, although, in the additional presence of $G\alpha_s$, other subtypes (e.g. types II and IV) may be stimulated by this moiety. Types I and VIII are also stimulated by $Ca^{2+}/$ calmodulin (CaM) but the others are not. It is not presently known whether adenylyl cyclase self-regulates its activity by autophosphorylation but the membrane-bound receptors which trigger the response may themselves be down-regulated through phosphorylation by, for example, protein kinase A, protein kinase C or CaM kinase (see below).

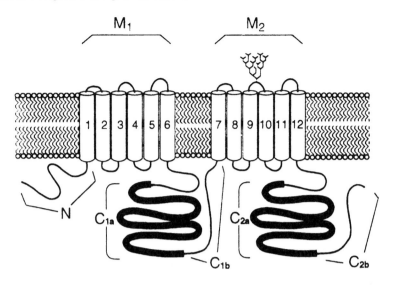

Figure 4.4 Structure of adenylyl cyclase. The predicted topology of membrane-bound adenylyl cyclases is shown. Cylinders represent membrane-spanning regions, while bold-face lines indicate regions of high amino acid similarity among all members of the family. Nomenclature is as follows: N, amino-terminal domain; M1, first set of membrane-spanning regions; C_{1a} and C_{1b}, the first large intracellular cytoplasmic domain; M_2, second set of transmembrane spanning regions; and C_2 and C_{2b}, second large intracellular domain. (Reproduced from Taussig R., Gilman A. G., *Journal of Biological Chemistry* 1995, **270**: 1–4, by permission of The American Society for Biochemistry and Molecular Biology)

Phospholipase C

As indicated above, the activation of phosphoinositide-specific PLC by G-protein linked receptors is another important route through which intracellular signals are generated. Activated PLC catalyses the hydrolysis of phosphatidyl inositol-bisphosphate to generate two second messengers, IP_3 and DAG, whose actions are described on pages 106 and 113 (Fig. 4.10). Seven mammalian subtypes of PLC have been identified; these fall into three main classes which are typified respectively by PLC-β1 (150 kDa), PLC-γ1 (145 kDa) and PLC-δ1 (85 kDa). All species of the enzyme contain two highly conserved sequences of about 170 and 260 amino acids which are designated X and Y respectively. Their catalytic properties are dependent on Ca^{2+} and it has been proposed that the Ca^{2+} binding site resides in the carboxyl-terminal half of the Y region. While activation of PLC may be consequent upon the stimulation of G-protein coupled receptors, it is important to note that the enzyme may also be activated by other mechanisms. Indeed, to date four distinct modes of PLC activation within the cell have been described, only two of which are dependent on G-protein coupled receptor stimulation. (a) In studies with PLC-β isozymes activation by the G-protein α-subunits α_q and α_{11}, but not by other α-subunits, has been described. (b) Equally, combinations of β_1 with $\gamma_{2,3}$ or γ_5 or β_2 with γ_2 have similar activating potencies on PLC-β isozymes, whereas $\beta_1\gamma_1$ or $\beta_2\gamma_3$-subunit combinations are only weakly active. (c) Growth factors stimulate PLC by G-protein independent mechanisms which involve phosphorylation through activation of intrinsic receptor tyrosine kinase activity (see Section 4.3.3 below). In the case of studies with PLC-γ_1, for example, activation has been shown to depend specifically on phosphorylation at Tyr-783. (d) Finally, several non-receptor protein kinases have been shown to phosphorylate and hence to activate PLC-γ isozymes.

Inositol Trisphosphate and Ca^{2+} Ions

Inositol trisphosphate (IP$_3$) is released from the cell membrane through the actions of PLC-β (G-protein linked receptors) or PLC-γ (tyrosine kinase linked receptors, see Section 4.3.3) on phosphatidyl inositol and subsequently binds to specific IP$_3$ receptors. These are located at sites in the smooth endoplasmic reticulum that are modified to form Ca^{2+} stores by the presence of pumps, which accumulate the ion against a concentration gradient, and specific binding proteins (e.g. calsequestrin or calreticulin) which bind and hence sequester Ca^{2+}. When stimulated IP$_3$ receptors function as Ca^{2+} channels and release Ca^{2+} into the cytosol. The IP$_3$ receptor is tetrameric (Fig. 4.5) and has a high degree of structural homology with the ryanodine receptor of smooth muscle which fulfils a similar role in releasing Ca^{2+} but is stimulated either by direct contact with a membrane dihydropyridine receptor (which detects small changes in membrane potential) or by Ca^{2+} (which enters the cell by voltage-gated Ca^{2+} channels). In a similar manner IP$_3$ receptors are also sensitive to Ca^{2+}. Thus, in the absence of cytosolic Ca^{2+}, IP$_3$ fails to mobilise Ca^{2+} from its stores but as the cytosolic Ca^{2+} is raised it induces an increasing degree of Ca^{2+} release, with a maximal effect emerging at a Ca^{2+} concentration of 300 nmol/l (beyond which the effects of the ion become inhibitory). As a result of this positive feedback Ca^{2+} release has an "all-or-nothing" character and Ca^{2+} fluxes may be propagated in all directions from the specific sites at which the response was initiated. These may be readily visualised by appropriate imaging devices and appear as a succession of waves propagated on spherical points. IP$_3$ may also regulate Ca^{2+} intake at the cell membrane; this may depend on the repletion state of the intracellular stores but the mechanisms involved remain to be explained.

Ca^{2+} release into the cytosol generally occurs as an oscillatory signal due to the periodicity of Ca^{2+} release from cytosolic stores and Ca^{2+} entry via cell membrane voltage gated Ca^{2+} channels (Fig. 4.6). Periodicity is frequently encountered in biological systems, though its measurement often depends on

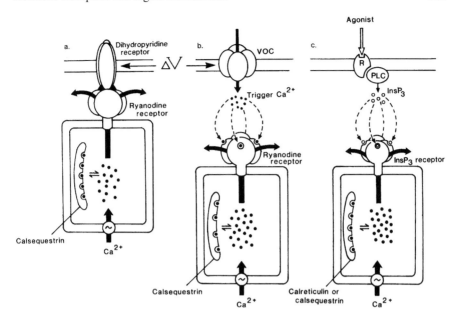

Figure 4.5 Control of calcium release by intracellular tetrametric calcium channels. **a** Ryanodine receptors (RYRs) located in the sarcoplasmic reticulum of skeletal muscle contribute to the T-tubule foot structure responsible for excitation–contraction coupling. The dihydropyridine receptor in the surface membrane senses a change in voltage (ΔV) and undergoes a conformational change which is transmitted through the bulbous head of the RYR to open the calcium channel in the sarcoplasmic reticulum. **b** Calcium-induced calcium release in cardiac muscle and perhaps also in neurones. A voltage-operated channel (VOC) responds to ΔV by gating a small amount of trigger calcium, which then activates the RYR to release stored calcium. **c** Agonist-induced calcium release. Signal transduction at the cell surface generates inositol trisphosphate ($InsP_3$) which diffuses into the cell to release calcium by binding to $InsP_3$ receptors. (Reprinted with permission from Berridge M. J., *Nature*, 1993, **361**: 315–325; Copyright 1993, Macmillan Magazines Limited)

sophisticated methodology for the real time evaluation of rapidly changing events. Clearly, it arises in any system in which an early, rate-limiting step is positively enhanced either by specific stimulation or by a low concentration of end product, but is inhibited at higher end product concentrations. It also requires a constant utilisation or drain of end product from the system. It follows that all important metabolic events (including hormone secretion) are intrinsically oscillatory in this way. In the case of cytosolic Ca^{2+}, the inhibitory events which occur at high Ca^{2+} concentrations include the inhibition of Ca^{2+} entry through voltage operated channels or by the blockade of Ca^{2+} release from replete stores. Intracellularly, oscillatory release of Ca^{2+} from intracellular stores may simply reflect oscillatory release of IP$_3$ which, though stimulated by the presence of

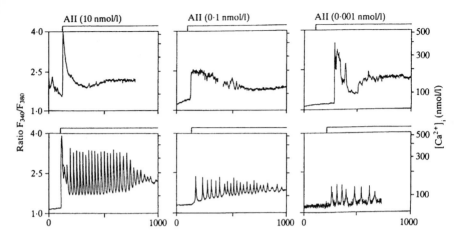

Figure 4.6 The two types of cytosolic free Ca^{2+} ($[Ca^{2+}]i$) response to various angiotensin II (AII) concentrations. Individual bovine adrenal glomerulosa cells were loaded with the Ca^{2+} indicator fura-2 and microperfused with AII at 10, 0.1 or 0.01 nmol/l as indicated. The time and the duration of the AII microperfusion is shown by the horizontal bar at the top of each panel. In all panels, extracellular $[Ca^{2+}]i$ are shown in the upper panels and oscillatory $[Ca^{2+}]i$ responses are shown in the lower panels. F_{340}/F_{380} is the ratio of fluorescence emitted at 340 and 380 nm excitation. (From Johnson E. M. I., Capponi A. M., Vallotton M. B., *Journal of Endocrinology*, 1989 **122**: 391–402; reproduced by permission of the Journal of Endocrinology Ltd.)

agonist, is inhibited by the accumulation of the other end product of PLC action, DAG. In these cases, the Ca^{2+} "drain" is the pumping of Ca^{2+} out of the cell or into the intracellular stores.

Protein Kinases

The discussion so far has shown that stimulation of G-protein linked 7-transmembrane domain receptors frequently results in the activation of specific enzymes which liberate signals such as cAMP, IP_3/Ca^{2+} ions and DAG into the cytosol. These "second messengers" act, in turn, to stimulate specific protein kinases which then phosphorylate various target proteins within the cell to bring about the biological response. These kinases are not specific in their protein targets but interact with substrates as diverse as hormone receptors, enzymes (including other protein kinases) and components of other signalling pathways, thus providing opportunities for significant intracellular "cross-talk" between signals generated by membrane events.

Protein Kinase A. Like other protein kinases, protein kinase A (PKA) normally requires activation by a specific signal. In the resting state, PKA is inhibited by a negative regulatory subunit (R) which contains a pseudosubstrate region that competitively inhibits protein phosphorylation. Cyclic AMP binds to the regulatory subunit which then dissociates, allowing access of substrate. Structural studies have revealed that the kinase contains two "lobes", the smaller being located in the N-terminal region and the larger one in the C-terminus. ATP binds in the deep cleft between these lobes, while the protein substrate interacts with residues on the surface of the larger C-terminal lobe. These substrates are characterised by a consensus recognition sequence, Arg-Arg-X-Ser-/Thr-Y, where X is any small residue and Y is a large hydrophobic residue. Binding the substrate produces a conformational change which is associated with closure of the active site cleft and is followed by rapid transfer of the γ phosphate of ATP to the hydroxyl group of a serine or threonine of the substrate.

Calcium/Calmodulin Protein Kinase. In most cells the major Ca^{2+} binding protein is calmodulin, a heat stable protein of approximately 17 kDa which binds four Ca^{2+} ions with an overall K_d of about 1 μmol/l. The formation of the Ca^{2+}/calmodulin complex leads to the activation of one or more of a family of protein kinases collectively termed calcium/calmodulin dependent protein kinases (CaM kinases). These enzymes are involved in an extremely wide variety of processes in many different types of cells. Four classes of CaM kinase (termed α, β, γ and δ) have been identified, each of which is encoded by a separate gene. The α and β classes are restricted to nervous tissue but the γ and δ subtypes are present in most tissues. Irrespective of the class, the enzymes comprise an N-terminal catalytic domain, a regulatory domain with a CaM binding site and a C-terminal "association" domain which may have a role in intracellular targetting of CaM kinase activity (Figs 4.7 and 4.8). Differential mRNA splicing in the region encoding this latter region accounts for much of the further variation within each class of CaM kinase. The enzyme exists as a complex (termed a "holoenzyme") which appears to be composed of a multimeric assembly of monomeric enzyme units. The complex may comprise members from the same or different classes, with the N-termini extending as spokes from a hub formed by the C-terminal association domains.

Activation of CaM kinase is triggered by binding of calmodulin to the C-terminal region of the regulatory domain which disrupts the auto-inhibitory site at its N-terminus. This effect is potentiated by autophosphorylation (by adjacent subunits in a single holoenzyme) which increases the enzyme's affinity for calmodulin even if the Ca^{2+} concentrations are subsequently reduced. While phosphorylated, the enzyme also remains partially activated when calmodulin eventually dissociates (Figs 4.7 and 4.8). This positive co-operation thus has a signal amplification effect, which may also distinguish Ca^{2+} oscillations of different frequencies.

Protein Kinase C. The Ca^{2+} and phospholipid-dependent protein kinase C

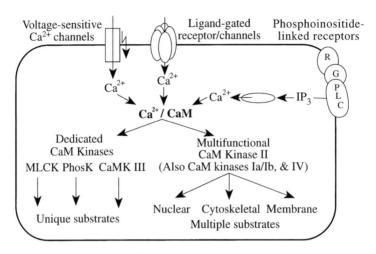

Figure 4.7 Elevation of intracellular calcium by a variety of extracellular stimuli can lead to the activation of the multifunctional CaM kinase II, along with other multifunctional and dedicated calcium/calmodulin-dependent protein kinases. PLC, phospholipase-C; R, receptor; G, G-protein. (From Braun A. P. and Schulman H., 1995. Reproduced, with permission, from the *Annual Review of Physiology* **57**, 417–45. © 1995 by Annual Reviews Inc.)

(PKC) is a key regulatory kinase and is involved in multiple cell processes, including growth and differentiation, neural and smooth muscle functions and cancer, as well as in endocrine signal transduction. Eleven subtypes have been recognised which fall broadly into four subclasses, the conventional Ca^{2+} dependent form (cPKC), a Ca^{2+} independent form (nPKC), "atypical" (aPKC) and PKCμ. Of these, the first is primarily involved in cellular responses to hormonal stimulation. PKCs typically comprise a single peptide chain with a regulatory domain of about 30 kDa and a catalytic domain of about 50 kDa; up to four conserved (C1–4) and five variable (V1–5) regions may be included in the sequence (Fig. 4.9). The C1 domain contains a tandem repeat of cysteine-rich sequences and forms zinc fingers by binding zinc atoms through co-ordinate bonding to three cysteines and one histidine; this stabilised conformation is required for the binding of phorbol esters, lipid and DAG. The C2 region (not present in the Ca^{2+} independent forms) is required for the binding of both phorbol ester and Ca^{2+}. In addition, the C1 domain contains a pseudosubstrate site which blocks the substrate binding site in the C4 domain when the enzyme is in the unactivated state.

Activation of PKC (Fig. 4.10) by second messengers depends on prior phosphorylation of the catalytic subunit by a PKC kinase, itself possibly another PKC isoform. Activation by DAG or by phorbol ester also requires translocation of the enzyme from the cytoplasm to the cell membrane. This process is

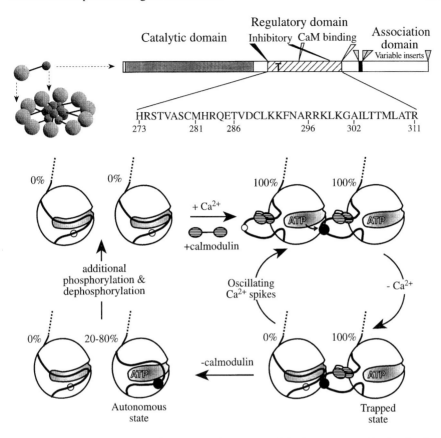

Figure 4.8 CaM kinase: the hub-and-spoke pattern of the holoenzyme. Each subunit of CaM kinase contains an autoregulatory region, whose displacement is critical in maintaining autonomous catalytic activity and calmodulin trapping. It is also the site from which inhibitory peptides have been derived. (From Braun A. P. and Schulman H., 1995. Reproduced, with permission, from the *Annual Review of Physiology* 1995, **57**, 417–45. © 1995 by Annual Reviews Inc.)

frequently used as a measure of activation because the proportions of enzyme found in the cytoplasm (70–90%) and in association with the membrane (10–30%) in control conditions are reversed after stimulation. PKC may be activated by Ca^{2+} alone, but only when the intracellular Ca^{2+} concentration is raised some 100-fold. DAG increases the affinity of PKC for phospholipid binding and reduces the requirement for Ca^{2+} to the micromolar range. The activated PKC thus requires the formation of a quaternary complex with phospholipid, particularly phosphatidyl serine, Ca^{2+} and DAG. Phorbol esters, by contrast, achieve activation by effecting translocation alone. In both cases activation results in a conformational change which removes the pseudosubstrate domain from the

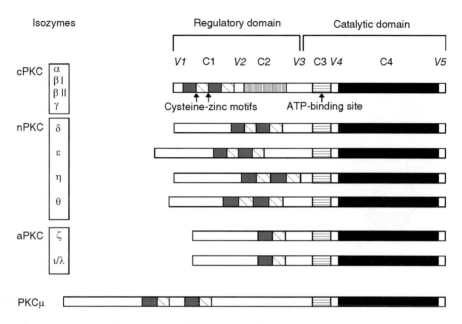

Figure 4.9 Domain structure of the protein kinase C (PKC) family. Eleven PKC isoforms of the PKC family are depicted in four groups cPKC, nPKC, aPKC, and PKCμ. The conserved (C1–C4) and variable (V1–V5) regions of PKC are indicated in the regulatory and catalytic domains. The cysteine-zinc motifs and ATP-binding site are pointed by arrows. (Reprinted from *Molecular and Cellular Endocrinology*, Vol. **116**; J.-P. Liu: Protein kinase C and its substrates, pp 1–29, 1996; with kind permission from Elsevier Science Ireland Ltd, Bay 15K, Shannon Industrial Estate, Co. Clare, Ireland)

substrate binding site and thus allows access of the substrate. Further inhibition or activation of PKC activity may be achieved by autophosphorylation, proteolytic degradation, regulation by sphingolipids or ceramide and other factors.

4.3.3 Tyrosine Kinase Receptors

The tyrosine kinase receptor family includes receptors for insulin, insulin-like growth factor (IGF) and other growth factors. These transmembrane receptors comprise four domains (Fig. 4.11):

(a) an extracellular ligand binding domain which contains one, two or more cysteine rich regions,

(b) a comparatively small single α-helical transmembrane domain,

(c) an intracellular region which includes a functional tyrosine kinase, and

(d) a cytoplasmic C-terminus which may itself contain several phosphorylation sites.

The insulin receptor is slightly modified from this general pattern in that it exists as a dimer with each subunit comprising an α- and a β-chain. The two α-chains are linked by a disulphide bridge and are entirely extracellular. A further set of disulphide bridges links the α-chains to the two β-chains which span the membrane and extend into the cytoplasm. The cytosolic regions contain the tyrosine kinase domain together with clusters of tyrosine residues which are available for phosphorylation. A similar structure characterises the closely related IGF receptor and also the so called IRR receptor for which no ligand has been identified (i.e. an orphan receptor).

Although the other receptors which are members of this family are monomeric

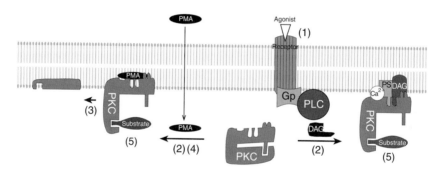

(1) Receptor activation
(2) Translocation
(3) Down-regulation
(4) Membrane insertion
(5) Substrate phosphorylation

Figure 4.10 Schematic representation of proposed mechanisms of PKC activation in eukaryotic cells. There are two pathways to activate intracellular PKC from extracellular environment: receptor-mediated production of diacylglycerol (DAG) through G-protein-coupled phospholipase C (PLC) and phorbol ester-induced direct pharmacological activation. Both DAG and phorbol esters (such as PMA, phorbol 12-myristate 13-acetate) bind to PKC C1 region of the regulatory subunit to cause a physical association of PKC with the plasma membrane (translocation) but, whereas DAG promotes a complex formation of PKC, phosphatidylserine (PS) and Ca^{2+} phorbol esters induce a plasma membrane insertion of PKC and then down-regulation. Both DAG and phorbol esters induce a conformational change of PKC structure so that the inhibitory pseudosubstrate sequence moves away from the substrate binding site to allow binding and phosphorylation of PKC substrates to occur. (Reprinted from *Molecular and Cellular Endocrinology*, Vol. **116**; J.-P. Liu: Protein kinase C and its substrates, pp 1–29, 1996; with kind permission from Elsevier Science Ireland Ltd, Bay 15K, Shannon Industrial Estate, Co. Clare, Ireland)

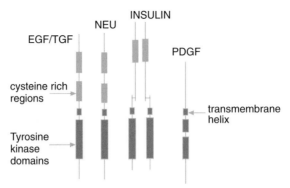

Figure 4.11 Domain structures of tyrosine kinase receptors: epidermal growth factor (EGF), transforming growth factor (TGF), protein product of the *neu* oncogene (NEU), platelet derived growth factor (PDGF)

in their basic structure, their activation requires the formation of dimers via a reversible, non-covalent, association (Fig. 4.12). The requirement for dimerisation arises because the receptors are themselves the substrates for the receptor tyrosine kinase: thus, the formation of the dimer which occurs on ligand binding

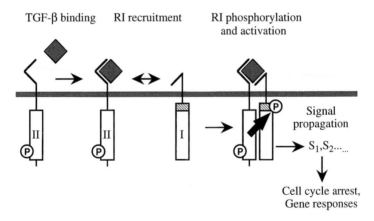

Figure 4.12 A general model for the initiation of signalling by the transferring growth factor β (TGF-β) receptor. Receptor II is the primary TGF-β receptor and is a constitutively active serine-threonine kinase that recruits receptor I by means of bound TGF-β (diamond). Subsequent phosphorylation of the GS domain (striped box) by receptor II allows the receptor I kinase to propagate the signal to downstream substrates that mediate antiproliferative as well as gene responses. (Reprinted with permission from Wrana J. L., Attisano L., Wiesser R., Ventura F., Massagué J. *Nature*, 1994, **370**: 341–347; Copyright 1994, Macmillan Magazines Limited)

leads to the alignment of phosphorylation sites on one receptor subunit with the tyrosine kinase domain on the other (Fig. 4.12). In the case of insulin, the binding of one insulin molecule to the holoreceptor appears to be sufficient to initiate signalling and thus to phosphorylate the major substrate, insulin receptor substrate 1 (IRS1); a second insulin molecule will bind to the receptor only if the concentration of the ligand is supraphysiological. Insulin binding causes rapid receptor autophosphorylation (an essential step for insulin action) but thereafter the signalling pathways used by the insulin receptor and by other members of the tyrosine kinase receptor family diverge.

For other tyrosine kinase receptors, activation results in sequential activation of a series of binding proteins and protein kinases which effectively amplifies the signal and provides the opportunity for multiple interactions (i.e. "cross-talk") between different signalling pathways. Finally, specific nuclear transcription factors and proto-oncogenes, particularly those associated with the mitogenic responses to growth factors, are activated. A model for tyrosine kinase receptor transduction through the Ras activated protein kinase cascade is shown in Fig. 4.13 and important components of this sequence are detailed below, although it must be noted that substantial variation may occur in different circumstances:

(a) Activation of a receptor tyrosine kinase leads to phosphorylation of tyrosine residues, allowing the receptor to interact with the rSH2 (src-homology 2) domain of proteins such as Grb2. Grb2 then binds to an adapter protein, termed Sos, which recruits a Ras protein to the receptor.

(b) Ras is a monomeric proto-oncogene product which occupies a key position in the sequence. It has a molecular weight of about 21 kDa (three subtypes have been identified in man) and is linked to the inner surface of the cell membrane; Ras binds guanine nucleotides (i.e. it is a G-protein) and possesses weak GTPase activity. The transmission of a signal causes GTP to bind to Ras and activates components downstream in the sequence. In particular, activated Ras interacts directly with the regulatory domain (CR-1) of Raf protein. Ras signalling is terminated by proteins which stimulate Ras GTPase.

(c) Raf is another proto-oncogene product with a molecular weight of about 70–75 kDa. It possesses a protein kinase domain at the C-terminus and the CR-1 domain is positioned at the N-terminus. As well as being stimulated by Ras, the activity of Raf is greatly enhanced by phosphorylation; this may possibly be effected by PKC or, alternatively, tyrosine kinases may be involved. Raf has a highly specific substrate, namely mitogen activated kinase kinase (MAPKK or MEK).

(d) In mammals MAPKK comprises a family of three conserved protein serine-threonine kinases (41–45 kDa). These in turn have a highly specific set of substrates termed the mitogen activated kinases (MAPK or ERK1 and ERK2)

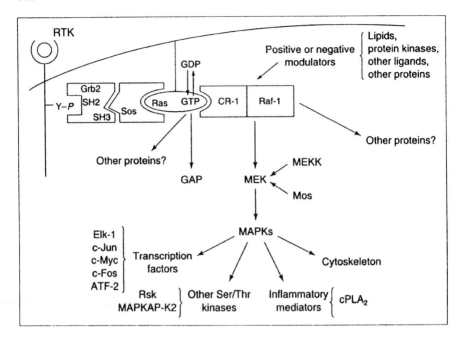

Figure 4.13 Model for receptor tyrosine kinase (RTK) signal transduction through the Ras-activated protein kinase cascade. Activation of an RTK leads to its phosphorylation on tyrosine residues (Y-P), allowing the receptor to interact with SH2-domain-containing proteins such as Grb2. In turn, Grb2 binds to an adapter protein, Sos, which recruits Ras to the receptor. As explained in the text, Ras recruits Raf to the complex, allowing Raf activation and providing a means of activating the MAPK cascade. MAPKAP-K2, MAPK-activated protein kinase 2; cPLA$_2$, cytoplasmic phospholipase A$_2$. (Reproduced from Avruch J., Zhang X.-F., Kyriakis J. M., *TIBS*, 19 July 1994, 279–283; by permission of Elsevier Trends Journals, Cambridge, UK)

with molecular weights in the region of 40–44 kDa. Activation of these kinases results from a double phosphorylation at threonine and tyrosine residues in a TXY motif. The ERKs phosphorylate serine or threonine residues which are adjacent to prolines; their major substrates include transcription factors, such as c-*jun*, c-*fos*, c-*myc* and probably many others, thus providing a complete pathway from the growth factor receptor to the mitogenic events in the nucleus. Other important substrates include other ser-thr protein kinases (e.g. MAPK-activated protein kinase 2), cytosolic phospholipase A$_2$, which gives rise to inflammatory mediators, and various cytoskeletal proteins.

4.3.4 Cytokine Receptors

The cytokines form a large group of intercellular mediators and include interleukins (ILs), colony-stimulating factors (CSFs), interferons (IFNs), tumour necrosis factor (TNF) and others (see Chapter 3). Their receptors, which have no intrinsic tyrosine kinase activity, are grouped into two classes: Class I, the cytokine-prolactin growth hormone receptor and Class II, the IFN receptor family. The general scheme of their structures is illustrated in Fig. 4.14. In Class I receptors, the major sites of homology are a group of four cysteines (shown as "c" in Fig. 4.14) and a Trp-Ser-X-Trp-Ser (WSXWS) motif in the barrel-shaped extracellular regions close to the cell membrane. Two intracellular sequences,

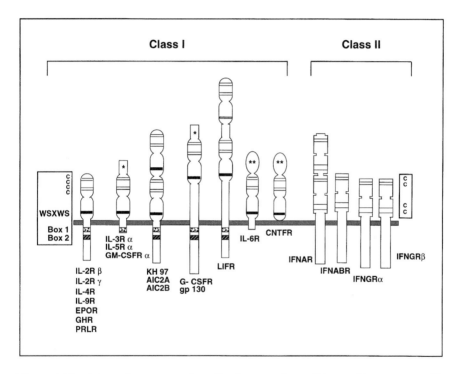

Figure 4.14   Schematic representation of various members of the cytokine receptors. The structural features of Class I and Class II families are shown in the left and right insets respectively. Key: * fibronectin type III; ** immunoglobulin-like region; IL, interleukin; LIF, leukaemia inhibitory factor; G-CSF, granulocyte-macrophage colony stimulating factor; CNTF, ciliary neurotrophic factor; G-CSF, granulocyte colony stimulating factor; OSM, oncostatin M; EPO, erythropoietin; GH, growth hormone; PRL, prolactin; IFN, interferon. KH97 and AIC2B are the human and mouse β-subunits common to IL-3, IL-5 and GM-CSF receptor heterodimers. (From Finidori J., Kelly P. A., *J Endocrinol*, 1995, **147**: 11–23. Reproduced by permission of the Journal of Endocrinology Ltd.)

Box 1 and Box 2, also show some degree of conservation. The Class II receptors also show homology in the extracellular region with the positioning of four cysteines, but they lack the WSXWS motif found in Class I receptors.

Both classes of receptors form either homo- or hetero-dimers on cytokine binding. Intracellular signalling involves activation of a sequence of protein kinases (see Fig. 4.15), starting with a tyrosine kinase of the janus kinase (JAK) family. Substrates for JAKs include the JAKs themselves, the cytokine receptors and members of the STAT (signal transduction and activation of transcription) family of proteins. Once phosphorylated, STAT proteins dissociate from the JAK complex and form homo- or hetero-dimers which are translocated to the nucleus

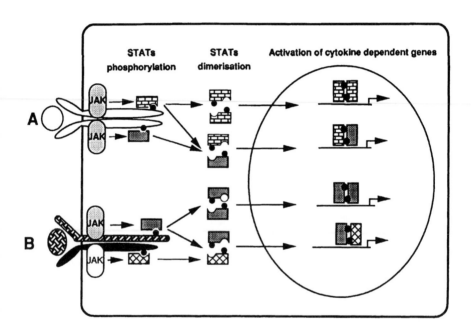

Figure 4.15 Diagram of the known steps of cytokine receptor signalling via STATs (signal transduction and activation of transcription) proteins. Ligand binding induces (A) homodimeric or (B) heterodimeric association of cytokine receptor subunits and activation of (A) two of the same or (B) two different janus kinases (JAKs). Recruitment of STAT proteins could occur via their SH2 domains and the tyrosine phosphorylated residues of the receptor subunits. Different STAT proteins can be stimulated by the same receptor and, conversely, different receptors can stimulate the same STAT protein. The various STATs are subsequently phosphorylated on their conserved carboxy-terminal tyrosine residue, allowing dissociation from the receptor and homo- or heterodimerisation. The complexes formed are then able to translocate to the nucleus and activate the transcription of cytokine-dependent genes. (From Finidori J., Kelly P. A., *J Endocrinol*, 1995, **147**: 11–23. Reproduced by permission of the Journal of Endocrinology Ltd.)

where they directly activate transcription of cytokine dependent genes (Fig. 4.15). In addition, other signalling pathways, including the Raf-Ras, MAPK pathways may be activated.

4.4 NUCLEAR RECEPTORS

This major class of receptors recognises hormones, such as the steroids, thyroid hormones or retinoic acid, which enter the cell by simple diffusion through the cell membrane. Their primary site of action is within the nucleus where, once activated by hormone binding, they act as transcription factors and promote transcription of specific target genes. Because of this, and because they are generally located in the nucleus even prior to activation, they are grouped together as the "nuclear receptors". Although this term is useful, it is not always entirely accurate as unactivated receptors are only loosely associated with the nucleus and some may also be found within the cytoplasm, for example the glucocorticoid and mineralocorticoid receptors (GR and MR).

All members of this receptor family have a similar structure (see Fig. 4.16 for schematic diagram). They thus comprise a variable N-terminal domain (usually designated A/B), a highly conserved DNA binding domain (DBD) (C), a variable "hinge" region (D), a conserved ligand binding domain (LBD) (E) and a variable C-terminal region (F). The total number of amino acids in the chain varies from 448 for retinoic acid receptor β to 984 for the MR. Most of this variation arises from differences in the A/B domain and the others are remarkably consistent in length (Fig. 4.16). Each of the domains has more than one functional role; thus, both receptor dimerisation (see below) and translocation (i.e. localisation of activated receptors in the nucleus) depend on regions in the C, D and E domains, the binding of heat shock proteins requires the E domain, while transactivation depends primarily on two regions, one (termed AF1) located in the A/B domains and the other (AF2) in the E domain (Fig. 4.17). The conservation of cysteines and basic and hydrophobic amino acids in the DNA binding domain confers special properties. At two sites, two pairs of cysteines co-ordinately bind a zinc ion thus forming "zinc fingers" which interact with the DNA helix (see Figs 4.18 and 4.19). In addition to the well-defined hormone receptors, other members of this receptor family exist for which there is no known ligand—so called "orphan" receptors. Some may act as homodimeric transcription factors, such as RXR or COUP homodimers, others, apparently, as monomers (e.g. SF-1, DAX-1).

Dimerisation of the nuclear receptors is a universal property. Dimers may be homodimers, as in the case of steroid receptors, in which both units take part in binding to DNA at palindromic hormone response element (HRE) sites separated by three nucleotides (see Fig. 4.19). Other receptors, including those for thyroid hormone, retinoic acid and vitamin D, require the presence of accessory factors with which they form heterodimers. The only proteins known to perform this accessory function are three isoforms of an orphan nuclear receptor designated RXR. The formation of the heterodimers depends on specific sites

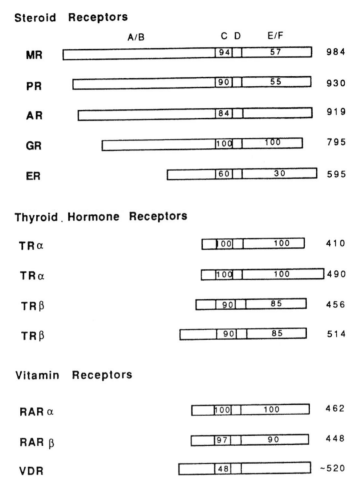

Figure 4.16 Schematic diagram of the structure of nuclear receptors. The receptors, which are divided into regions A to F, are as follows: mineralocorticoid (MR), progesterone (PR), androgen (AR), glucocorticoid receptor (GR), oestrogen (ER), vitamin D (VDR), thyroid (TR) and retinoic acid (RAR). The number of amino acids for each receptor in humans is shown on the right. They have been compared in region C, the DNA binding domain, and region E, the ligand binding domain, and the percent homologies, where known, are shown for the steroid receptors relative to GR, thyroid receptors relative to TRα and retinoic acid receptors relative to RARα. (From Parker M. G. *J Endocrinol*, 1988, **119**: 175–177. Reproduced by permission of the Journal of Endocrinology Ltd.)

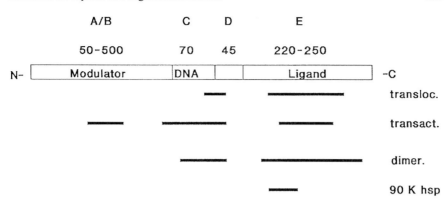

Figure 4.17 Functional organisation of nuclear receptors. Transloc, nuclear translocation region; transact, transactivation domain; dimer, dimerisation domain; 90 K hsp, 90 kDa heat shock protein binding region. (Reproduced by permission from Beato M. *Cell*, 1989, **56**: 335–344; copyright Cell Press)

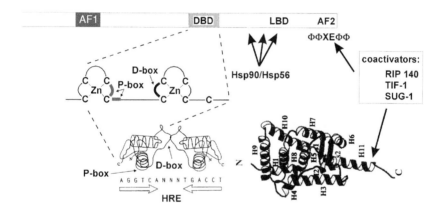

Figure 4.18 Domain structure of steroid hormone receptors (SHRs). The glucocorticoid receptor is taken as a model to visualise general features: the core transactivation domains AF1 (also called τ1, which is hormone independent) and AF2 (which is hormone dependent). AF2, to which the putative coactivators bind, is located in the C-terminal portion of helix 11 of the ligand binding domain (LBD). The backbone drawing is derived from the crystal structure of the RXRα LBD, possibly resembling those of SHRs. The DNA-binding domain (DBD) of the glucocorticoid receptor is assembled as a dimer on the palindromic hormone response element (HRE). The organisation by the zinc-binding motifs is made visible by the expanded drawing. Φ stands for hydrophobic amino acid in the putative AF2 consensus sequence. The scheme presented here is being added to continually and the number of coactivators is increasing continuously. Coreceptors, which also have a role, are not included here. Coactivator SUG1 may not be correct in that it has been found to be involved in receptor turnover. (Reproduced by permission from Beato M., Herrlich P., Schütz G., *Cell*, 1995, **83**: 851–857; copyright Cell Press)

Nuclear Receptor Superfamily

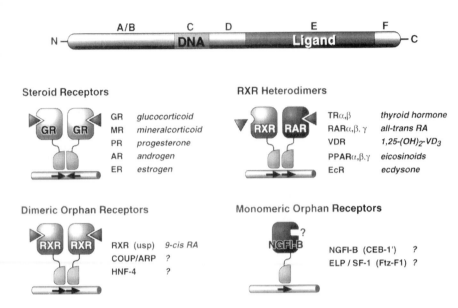

Figure 4.19 Nuclear receptors share common structure-function domains. A typical nuclear receptor contains a variable N-terminal region (A/B), a conserved DNA-binding domain (C), a variable hinge region (D), a conserved ligand-binding domain (E) and a variable C-terminal region (F). Nuclear receptors can be grouped into four classes according to their ligand binding, DNA binding, and dimerisation properties: steroid receptors, RXR heterodimers, homodimeric orphan receptors and monomeric orphan receptors. Shown are representative receptors for each group. Question marks refer to orphan receptors for which ligands are not known. (Reproduced by permission from Mangelsdorf D. J., Thummel C., Beato M., Herrlich P., Schtz G., Umesono K., Blumberg B., Kastner P., Mark M., Chamon P., Evans R. M. *Cell*, 1995, **83**, 835–839; copyright Cell Press)

within the receptor DNA binding and ligand binding domains. The hormone response elements for these heterodimers consist of direct repeats of the core AGGTCA half site, separated (depending on the receptor) by three, four or five nucleotides.

In the unactivated state, it is likely that the nuclear receptors exist in an oligomeric assembly of a receptor dimer attached to two heat shock protein molecules (hsp 90 or hsp 65) which dissociate on binding of hormone to its receptor. Structural studies of the unliganded $RXR\alpha$ and liganded $RAR\gamma$ subtypes suggest that a model of the ligand binding domain and its transformation that leads to receptor activation may be generally applicable to all nuclear receptors. In this model, a conserved 20 amino acid region constitutes a nuclear receptor specific sequence which stabilises a fold in the ligand binding domain. Ligand binding induces a more compact structure (with increased resistance to proteases) in which AF2 is activated. The integrity in one particular amphipathic α-helix (H12), which is located in a weak autonomous activating domain within AF2 (AF2-AD), is essential for AF2 activation and may play a role in the binding of putative transcriptional mediators-coactivators or transcriptional intermediary factors (TIFs). One function of the conformational change induced by ligand binding is therefore to create an interaction surface to which TIFs may bind; this may be accompanied by destruction of the interaction surface for repressor binding.

There may well be ways in which individual receptors do not wholly conform to this general description. For example, in some instances specific steroid receptors form heterodimers with other members of the nuclear receptor family (for example GR and MR); such conformations may provide a further means of fine-tuning the genomic response. In addition, some receptors (e.g. progesterone or oestrogen receptors) may exist as two or more isoforms. These may be of different sizes, resulting from the existence of more than one promoter (the progesterone receptor) or from differential RNA splicing (the oestrogen receptor). Alternatively, the receptors may be phosphorylated, again, presumably, leading to changes in biological activity. The different roles of these isoforms have not been entirely explained, but it is certainly possible that they too combine to form heterodimers with distinct biological functions.

Further important aspects of steroid action must also be considered. Importantly, while steroid-receptor complexes frequently act as transcription factors and thereby up-regulate the expression of specific target genes, there are many examples of instances where the complexes depress transcription and, thus, the synthesis of specific protein; for example, the glucocorticoids inhibit the synthesis of several pro-inflammatory cytokines (e.g. IL-1) and enzymes which cause the release of inflammatory mediators (e.g. the inducible forms of cyclooxygenase and nitric oxide synthase, see also Chapter 8). This may be brought about by direct interactions of the steroid–receptor complex with the genome or by interference with the access or activity of other transcription factors. Increasing evidence also suggests that steroids also exert important regulatory actions by mechanisms which are independent of the classical nuclear receptor–genomic route. For example, progesterone activates sperm function through a cytoplasmic calcium signal; since there is no DNA transcription in sperm there can be no nuclear mode of action. Another example is aldosterone which has non-genomic effects on mononuclear leukocytes, vascular smooth muscle cells and kidney cells, again through a cytoplasmic calcium signal. A further non-genomic mechanism involves the interaction of steroid metabolites of the pregnane series with the $GABA_A$ receptor–chloride ion channel complex as allosteric modulators, in a manner analogous to the actions of benzodiazepines or barbiturates (see Section 4.3.1).

4.5   CONCLUSIONS

It can be seen from this brief review that the ability of a cell to transduce a simple chemical stimulus into a specific physiological response depends on the integrity of complex biochemical machinery within the cell. Our knowledge of the diverse signalling systems employed by eukaryotic cells is developing rapidly and leading to significant advances, not only in fundamental cell biology but also in our understanding of the pathogenesis of a variety of diseases such as cancers, immune-inflammatory disorders and degenerative disease. Several potential therapeutic targets have been identified (for example inhibitors of type 4 phosphodiesterase—the enzyme which degrades cAMP—are presently being developed as anti-asthma drugs) and it may be expected that a new generation of drugs will emerge in the future.

COMMONLY USED ABBREVIATIONS AND DEFINITIONS

Receptors

GPCR   G-protein coupled receptor
RTK   Receptor tyrosine kinase,
            e.g. EDGF, insulin receptors

Oncoproteins

fos }   DNA activation factors
jun }
Grb   Adapter protein
Ras   Membrane located by prenylation, binds to RTK/Grb/Sos complex
Raf   Cytosolic kinase, recruited to membrane by binding to Ras
Sos   Ras guanine nucleotide exchange factor
            Link RTK to Ras by protein–protein interactions involving Src homologous ("SH2") domains, having multiple tyrosine residues which are phosphorylated and provide docking sites

Cellular kinases

CaM kinase Calcium/calmodulin dependent protein kinase
GRK   G-protein coupled receptor kinase, e.g:
βARK β-adrenoceptor kinase
            Activated by binding to G-subunits, phosphorylates, and thus deactivates GPCR

JAK	Janus kinase (or . . . just another kinase)
MAPK	Mitogen activated protein kinase
(= ERK)	(Extracellular signal regulated kinase)
MEK	MAPK/ERK kinase
MEKK	MEK kinase
	Involved in transmitting phosphorylation cascade from receptor to nucleus
PLC	Phospholipase C
STAT	Signal transduction and activation of transcription
	Transmit signal from cytokine/interferon type receptors to nucleus

General

ACTH	Adrenocorticotrophic hormone, corticotrophin
AF1,2	Transactivating domain 1,2
ATP, ADP, AMP	Adenosine triphosphate, diphosphate, monophosphate
CRE	Cyclic-AMP response element
CREB	CRE binding protein
CRH	Corticotrophin releasing hormone
CSF	Colony stimulating factor
cyclic-AMP	$3',5'$-cyclic adenosine monophosphate
DAG	Diacylglycerol
FSH	Follicle stimulating hormone
GABA	Gamma-aminobutyric acid
GAP	GTPase activating protein
	Activates G protein αq GTPase activity (as does binding to PLC-β), allowing reassociation of G-protein $\alpha\beta\gamma$ subunits, i.e. reassembly of non activated form
GTP, GDP	Guanine triphosphate, diphosphate
HRE	Hormone response element
IGF	Insulin-like growth factor
IFN	Interferon
IL	Interleukin
IP_3	Inositol trisphosphate
IRS	Insulin receptor substrate
K_d	Dissociation constant
LH	Luteinising hormone
Prenylation	Covalent modification by isoprenoid lipids (e.g. farnesylation, geranylgeranylation)
TIF	Transcriptional intermediary factors
TSH	Thyroid stimulating hormone, thyrotrophin

FURTHER READING

Avruch J., Zhang X.-F., Kyriakis J. M. Raf meets Ras: the framework of a signal transduction pathway. *Trends Biochem Sci*, 1994, **19**: 279–83.

Beato M., Herrlich P., Schütz G. Steroid hormone receptors: many actors in search of a plot. *Cell*, 1995, **83**: 851–7.

Berridge M. J. Inositol trisphosphate and calcium signalling. *Nature*, 1993, **361**: 315–325.

Boege F., Neumann E., Helmreich E. J. M. Structural heterogeneity of membrane receptors and GTP-binding proteins and its functional consequences for signal transduction. *Eur J Biochem*, 1991, **199**: 1–15.

Braun A. P., Schulman H. The multifunctional calcium calmodulin-dependent protein-kinase—from form to function. *Ann Rev Physiol*, 1995, **57**: 417–45.

Hepler J. R., Gilman A. G. G proteins. *Trends Biochem Sci*, 1992, **17**: 383–7.

Lee J. S., Pilch P. F. The insulin-receptor—structure, function, and signalling. *Am J Physiol*, 1994, **266**: C319–C334.

Liu J.-P. Protein kinase C and its substrates. *Mol Cell Endocrinol*, 1996, **116**: 1–29.

Mangelsdorf D. J., Evans R. M. The RXR heterodimers and orphan receptors. *Cell*, 1995, **83**: 841–50.

Mangelsdorf D. J., Thummel C., Beato M., Herrlich P., Schütz G., Blumberg B., Kastner P., Mark M., Chambon P., Evans R. M. The nuclear receptor superfamily: the second decade. *Cell*, 1995, **83**: 835–39.

Morgan D. O., De Bondt H. L. Protein kinase regulation: insights from crystal structure analysis. *Current Opinion in Cell Biology*, 1994, **6**: 239–46.

Neer E. J. Heterotrimeric G proteins: organisers of transmembrane signals. *Cell*, 1995, **80**: 249–257.

Noh D. Y., Shin S. H., Rhee S. G. Phosphoinositide-specific phospholipase-C and mitogenic signalling. *Biochimica et Biophysica Acta: Reviews On Cancer*, 1995, **1242**: 99–113.

Panayotou G., Waterfield M. D. The assembly of signalling complexes by receptor tyrosine kinases. *Bioessays*, 1993, **15**: 171–7.

Parker M. G. (vol. ed.). Steroid Hormone Action. In Hames B. D., Glover D. M. (series eds) *Frontiers in Molecular Biology*. New York, Oxford University Press Inc., 1993 1–209.

Rang H. P., Dale M. M., Ritter J. M. *Pharmacology*. New York, Churchill Livingston, 1995, 22–46.

Ross E. M. Pharmacodynamic mechanisms of drug action and relationship between drug concentration and effect. In Hardman J. G., Limbard L. E. *Goodman and Gilman's The Pharmacological Basics of Therapeutics* (9th edition). New York, McGraw-Hill, 1996, 29–42.

Seger R., Krebs E. G. The mapk signaling cascade. *FASEB Journal*, 1995, **9**: 726–35.

Taussig R., Gilman A. G. Mammalian membrane-bound adenylyl cyclases. *J Biol Chem*, 1995, **270**: 1–4.

Vinson G. P., Whitehouse B. J., Hinson J. P. *The Adrenal Cortex*. Englewood Heights, NJ, Prentice-Hall, 1992.

Wrana J. L., Attisano L., Wieser R., Ventura F., Massagué J. Mechanism of activation of the TGF-β receptor. *Nature*, 1994, **370**: 341–7.

Wurtz J.-M., Bourget W., Renaud J.-P., Vivat V., Chambon P., Moras D., Gronemeyer H. A canonical structure for the ligand-binding domain of nuclear receptors. *Nature Structural Biology*, 1996, **3**: 87–94.

Methods of Assessing Neuroendocrine, Autonomic and Immune Function and of Monitoring Behavioural Responses to Stress

Chapter 5

In Vivo and *In Vitro* Methods for Assessing Neuroendocrine Function

Anne-Marie Cowell, Julia C. Buckingham and Glenda E. Gillies

Imperial College School of Medicine, London, UK

5.1 INTRODUCTION

The hypothalamo–pituitary axis plays an essential role in the maintenance of homeostasis. Its activity is tightly regulated by a variety of mechanisms, including ascending and descending neural inputs to the hypothalamus, local regulatory mechanisms operating within the hypothalamus and pituitary gland and blood borne factors acting at the level of the hypothalamus and adenohypophysis. Dysfunction of this system invariably results in a spectrum of disorders of physical and mental development, growth, osmotic balance, metabolism and reproductive function as well as an impairment in the ability of an individual to respond appropriately to acute or long-term stress. Clinically, such conditions may be precipitated by pathological lesions or by drugs and other xenobiotic agents such as environmental pollutants (1). Thus, there is growing awareness of the importance of assessing neuroendocrine function and the present chapter

Stress, Stress Hormones and the Immune System. Edited by J. C. Buckingham, G. E. Gillies and A.-M. Cowell
© 1997 John Wiley & Sons, Ltd.

aims to outline the principles underlying the *in vivo* and *in vitro* methods currently available for this purpose. The advantages and limitations of each preparation will also be discussed. In addition, the indices used to measure hypothalamic and pituitary function will be described.

5.2 *IN VIVO* MODELS

In vivo methods may be used to examine both the acute and long-term effects of pharmacological, surgical or pathophysiological experimental manipulations (e.g. antigenic challenge) on neuroendocrine function. These studies often involve measuring changes in blood concentrations of the pituitary hormones or those of their peripheral target organs (e.g. thyroid hormones, steroids of the gonads or the adrenal cortex) induced by acute or repeated treatments. Following long-term manipulation, indirect indices of pituitary activity—such as body weight, urine volume and osmolarity, the weight and histological appearance of the pituitary gland, the peripheral target organs (e.g. thyroid, gonads, adrenal glands) and appropriate target tissue (e.g. thymus)—may also provide an accurate picture of neuroendocrine function.

Several points must be considered when designing these studies. Firstly, neuroendocrine function may be influenced by diet, housing, lighting and handling regimes as well as by the type and sex of the experimental species used. Secondly, techniques of blood sampling are important; in some cases animals may be bled intermittently via indwelling cannulae, while in others the combined stressful effects of the sampling procedure and volume depletion may necessitate collection *post mortem*. Thirdly, since the effects of drugs and other experimental manipulations on the neuroendocrine system are not often manifested by marked changes in "basal" hormone secretion, it is also important to examine the impact on the normal rhythmic patterns of secretory activity (e.g. circadian, those related to the ovarian cycle) and on the critical responses to pathological challenge (e.g. stress, cold, hypoglycaemia, immune challenge) or pharmacological stimuli (e.g. target organ response to appropriate secretagogues).

These studies inevitably provide only limited information regarding the mechanisms through which a stimulus effects changes in neuroendocrine activity. For example, the responses observed to a peripherally administered substance could be due to an action at higher centres in the central nervous system (CNS), assuming it crosses the blood–brain barrier, at the hypothalamus, at the anterior pituitary gland or at the peripheral endocrine system (see Chapter 1). Alternatively, they could reflect an indirect response to a peripheral action of the drug, for example a prompt drop in blood pressure or blood sugar is a potent stimulus to the hypothalamo–pituitary–adrenal axis. Although the direct actions on the peripheral endocrine system could be largely detected by measuring circulating pituitary hormones, it remains a possibility that an alteration at the peripheral organ could alter the feedback signal and thus anterior pituitary hormone secretion (see Chapter 1). This effect is more likely to be apparent in long-term studies and experiments where the peripheral organ is removed might be considered. It may, however, be more appropriate to check this possibility *in vitro* (see below). A number of *in vivo* models have also been developed in attempts to identify more clearly the sites at which drugs might affect the hypothalamo–pituitary axis.

5.2.1   Investigations of Hypothalamic Function *In Vivo*

Implantation and electrical stimulation or lesion techniques are often used to examine hypothalamic function *in vivo*. One of the most widely used techniques is administration of drugs which alter the synthesis, release, activity or metabolism of neurotransmitters/neuromodulators. The drugs are frequently administered into the third ventricle via an indwelling cannula (implanted stereotaxically under anaesthesia) with subsequent measurement of pituitary hormone in the plasma—for review see (2). This technique provides a direct means of introducing the drug into the CNS and may therefore circumvent some of the problems associated with peripheral administration. However, although the drug is likely to produce its effects via an action in the hypothalamic tissue surrounding the third ventricle, the possibility that small quantities of the agent may diffuse to other brain areas or perhaps to the anterior pituitary gland cannot be ignored. Similarly, drugs injected stereotaxically into the hypothalamus, particularly in areas near the capillary plexus, may reach the adenohypophysis. The impact of this problem may be reduced or avoided by measuring transmitter/peptide release within the hypothalamus, using *in vivo* sampling techniques such as push-pull cannulae, microdialysis or collection of hypophyseal portal blood.

The push-pull technique is used mainly to measure the basal and stimulated release of neuroactive substances from localised brain areas but it also has the capacity to measure synthesis and metabolism. Its application to neuroendocrinology has recently been reviewed by Dluzen and Ramirez (3). Briefly, the push-pull cannula consists of two concentric tubes which may be stereotaxically implanted, for example, in the median eminence. Fluid is introduced by a perfusion pump through the inner tube and is in direct contact with the brain tissue which surrounds the tip of the cannula. Endogenous substances are taken up in the perfusion fluid and removed by a second pump through the outer tube. The main disadvantages of push-pull cannulation are clogging of the tube and progressive damage to the tissue surrounding the probe which may be exacerbated when small pieces of tissue block the pull line, producing an imbalance where more liquid is being pumped into the brain than is being removed. There is also a risk that blood vessels will be damaged, resulting in contamination of samples.

Microdialysis is an extension of the push-pull technique and its use in the field of neuroendocrinology has been widely discussed (4, 5). As with the former technique, a moving pool of fluid is brought into contact with a relatively stationary pool of extracellular fluid but, unlike the push-pull cannula, the microdialysis probe has a length of semipermeable tubing covering the inflow and outflow cannulae which provides a barrier between the tissue and the fluid pumped through the probe. Larger animals are best suited to microdialysis because their brain size permits the use of longer or wider diameter membranes, resulting in improved recovery of substances (see also Chapter 6). Microdialysis has a number of advantages over the push-pull cannula technique. Firstly, tissue damage is less since no fluid is pumped into the tissue and damage is caused only by insertion of the probe and not by the sampling procedure. Secondly, the dialysis membrane prevents the passage of proteins and other large molecules present in the extracellular fluid. This means that the sample does not require to be extracted prior to analysis and that enzymatic degradation of the sample is eliminated once the material has passed into the probe. It also minimises perturbation of the neural environment, although removal of ions and small molecules may affect the homeostatic balance of the extracellular medium. However, one of the main problems with microdialysis is that, although it tends to be useful for recovering small molecular weight substances such as the decapeptide gonadotrophin releasing hormone (GnRH), the physical cut off of the membrane prevents the adequate penetration of high molecular weight compounds (e.g. large polypeptides such as cytokines) and recoveries are so low that extracellular concentrations are difficult to detect. In this instance the push-pull cannula technique would prove more useful.

Push-pull cannulae and microdialysis can be used repeatedly in anaesthetised or conscious unrestrained animals. Performance in conscious free-moving animals will eliminate any artificial suppression of neurohormone and neurotransmitter release that is known to result from use of anaesthetics. However, the push-pull technique is more suitable for acute experiments and cannot be used continuously to monitor neurochemical release over prolonged periods. In contrast, microdialysis can be successfully employed for sampling in conscious animals over extended periods, although for chronic sampling methods restraint may be used. When using conscious animals however, one must allow a recovery period of several days before sampling is carried out since the surgical procedures required are severe and may thus precipitate non-specific effects due to trauma in the experimental animal as well as a degree of glial reaction in the path of the cannula immediately after its insertion.

Collection of hypophyseal portal blood is another powerful technique for monitoring changes in the hypothalamic signals to the anterior pituitary gland but it is not used routinely since it requires great skill. There are two main methods of obtaining pituitary portal blood, described in detail by Sarker and Minami (6). The first involves a transpharyngeal approach to expose the pituitary and stalk followed by periodical aspiration of pituitary blood as it accumulates around the transected stalk. In the other method the pituitary stalk is exposed by a parapharyngeal approach, after which a close-fitting polyethylene cannula is placed over the bleeding stump and the blood is withdrawn with the aid of a pump. The latter method eliminates possible contamination of the sample by extraneous blood and allows the collection of virtually pure portal blood. In contrast, the aspiration method has been criticised since the blood collected contains 68% pure portal blood, 21% extraneous peripheral blood and 11% pituitary blood from the distal end of the transected stalk (7). However, removal of the pituitary does eliminate the latter contamination. Moreover, it has been suggested that the aspiration method causes less trauma to the stalk and median eminence and less interference with normal blood flow in the portal vessels due to the absence of a tightly fitting cannula. The method of collection used will depend on the hypothalamic hormone to be measured. The aspiration method is useful for measurement of labile substances such as catecholamines because appropriate preservatives can be added within seconds of collection of the blood. In contrast, the stalk cannulation method is preferred for collection of blood over longer intervals for less labile hormones and for hypothalamic hormones which are also found in the pituitary gland (e.g. β-endorphin) since, in this instance, contamination of the blood sample by pituitary backflow makes the aspiration technique unsuitable. Portal vessel measurements in most species require the use of anaesthetics. The choice of anaesthetic depends on the particular hormone under study and the appropriate anaesthetics for various hypothalamic hormones have been summarised by Sarker and Minami (6). One must also remember that, with this and the other sampling and implantation techniques described previously, the most sensitive analytical methods are required to ensure detection of basal release of substances since only very low concentrations are recovered.

Electrophysiology has not been widely applied to the study of neuroendocrine function, largely because of the difficulties in identifying the cell type from which recordings are made. The most successful studies have focused on the magnocellular system where the cells can be identified by antidromic stimulation of the nerve terminal in the posterior pituitary gland. This method has the disadvantage that the animals are anaesthetised and undergo substantial surgery. Nonetheless, the technique provides a valuable tool with which to examine pathophysiological and pharmacological factors that influence the activity of the vasopressinergic and oxytocinergic neurones.

5.2.2 Investigations of Pituitary Function *In Vivo*

Evidence for an action of a drug at the pituitary level may be obtained by measuring plasma pituitary hormone concentrations following direct intrapituitary cannulation and implantation of the drug. This type of experiment is technically complex and more frequently the effects of peripherally administered agents on plasma pituitary hormone concentrations are studied. In these studies a central site of action may be eliminated by blocking the activity of the endogenous hypothalamic hormones pharmacologically (administration of antagonists) or immunologically (administration of antisera) or by lesioning the median eminence electrically or pharmacologically (e.g. using a cocktail of chlorpromazine, morphine and phenobarbitone). This type of experiment is especially important in investigating the stress axis where not only the test substance itself but also the experimental manipulations could activate responses centrally. These approaches reveal direct actions of the drug on the secretory activity of the pituitary cells. Further studies, in which the pituitary responses to each of the hypothalamic hormones are examined in drug treated median-eminence lesioned animals, are therefore necessary to verify whether the drug modulates the pituitary response to neurochemical stimulation (e.g. corticotrophin, ACTH, response to corticotrophin releasing hormone, CRH).

5.3 *IN VITRO* MODELS

Investigations of the wide array of mechanisms regulating the hypothalamo–pituitary axis *in vivo* are complicated by the inaccessibility and sensitivity of the tissues to experimental manipulation. These difficulties have led to the development of a number of *in vitro* methods to study hypothalamic and adenohypophysial activity which, unlike their *in vivo* counterparts, allow examination of the responses at cellular and molecular levels to be conducted in a precisely controlled environment. However, such methods have the inherent disadvantage that the tissue is removed from its endogenous environment and may therefore exhibit a difference in sensitivity to various secretagogues.

As with *in vivo* studies the diet, housing, lighting and handling regimes should be stringently controlled since these may affect the subsequent activity of hypothalamic and pituitary tissue *in vitro*. Moreover, the tissue should be obtained from animals of the same strain, weight, age and sex and, if female, stage of the oestrous cycle. In principle, the animals may be exposed to a drug or other experimental manipulation *in vivo* and the respective tissues removed and their functional activity assessed *in vitro*; alternatively, the glands may be removed from the normal animal and subjected to appropriate experimental manipulations *in vitro*. The latter method lends itself to precise pharmacological studies although particular care should be taken to include appropriate vehicle controls because several solvents, such as ethanol and dimethylsulphoxide, can produce pronounced effects on the secretory activity of hypothalamic and pituitary tissue *in vitro*.

The techniques used to maintain hypothalamic and adenohypophysial tissue *in vitro* fall into two main categories, short- and long-term. The choice of method will depend on whether acute or chronic experimental paradigms are to be studied, although, ideally, for pharmacological studies the responses to a wide range of doses or concentrations of drugs should be examined in more than one preparation to obtain the most accurate results. In each case the function of the tissue is assessed by measuring the output of the hormone under investigation using well-validated, specific, precise immunological or biological assays, the most common of which are described later (see Section 5.5).

5.3.1   Investigations of Hypothalamic Function *In Vitro*

Short-Term Hypothalamic Preparations

Short-term hypothalamic preparations include synaptosomes, whole hypothalami, hypothalamic fragments and hypothalamic slices. These preparations lend themselves to pharmacological manipulations and to the measurement of a wide range of biochemical indices. Synaptosome and slice preparations are also suitable for electrophysiological studies including, in the case of synaptosomes, patch clamp work.

Synaptosome preparations primarily comprise sealed nerve endings which maintain many of the metabolic characteristics of intact cells when incubated under carefully controlled conditions *in vitro*. However, one should be aware that the initial trauma of homogenization and centrifugation may damage the membrane and its receptors. The hypothalamic synaptosome preparation was first developed by Edwardson and colleagues (8) and has provided a useful means for examining the mechanisms controlling release processes at the nerve terminal. It is however unsuitable for studying aspects of neurotransmission, such as synthesis and processing of peptides, since the perikarya and axons are absent.

One of the most widely used short-term preparations is the whole hypothalamus which was first developed by Bradbury and colleagues (9). This method has been successfully employed to examine the physiology, pharmacology and biochemistry of the hypophysiotrophic neurones and has generated data which are largely concordant with the findings of *in vivo* studies where indirect indices of hypothalamic function were measured. The preparation has the advantage that it resembles closely the *in vivo* situation in that the three-dimensional relationships between neurones and non-neuronal supporting cells are maintained and normal autocrine and paracrine interactions are not disrupted. However, it has the disadvantage that the cells in the centre of the tissue may undergo necrosis. The volume of the tissue block is considerably greater than the maximum volume of brain tissue (1 mm^3) reported to allow adequate diffusion of nutrients, metabolites and secretory stimulants and products into and out of the tissue (10).

Trypan blue exclusion studies have demonstrated reduced cell viability in hypothalamic blocks after 1 h *in vitro* (11) but other studies have demonstrated stable oxygen consumption for up to 3 h (9). Thus the preparation is only suitable for short-term studies, although one group (12) has successfully maintained the "explants" for more than 24 h.

The viability of hypothalamic tissue may be prolonged by the use of smaller fragments which improves the diffusion of nutrients and metabolites to and from the tissue. These preparations include hypothalami bisected by a mid-saggital incision, quartered by perpendicular midsaggital and coronal cuts or sliced in the saggital plane. Alternatively, a smaller total hypothalamic mass, such as the medial basal hypothalamus and the median eminence, may be used. The main disadvantage of these systems is that neuronal connections and connections between neuronal and non-neuronal supporting cells are disrupted. Thus, an effective compromise is the bisected organ in which the improvements in diffusion are coupled with a high degree of cellular integrity (13). Superfusion procedures, which have been applied to whole hypothalami, fragments or slices, also improve viability, with little deterioration occurring for periods of up to 4–5 h. In theory, therefore, such preparations could be subjected to repeated stimulation but in practice they often display marked tachyphylaxis. In addition, since very small amounts of neuropeptide are released, it may be necessary to incubate as many as 12 hypothalami in one perifusion chamber and to concentrate or lyophilise the eluate fractions, even when using the most sensitive assay procedures (13).

Long-term Hypothalamic Preparations

The principal long-term hypothalamic preparations which have been developed are organotypic cultures (14) or primary dissociated cell cultures (15), although increasingly immortalised neuronal cell lines such as the GT1 GnRH secreting cells (16) are becoming available.

Organotypic cultures can be prepared from fragments of hypothalami from fetal, neonatal or adult tissue (but survival is improved when the tissue is taken from fetuses or neonates) and slices (200–400 μm) containing the area of interest are allowed to grow on cover slips or other appropriate supports. Such preparations can be used to study maturation processes, the electrophysiological properties of neurones, hormone localisation and biosynthesis and release mechanisms (13). They possess the advantage that the normal intimate relationships between neurones, supporting glia and other non-neuronal cells are preserved although, with time, glial cell proliferation and migration is likely to occur. However, as with short-term hypothalamic block preparations, poor diffusion of nutrients and metabolites through the tissue results in neuronal and non-neuronal damage, although morphological and biochemical studies indicate that at least some neurones maintain their integrity for periods of up to three weeks (17). A further disadvantage of this preparation is the necessary presence of serum in the medium to provide the hormones, growth factors, nutrients and attachment factors essential for survival and growth *in vitro*. Serum is a variable, undefined cocktail of bioactive substances, some of which do not normally come into contact with brain cells and may interfere with the potential influence of any substances under test.

Cultures of dispersed hypothalamic cells also provide a useful technique for investigating hypothalamic functions. They are prepared from fetal or neonatal tissue (since adult tissue does not show the same ability to survive in culture) and are, therefore, particularly useful for the study of factors that influence the development of the neuroendocrine system. Dispersed hypothalamic neurone cultures have the advantage that isolated cells from a number of animals are pooled before plating, resulting in a homogeneous population which can be divided into individual dishes or wells to yield a number of replicate cultures. Biological variation is therefore minimised and standard errors are small. However, the results are representative only of a single pool of cells and demonstration of the reproducibility of statistically significant effects on several pools is imperative. It is possible to maintain these cultures *in vitro* for several weeks in chemically-defined serum-free medium (15). Problems with diffusion are essentially eliminated and there is rapid exchange of nutrients, secreted products and catabolites between cells and bathing medium. This method can therefore be used to investigate repeated responses over many weeks *in vitro* as well as the effects of prior treatments (acute compared to chronic) on subsequent responses. In addition, the cultures are better suited than whole organ cultures and short-term hypothalamic preparations for studying the localisation of peptides by immunocytochemical techniques since the cells are readily accessible to antisera (18). Using this preparation it is possible to study functional maturation of many hypothalamic neuronal populations including those producing CRH, arginine vasopressin (AVP), somatostatin (SRIH), γ-amino butyric acid and dopamine. In some cases, for example CRH and AVP, perinatal tissue levels are low and require exceptionally sensitive methods, or the use of a concentration step, for their detection. It should also be appreciated that not only are the hypothalamic cell cultures heterogeneous in terms of their neurochemical identity but some populations may be further subdivided in terms of their function and biochemical features. For example sub-populations of dopamine and SRIH-producing neurones can be identified by their discrete location within the hypothalamus and their expression of oestrogen receptors (19). In this respect slice cultures offer some advantages, in that discrete hypothalamic regions may be selected. A further disadvantage of isolated cell cultures is that it is difficult to ensure that responses resemble those of normal cells *in situ*, since the cultures never attain the normal cytoarchitecture found *in vivo*, although cell interactions and patterns of organisation are visible. In addition, the secretory responses of the cells may be altered by their static environment and by feedback regulation by secreted cell products and metabolites. Generally, however, cultured hypothalamic cells behave in many ways as would be expected *in vivo*, exhibiting both a morphological and functional maturation (18, 20) as well as electrical activity, synaptogenesis and Ca^{2+} dependency of their secretory activity.

5.3.2   Investigations of Anterior Pituitary Function *In Vitro*

Short-term Pituitary Preparations

Short-term pituitary preparations utilise tissue segments or enzymatically dispersed cells maintained in static or dynamic conditions. The tissue is usually obtained from rats but bovine and ovine pituitary tissue is sometimes used.

The static incubation system using rat pituitary glands, typically cut into four segments, is well established (21) and has several advantages. Firstly, it reflects the *in vivo* situation as the tissue retains its three-dimensional structure and, hence, the cell–cell communication inherent to the tissue as a whole. Secondly, the system is highly precise and is therefore useful for the quantitative analysis of drug actions. Thirdly, it is simple and inexpensive to perform. Diffusion of nutrients into and metabolites out of the tissue may be limited, however, leading to necrosis at the centre of the segment. This problem is minimised by the use of small segments ($<$ 1 mg) but nonetheless experiments should not continue for longer than 3 h. Because of inter-animal variation, it is important to randomise segments throughout the treatment groups, such that no one treatment group contains more than one segment from the same animal.

The problems of poor diffusion and inter-animal variation are minimised in models using enzymatically dispersed cells maintained in static conditions (22). Furthermore, only a small number of animals is required to produce a cell pool which can be divided into an appropriate number of aliquots to permit the simultaneous comparison of several variables in one experiment. However, the ability to reproduce statistically significant results in several experiments is essential, as discussed above. Moreover, with this method the normal cell–cell communication network may be compromised or lost and the opportunity for transmission of autocrine and paracrine influences, which are increasingly being recognised as important factors in regulating anterior pituitary hormone release, is lost. It is also important to ensure that the enzymes used during the dispersion procedure do not damage receptors on the cell membrane and thus affect the secretory responses. However, dispersed cells do respond to known secretagogues although they are relatively insensitive (23).

Perfusion and superfusion systems both for pituitary segments (24) and dispersed cells have also been developed, with the latter preparation being the most sensitive of all the *in vitro* preparations described here (25). These methods permit the continuous clearance of secretory products and metabolites from the cellular environment, thereby minimising the possible effects of these substances on the release of the pituitary hormones. The test material can be introduced in a pulsatile manner which mimics more closely the pattern in which the hypothalamic regulatory factors are secreted; the sampling is much easier and consequently the timing and the subtle changes in responsiveness may be easily analysed. Thus, such preparations may provide valuable information about the dynamics of pituitary hormone release and permit detailed examination of the rate of onset, intensity and duration of acute responses to drugs. They are also invaluable in studies on drugs which may exert biphasic actions, for example steroids. Moreover, in contrast to a static incubation, the responses of the perifused anterior pituitary cell column are almost immediate and because the pituitary gland contains large stores of hormones the cells may be stimulated repeatedly for periods of up to 8 h. Thus several compounds can be tested on the same column. However, because perifused cells exhibit pronounced variations in the magnitude of the secretory responses to repeated stimulation (26) and one stimulus could possibly influence the magnitude of a subsequent response, it is crucial to randomise doses with at least four replicates per dose per study.

Long-term Pituitary Preparations

Long-term preparations include primary cultures of isolated anterior pituitary cells (i.e. a mixed population) and heterogeneous or homogeneous cell lines such as the growth hormone(GH)–prolactin producing GH_3 cells and the corticotrophin producing AtT20 cells, respectively. In addition, techniques for separating specific pituitary cell subpopulations by, for example, fluorescence activated cell sorting (see Chapter 7) or counterflow centrifugation (27) are being increasingly exploited in attempts to establish primary cultures of "enriched" cell populations. Cell cultures allow examination of both the acute and more long-term effects of drugs on pituitary hormone secretion in tightly controlled conditions. In many respects the advantages and limitations of cultured pituitary cells (primary culture or cell lines) resemble those of static incubates of acutely dispersed pituitary cells, although a three-dimensional aggregate cell culture system, in which cell–cell communication is at least partly restored, has been developed (28). It should also be borne in mind that the sensitivity of cultured cells may alter over a period of time and that both primary cultures and tumour cells may exhibit properties which differ from normal anterior pituitary cells in acute *in vitro* or *in vivo* experiments. Thus extreme care should be taken in extrapolating findings from these cells to normal cells.

5.4   MODELS INVOLVING GENETIC MANIPULATIONS

Advances in molecular biology have led to the development of a variety of techniques which enable the expression of specific genes to be precisely manipulated either *in vivo* or *in vitro*. It is thus possible to create experimental models in which the expression of a target protein (e.g. a polypeptide hormone, a receptor or an enzyme) is permanently or transiently up- or down-regulated. Such models provide opportunity for detailed examination of the roles of specific genes and their products in physiological processes and in disease.

5.4.1   *In Vivo* Techniques

Long-term over-expression of a gene *in vivo* is achieved by incorporating an appropriate DNA sequence into the genome and thus producing a "transgenic" strain of animal (29). This is normally done in mice, although the technology may also be applied to other species. Briefly, the DNA construct (ideally genomic DNA), including a promoter sequence, is micro-injected into fertilised eggs obtained from "super-ovulated" females. The eggs are then implanted in the uterus of pseudopregnant females and the consequent pregnancy allowed to go to term. The offspring are screened for expression of the transgene by detection of DNA (southern blots, polymerase chain reaction, PCR), mRNA (northern blots, RNase protection or reverse transcriptase-PCR, RT-PCR) and protein (western blots, immunostaining) as described in Section 5.5.1. Success is variable and depends on a variety of factors which influence the integration of the transgene into the genome (e.g. the quality and concentration of the DNA construct), the expression of the DNA (e.g. characteristics of the DNA construct, such as the promoter and the presence of introns and specific enhancer sequences) and the transmission of the transgene to the next generation (failure may, for example, be due to the production of chimaeras which do not contain the transgene in their germ cells or the generation of transgenes which are lethal to the host before it attains reproductive competence).

The generation of strains of animal in which the expression of a target gene is specifically deleted (i.e. "knocked out") involves a technique of homologous recombination in pluripotent embryonic stem (ES) cells (30). Again, this is normally done in mice, although there are examples of the technology being applied to rats. In essence, a homologous sequence of genomic DNA (derived from the same mouse strain as the ES cells) is modified by interruption of the exon so as to produce a nonsense or prematurely truncated protein; this construct is transfected into ES cells which are then plated out in conditions which prevent differentiation. A cell clone which has successfully undergone homologous recombination is selected and introduced *in vitro* to mouse embryos which are then implanted into pseudopregnant mice. The modified embryos give rise to chimaeric mice which are then crossed with normal mice to produce hetero-zygotes; these, in turn, are cross bred to yield the homozygotes. Careful genomic screening is again essential. Assuming homologous recombination has been successful, the most common pitfall is failure of the ES cells to contribute to the germ cells of the chimaeras and, thus, for the mutant DNA construct to be transmitted to the next generation to yield the heterozygotes.

There are many examples in the literature of the successful development of strains of "transgenic" or "knockout" animals and many of these are being used extensively both for *in vivo* physiological experiments (see Section 5.2) and for studies in which the pathophysiology of specific tissues is examined *ex vivo*, using either acute incubations or cell culture techniques (see Section 5.3). In some cases, particularly in knockouts, the results have been disappointing for, although the genetic manipulation has been successful, no obvious phenotype has emerged; this may be because the experimenters have failed to address the "right" physiological questions or possibly because compensatory mechanisms have developed which overcome the pathology induced by the genetic lesion. In other instances, the phenotype has been surprising and provided important new insight to the physiological role of the targeted protein.

Techniques for the short-term manipulation of gene expression *in vivo* are in their infancy. Acute gene transfer (gene therapy) which involves administration at a discrete locus (e.g. lungs, muscle) of cDNA in an appropriate vector (e.g. adenovirus, liposome or simple plasmid) has met with limited success, partly because expression of the protein has been limited and partly because the procedure often triggers a significant immune response. Attempts to attenuate gene expression by administration of specific antisense oligonucleotides, which hybridise with specific mRNA sequences and thus prevent translation, have also met with only limited success (31). There are several reasons for this. Firstly, the chemical modifications (e.g. additions of phosphothiorate groups) necessary to protect the nucleotides from nuclease degradation render the molecules toxic, particularly in the CNS. Secondly, there are concerns about the accessibility of the nucleotides to their targets. Thirdly, there is controversy about the mode of action of antisense and, in addition to targeting specific mRNA sequences, there is increasing evidence that antisense nucleotides may also interfere with other aspects of gene expression (e.g. mRNA stability) and, more worryingly, produce effects which are unrelated to the expression of the target gene. Antisense experiments thus require rigorous control including:

(a) assurance that the base sequence is of an appropriate length (18–22 bases) and that it recognises a mRNA sequence unique to the target protein,
(b) mapping of labelled nucleotide to assure that it reaches its target,
(c) administration of control sequences (normally the corresponding sense and a "scrambled" sequence of the same bases),
(d) measurements of the expression of the target mRNA or protein and an

unrelated control protein, and
(e) screening for possible toxic effects.

Successful applications of this technology include transient ablation of the expression of neuropeptide Y receptors in the CNS, CRH and AVP—for review see (32).

5.4.2 *In Vitro* Techniques

Stable or transient transfection of cells with DNA sequences *in vitro* has been used widely to examine the factors which influence the expression of specific genes and to investigate the roles of target proteins at the cellular level—for review see (33). In many instances, small modifications are made to the DNA sequence (site directed mutagenesis) which result in the expression of a protein in which one (or more) amino acid at a locus of particular interest is substituted, thus permitting investigation of that specific part of the sequence. For example, the importance of potential phosphorylation sites (tyrosine or serine) may be readily examined by substitution of these residues with other amino acids. Cell transfection also has important commercial applications and the engineered expression of genes such as insulin, GH and the gonadotrophins in, for example, *E. coli* now provides an essential source of drugs for clinical use which avoids the risks associated with extraction of the proteins from human sources (and, in the case of insulin, the potential of antigenic responses to proteins of bovine or porcine origin).

For the reasons rehearsed above, transient attenuation of gene expression *in vitro* by the use of antisense probes has met with mixed success (31, 32). As for *in vivo* studies, experimental design is of paramount importance and rigorous control must be imposed at all levels. Moreover, even in the *in vitro* situation accessibility of the nucleotides to their intracellular targets cannot be assumed, particularly in cell lines some of which (notably those of lymphoid origin) may prove either to be impermeable to nucleotides or to sequester them in intracellular vesicles. Notwithstanding these reservations, when used appropriately antisense technology provides a powerful tool with which to examine the roles of specific proteins.

5.5 INDICES USED TO MEASURE HYPOTHALAMIC AND PITUITARY TISSUE RESPONSES

5.5.1 Measurement of Protein and mRNA

Much information can be gained regarding the function and activity of the neuroendocrine system by mapping the expression of various molecular components using a range of methods which detect either the peptide/protein itself or the mRNA transcripts which encode it. This section will summarise the principles underlying the most widely used methods along with their major advantages and limitations. Detailed consideration of the practicalities of these methods, which vary enormously from laboratory to laboratory, can be found in a number of recent texts—see (34–38).

Immunocytochemistry

Immunocytochemistry (ICC), or immunohistochemistry, relies on the use of specific antibodies to detect a given protein or peptide in cells or tissues, for example, hormones, enzymes, receptors (34, 35). Thus, in the first instance, it relies on the production of antibodies that are highly specific for the peptide or protein (antigen) under study. These may be polyclonal antibodies, typically produced by injecting the antigen (possibly coupled to a carrier molecule along with an adjuvant, to enhance immune activation) into animals such as rabbits or sheep. After an appropriate immunisation schedule, the serum may be collected and used directly, following appropriate dilution. To improve the performance (specificity and affinity) of the polyclonal antibodies, monospecific antibodies may be obtained by affinity purification with pure antigen. Alternatively, a monoclonal antibody, i.e. a single specific antibody, can now be produced in large amounts by immortalised antibody producing cell lines formed by the fusion of a normal antibody-producing B cell and a myeloma line (a monoclonal tumour derived from a B lymphocyte).

Prior to immunostaining it is essential to select optimal conditions for the preparation and fixation of the tissue to retain antigens *in situ* and to preserve tissue structure. Commonly used fixatives are aldehydes (formaldehyde, glutaraldehyde) which cross-link proteins. While preserving morphology and retaining proteins in the cells and tissues, these chemicals will also interfere with primary and tertiary protein structure which are important for antigenicity. The success of the procedure thus depends on getting the right balance of each of these parameters. It is possible to perfuse the anaesthetised animal with fixative via a cardiac cannula for optimal penetration of the fixative or, alternatively, the piece of tissue under study can be removed and placed directly into fixative. After the appropriate time the fixed tissue block may be embedded in paraffin wax and stored for long periods, if necessary, before slices are cut on a sledge microtome for ICC. Alternatively, the fixed tissue may be cryopreserved in sucrose, rapidly frozen (e.g. on dry ice or isopentane) and stored in the freezer until ready for slicing on a cryostat. Schedules may vary, however, and for certain antigens (e.g. lipocortin, dystrophin) the optimal signal may be obtained by fixing after sectioning frozen tissue on a cryostat.

Unless the ICC is to be carried out on cultured cells, cutting the tissue into thin slices is important so that it can be viewed under either the light microscope for resolution at the cellular level, or the electron microscope for ultrastructural studies. The specific antibody (often termed the first antibody) is then allowed to react with antigen. Occasionally this antibody may be visualised directly, but more generally a second antibody generated against the species-specific region on the Fc region of the first antibody is used as a link to the visible signal and seems to improve sensitivity and specificity of the method. In its simplest form the second antibody may be tagged with a fluorescent molecule (e.g. fluorescein, rhodamine) which can be viewed under fluorescence optics. Alternatively, it can be linked to molecules that subsequently react with various chemicals to give a coloured product that can be seen under light microscope, for example the peroxidase-antiperoxidase-diaminobenzidine method or the avidin-biotin method. At the ultrastructural level the visualisation method relies on the production of an electron-dense signal.

Good quality reagents for ICC are now widely available commercially and are often supplied in kit form. Increasingly the method has been developed not only to locate a single antigen but also a second or even a third simultaneously which provides the added power to investigate the co-localisation of biologically active molecules such as hormones, neurotransmitters, neuromodulators and receptors. Although variations in intensity of the immunocytochemical signal have been extrapolated to indicate changes in the level of antigen present in the cell, the method is, however, not truly quantitative but at best semi-quantitative. It is also prone to false positive reactions, especially with the use of polyclonal antibodies which may contain clones that react with antigens other than the one under investigation. In addition, even specific antibodies may cross-react with structurally related antigens. Careful controls, including the parallel use of a non- or pre-immune serum in place of the first antibody and quenching of the signal with excess antigen, should therefore be carried out to eliminate such possibilities.

Western Blot Analysis

Western blot analysis permits the separation and identification of a specific protein in a sample (biological fluid or tissue) that may contain several thousand proteins. After an initial extraction procedure, the component proteins are separated on the basis of size and charge by sodium dodecyl polyacrilamide gel electrophoresis (SDS-PAGE) and transferred electrophoretically to nitrocellulose paper. The protein of interest is detected by incubation with a primary antibody and visualised by addition of a second antibody conjugated with an agent (e.g. peroxidase) which will react with specific additives to yield a coloured precipitate (e.g. diaminebenzidine, see above and pages 149–51). The molecular weight is determined by comparison with the migration of molecular weight markers and, if available, a standard preparation of the protein. The density of the band may be determined by image analysis and compared with that of graded concentrations of standard. However, the technique is at best only semi-quantitative; moreover, like other methods based on measurements of tissue content of a substance, it gives no indication of turnover.

In Situ Hybridisation

The technique of *in situ* hybridisation (ISH) is performed on fixed tissue slices or cell cultures prepared in a manner similar to that for ICC (36, 37) but fixation is more usually carried out on cryostat sections. It is used, however, to detect a specific DNA or RNA sequence using DNA or RNA which is complementary in structure to the genetic signal under investigation (cDNA or cRNA) as the probe which may be visualised. ISH is typically used to monitor mRNA and hence gene expression. Alternatively, with increasing knowledge of intron sequences, it is possible also to synthesise probes that span exon–intron interfaces and thus are suitable for detection of primary transcripts. In view of the prevalence of RNase and its remarkable stability, it is essential to ensure a RNase-free environment. This is best achieved by wearing gloves, by autoclaving glassware, equipment and solutions and by treating solutions with RNase inhibitors (e.g. diethylpyro-carbonate) when possible. Initially, cDNA and cRNA probes were cloned by insertion of a double stranded DNA into a vector for amplification in a bacterium and thus required non-trivial skills in molecular biological techniques. However, the development of oligonucleotide probes which can be readily custom synthe-sised, along with the production of commercial kits for probe labelling has opened up this method to many more researchers.

Probes can be labelled with radioactive isotopes (e.g. ^{32}P, ^{35}S) but, increas-ingly, non-radioactive methods are being developed which use reporter groups such as digoxigenin or biotin. For the larger cDNA and cRNA probes, polymer-ase enzymes are used to incorporate labelled nucleotides whereas oligonucleo-tide probes (which are typically 30–50 bases long) are labelled using enzymes (e.g. transferase) which add on a tail of up to 100 labelled bases. Many factors govern the strength of binding i.e. the hybridisation of a nucleic acid probe to its target nucleic acid. These include the length of probe, its base composition, temperature and salt composition as well as the number of mismatches. The specificity of hybridisation will also depend on these parameters, with oligo-nucleotide probes designed towards specific individual members of a gene family being generally more specific than the larger nucleic acid probes. A complex series of buffers has been developed, both for the hybridising step as well as the subsequent washing steps to remove excess probe, and the optimal conditions must be determined empirically for each probe. Essential specificity controls include blocking the signal with excess cold probe and the absence of signal using a sense probe.

ISH is often used quantitatively to detect changes in gene expression after various physiological or pharmacological manipulations. With care and the use of an image analyser, autoradiographic methods for detecting radiolabelled probes may be used, for example, to estimate the number of copies of target mRNA per cell. However, comparisons should always be relative, not absolute, as there is no index of target loss during procedure. Increasingly ISH is being used in association with ICC to confirm that mRNA is translated into protein or peptide, which is an important step towards establishing whether intensity of an mRNA signal will truly reflect rate of synthesis.

Northern Hybridisation

Northern hybridisation (RNA blotting) allows determination of the size and relative amounts of specific mRNA molecules in preparations of total or poly(A)$^+$ RNA (37). The extracted RNA is first separated according to size by electrophoresis through a denaturing agarose gel. The separated molecules are then transferred and immobilised onto nitrocellulose or nylon membranes where one or several RNAs of interest can be located after hybridisation to appropriately labelled specific probes similar to those used for ISH as described above. Hybridisation of RNA immobilised on a solid support (without electrophoresis) with excess radiolabelled probe constitutes the techniques of dot and slot hybridisation. The intensity of signal, as determined for example by autoradiography followed by densitometry, gives a semiquantitative measure of gene expression in various tissues/experimental conditions providing a constant amount of RNA is loaded and the expression of "housekeeping" gene (for example β-actin, which would not be expected to change) is also monitored. Similar methods can be applied to RNA which has not been subject to electrophoresis first.

Reverse Transcription Polymerase Chain Reaction

The hybridisation methods described above require at least several micrograms of total RNA for detection of specific mRNAs. By use of the RT-PCR at least a thousandfold increase in sensitivity can be obtained (37, 38). Initially PCR was developed to amplify DNA. Thus, the first steps in the RT-PCR method involve the extraction of total RNA followed by the production of complementary single stranded DNA using reverse transcriptase enzyme.

The PCR is then used to amplify a segment of DNA which lies between two regions of known sequence using a DNA polymerase. The segment to be amplified (template DNA) is chosen to be specific for the protein or peptide under study and is defined by two oligonucleotides complementary to the sequences flanking the template which serve as primers for the polymerising enzyme. The reaction proceeds through repeated temperature controlled cycles of denaturation, annealing and DNA synthesis with the amount of the desired DNA product doubling at every cycle. Under the reaction conditions which are commonly used, the polymerase becomes limiting after approximately 30 cycles by which time an amplification of the order of 10^6 can be achieved. When separated by electrophoresis on an agarose gel, a single band should be obtained and the product should be identifiable by molecular size (typically designed to be 200–500 base pairs in length), by sequencing and by hybridisation with a specific probe after transfer to nitrocellular or nylon membranes (Southern hybridisation). This method is therefore extremely powerful for the detection of mRNA of very low abundance and from very small amounts of starting material (potentially a single cell). A great many controls and precautions are, however, necessary to eliminate contamination especially by amplification of genomic DNA sequences. To date this method is widely used for semi-quantitative analysis by reference to a housekeeping gene but much development is going towards truly quantitative methods (38).

5.5.2 Measurement of Hormones and Neurotransmitters

Immunoassays and high performance liquid chromatography (HPLC) are the most commonly used methods for the detection of hormones and neurotransmitters of the hypothalamo–pituitary axes and their peripheral endocrine organs.

Immunoassays

Immunoassays involve the interaction of a specific antibody with the antigen (hormone) and can be divided into two main classes, namely radioisotope assays (e.g. radioimmunoassay and immunoradiometric assays) and non-isotope assays (e.g. enzyme-linked immunosorbent assays). In an assay it is essential that a standard curve is set up under conditions identical to those of the samples and that low, medium and high quality control samples are also included in the assay. Standards and samples should always be prepared at least in duplicate and parallelism should be demonstrated between dilutions of the standards and samples. One of the main problems with immunoassay is the potential cross-reactivity of the antibody with biologically inactive fragments or precursors of the hormone under investigation, resulting in marked dissociations between the data from biological and immunological assays. This problem is minimised by the use of two-site assays (see below). In addition, structural similarities between different hormones, for example GH and prolactin, may result in immunologic cross-reactivity. Care should also be taken to ensure that substances (e.g. drugs) present in the sample for analysis do not interfere with the assay.

Radioimmunoassay. The principle of radioimmunoassay (RIA) is illustrated in Fig. 5.1. The unlabelled antigen (i.e. standard or sample) is mixed with a finite amount of corresponding radiolabelled antigen and a highly specific antibody.

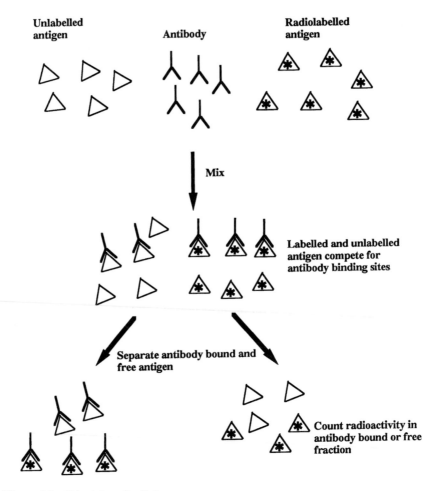

Figure 5.1   Principles of radioimmunoassay

The unlabelled and labelled antigen compete for the free binding sites on the antibody and soluble antigen-antibody complexes are formed. The amount of bound labelled antigen is inversely proportional to the amount of unlabelled antigen. Once equilibrium has been attained the antibody-bound and free antigen are separated and the radioactivity in one of the fractions is measured. Efficient separation of the bound and free radioactivity is essential. Separation methods include removal of free antigen by adsorption onto charcoal or silica, precipitation of antibody-bound using a second antibody capable of reacting specifically with the first antibody or non-specific precipitation of antibody-bound antigen with salt or organic solvent. The advantages and disadvantages of these separation techniques have been reviewed by Walker (39).

The advantages of RIA are that it is an extremely sensitive and specific method, with a precision that is comparable to that of other physio-chemical techniques and better than that of bioassays. In addition, RIA is highly automated and allows a large number of samples to be assayed with minimal handling. The major disadvantages of RIA are that the equipment and reagents are relatively expensive and the assays also usually take several days to complete. Moreover, operators are exposed to radiological hazards and since the antigens need labelling frequently due to the short half-lives (e.g. $t_{\frac{1}{2}}$ ^{131}I , 8 days; $t_{\frac{1}{2}}$ ^{125}I, 60 days) regular thyroid scans should be performed.

Immunoradiometric assay. Immunoradiometric assays (IRMAs) are used less frequently than RIAs but they have been successfully employed to measure hormones such as the hypothalamic hormone CRH. These assays have similar sensitivities to RIAs but require a much greater quantity of antibody (fiftyfold or more) than for the corresponding RIA. The principle of IRMA is similar to RIA but IRMAs differ from RIAs in that the antibody is radiolabelled rather than the antigen. The antigen (standard or sample) is incubated with an excess of radiolabelled antibody and the mixture is allowed to equilibrate. The subsequent separation of the immunocomplex from the free radiolabelled antibody is achieved by addition of an excess of immunoadsorbent which binds to any free labelled antibody. The antibody-immunoadsorbent complex is removed by centrifugation and the radioactivity in the supernatant, which is proportional to the amount of antigen in the standard or sample, is measured. Unless the antibody is effectively irreversible, removal of the free antibody from the initial equilibrium mixture will disrupt the equilibrium position and this assay is therefore potentially sensitive to timing and washing.

An extension of this assay is the two-site IRMA in which the major proviso is that the antigen has more than one immunological group available. The first step of this assay involves immobilisation of the target antigen by allowing it to bind to an unlabelled antibody which itself is bound to a solid phase (such as polyethylene centrifuge tubes). This complex is then reacted with a second labelled antibody which binds to a different site on the antigen. The free antibody is then decanted and the radioactivity of the solid phase measured. The main advantage of the two-site assay is that there is increased specificity and sensitivity compared to the one-site assay. Further details of these assays are provided by Mayer and Walker (40).

Enzyme-linked immunosorbent assay. Initially, enzyme-linked immunosorbent assays (ELISAs) were used in immunology to measure the titre and specificity of antisera but they have also been used for the detection and quantification of various antigens, including the anterior pituitary hormones prolactin, thyrotrophin and GH (41–43). The principle of ELISA is the same as that of RIA except that an enzyme, rather than a radioisotope, is used to label the antibody or antigen. The enzyme is readily detected on addition of the appropriate substrate and can be quantified by measuring the absorbance of the colour produced. The concentration of the unknown is then determined by comparison with a standard curve. A number of ELISAs, including competitive, double antibody and indirect competitive assays, have been developed and the principle of each one is summarised in Fig. 5.2.

In the competitive ELISA, a specific antibody is bound to a solid phase such as cross-linked dextran, polyacrylamide beads, cellulose discs, polypropylene tubes or polystyrene microtitration plates, the last of which are particularly convenient for large numbers of samples. The solid phase antibody is then reacted with samples containing a known amount of enzyme-labelled antigen and a known (standard) or unknown (test) amount of unlabelled antigen. Following an appropriate incubation period the complex is washed, the enzyme substrate is added and a coloured precipitate becomes visible. The enzyme activity is determined by measuring the absorbance of the precipitate which is proportional to the ratio of labelled to unlabelled antigen in the sample. Thus a high concentration of unknown antigen in the sample will result in a low absorbance detected from the coloured products of the enzyme reaction.

The double antibody method also involves a specific antibody bound to a solid phase but in this instance a sample containing a known (standard) or unknown (test) amount of unlabelled antigen is allowed to react with the antibody. The

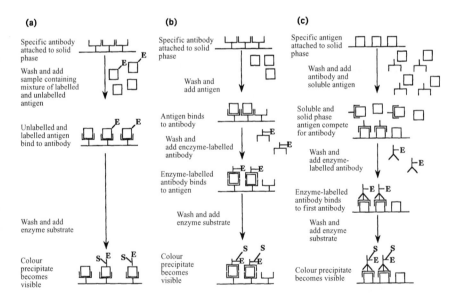

Figure 5.2 Principles of (a) competitive (b) double antibody and (c) indirect competitive enzyme-linked immunosorbent assays. E, enzyme; S, substrate

complex formed is then washed and an enzyme-labelled second antibody is added and allowed to react with it. After further washing the enzyme substrate is added and the amount of enzyme activity is determined as above. Under standard conditions this is directly proportional to the amount of antigen present in the sample.

More recently, indirect competitive ELISAs have been developed for the detection of anterior pituitary hormones (42, 43). In this approach the specific antigen is attached to the solid phase. A mixture of a known amount of first antibody and a known (standard) or unknown (test) amount of soluble antigen is added and the soluble and solid phase antigen compete for the antibody binding sites. Therefore a high concentration of soluble antigen in the sample results in a low concentration of antibody immobilised to the adsorbed antigen. The immobilised antigen–antibody complex is washed and exposed to an enzyme labelled anti-immunoglobulin antibody which binds to the primary antibody. This complex is then washed and the substrate for the enzyme added. The absorbance of the resulting coloured precipitate is indirectly proportional to the amount of antigen in the original sample.

As with RIA, a large number of samples can be tested at the same time in an ELISA. Moreover ELISAs have a number of advantages over RIAs, although the latter are extensively automated and sometimes more sensitive. Firstly, ELISAs are relatively cheap to operate, since the counting equipment is replaced by less expensive and less cumbersome absorbance detectors. Secondly, ELISAs can often be completed more quickly than RIAs and the analysis time is also considerably shorter since each ELISA plate takes only about 5 min to read. Thirdly, enzyme-conjugated reagents are stable upon storage for prolonged periods (i.e. they have a long shelf life) whereas radioactive isotopes of iodine have a short half-life. In addition, the reagents for ELISA are generally safe and the radiological hazards associated with RIA are eliminated. The main source of error is that in some ELISAs there is a large number of pipetting stages. Moreover, there are differences in absorbance values between well plates, although this discrepancy can be minimised by setting up a standard curve on each well plate within an assay. The perimeter wells also give a significantly higher absorbance value and for this reason only the inner wells of the well plate should be used.

High Performance Liquid Chromatography

HPLC is a separation technique which can be used to analyse samples derived from plasma and serum, urine, cerebrospinal fluid and various tissues. A variety of neurotransmitters, peptides and steroids can be detected by this method. The HPLC system consists of four major components, namely a solvent delivery system (i.e. a pump), an injection system (which may be manual or automatic), a column and a detector. In this method, a mixture of components in a liquid (mobile) phase is injected at the top of a column packed with a solid (stationary) phase. As the mixture of solutes travels down the column it is separated into component molecules, with the rate of migration of each component through the column being proportional to its distribution coefficient. Thus, components with a low distribution in the stationary phase will move more quickly through the column while those with a high distribution in the solid phase will elute more slowly. When measuring ionised compounds the stationary phase is more polarised than the mobile phase and the system is referred to as "normal phase" liquid chromatography. However, in some cases the sample binds so strongly to the stationary phase that even marked alterations in the polarity of the mobile phase fail to produce a sufficient decrease in retention time (the time of elution of the peak maximum). In this situation "reverse phase" chromatography would be used where the stationary phase is usually non-polar and the less polar solutes are retained on the column for a longer period of time than the ionised compounds. Following elution from the column individual solutes are monitored by a variable wavelength ultraviolet-visible spectrophotometer, a fluorimeter or an electrochemical detector and recorded as peaks on a chart recorder. Quantitative analysis can be carried out manually or electronically and involves comparing the heights or areas of the sample peaks in the elution chromatogram with those of standards. As many of the compounds analysed by HPLC are subject to temperature- and time-dependent decay, it is important to inject the external standard preparations between the unknown samples at regular intervals. Internal standards should also be added to samples (a process called "spiking") at the start of any extraction procedure so that recovery can also be monitored. See (44, 45) for further information about HPLC.

5.5.3 Detection and Characterisation of Receptors

Autoradiography

Autoradiography can be used to visualise the location of receptors within sections of whole cells or tissues and usually involves the use of soft β-emitting isotopes such as ^3H and ^{14}C. In this procedure tissue sections may be obtained from animals pretreated with a radiolabelled ligand selective for the receptor population of interest. More commonly, however, the tissue is removed from untreated animals and sectioned prior to incubation with the radioactive ligand *in vitro*, a procedure which obviates the need for complex *in vivo* experiments and is essential in the study of ligands that do not cross the blood–brain barrier readily. Following appropriate fixation and processing, the radiolabelled tissue is covered with a thin photographic emulsion and left in the dark, using an exposure period and ambient conditions (e.g. temperature) which depend upon the isotope, its level of activity, the sample type and the film type). During this time the radioisotope decays and the emitted particles are taken up by the photographic emulsion which consists of silver halide (usually silver bromide) crystals embedded, for example, in gelatin. Energy is transferred to the silver ions which are therefore reduced to silver atoms and a particulate latent image is formed. The emulsion is then developed and the location of radioactivity in the preparation is indicated by the position of the developed silver grains which cause a blackening of the film. The data can be quantified by recording the intensity of the image using a densitometer.

Radioligand Binding

Ligand binding studies also are used widely for detecting characterising and quantifying cellular receptors. They may be carried out on intact cells or tissues, tissue homogenates or purified membrane preparations. Briefly, the chosen preparation is incubated with graded concentrations of a radioactively labelled ligand (^{125}I and ^{3}H are the most commonly used radioisotopes) which is highly selective for the receptor population under investigation in the presence and absence of excess unlabelled ligand. The unlabelled ligand saturates the receptor and thus prevents binding of the radiolabelled ligand. Thus, any remaining bound label is a measure of non-specific binding. Incubation of the labelled ligand alone represents total binding and subtraction of the non-specific binding from this value is used to determine specific binding. Following an appropriate time for equilibration, the radiolabelled ligand-receptor complex and free labelled ligand are separated by equilibrium dialysis, filtration, centrifugation or precipitation and the amount of bound label is quantified. The data can be analysed using Scatchard analysis, which determines the number and binding affinity of the receptor. See (46, 47) for more detailed discussion of further aspects of ligand binding assays.

REFERENCES

1. Buckingham J. C., Gillies G. E. Hypothalamus and pituitary gland: xenobiotic induced toxicity and models for its investigation. In Flack J. D., Atterwill C. (eds) *Endocrine Toxicology*. Cambridge, Cambridge University Press, 1992, pp 83–114.
2. Forsling M. L., Wells T. Intracerebroventricular implantation and vascular cannulation in conscious unrestrained rats for neuroendocrine studies. In Greenstein B. (ed), *Neuroendocrine Research Methods*. Chur, Harwood Academic Publishers, 1991, pp 187–204.
3. Dluzen D. E., Ramirez V. D. Push-pull cannula—construction, application and considerations for use in neuroendocrinology. In Greenstein B. (ed), *Neuroendocrine Research Methods*. Chur, Harwood Academic Publishers, 1991, pp 163-86.
4. Levine J. E., Meredith J. M., Vogelsong K. M., Legan S. J. Microdialysis for the study of hypothalamic and pituitary function. In Robinson T. E., Justice Jr J. B. (eds),

Microdialysis in the Neurosciences. Amsterdam, Elsevier Science Publications BV, 1991, pp 305–25.

5. Kendrick K. M. *In vivo* measurement of amino acid, monoamine and neuropeptide release using microdialysis. In Greenstein B. (ed), *Neuroendocrine Research Methods*. Chur, Harwood Academic Publishers, 1991, pp 249–78.

6. Sarker D. K., Minami S. Pituitary portal blood collection in rats. A powerful technique for studying hypothalamic hormone secretion. In Greenstein B. (ed), *Neuroendocrine Research Methods*. Chur, Harwood Academic Publishers, 1991, pp 235–49.

7. Gibbs D. M. Collection of pituitary portal blood: a methodologic analysis. *Neuroendocrinology*, 1984, **38**: 97–101.

8. Edwardson J. A., Bennett G. W., Bradford H. F. Release of amino acids and neurosecretory substances after stimulation of nerve endings (synaptosomes) isolated from the hypothalamus. *Nature*, 1972, **240**: 554–6.

9. Bradbury M. W. B., Burden J., Hillhouse E. W., Jones M. T. Stimulation electrically and by acetylcholine of the rat hypothalamus *in vitro*. *J Physiol*, 1974, **239**: 269–83.

10. Lumsden C. L. Nervous tissue in culture. In Bourne G. H. (ed), *Structure and Function of Nervous Tissue*. New York, Academic Press, 1968, pp 67–140.

11. Grossman A., Costa A., Navarra P., Tsagarakis S. The regulation of hypothalamic corticotropin-releasing factor release: *in vitro* studies. In *Corticotropin-releasing Factor (Ciba Foundation Symposium 172)*. Chichester, J Wiley & Sons Ltd, 1993, pp 129–50.

12. Calogero A. E., Gallucci W. T., Bernadini R., Saoutis C., Gold P. W., Chrousos G. P. Effect of cholinergic agonists and antagonists on rat hypothalamic corticotrophin-releasing hormone secretion *in vitro*. *Neuroendocrinology*, 1988, **47**: 303–8.

13. Cowell A. M., Cover P. O., Gillies G. E., Buckingham J. C. *In vitro* models for examination of the mechanisms controlling the secretion of hypothalamic hormones. In Greenstein B. (ed), *Neuroendocrine Research Methods*. Chur, Harwood Academic Publishers, 1991, pp 111–30.

14. Dreifuss J. J., Gahwiler B. H. Hypothalamic neurones in culture. I. A short review of the literature. *J Physiol Paris*, 1979, **75**: 15–21.

15. Clarke M. J. O., Gillies G. E. Comparison of peptide release from fetal rat hypothalamic neurones cultured in defined media and serum-containing media. *J Endocrinol*, 1988, **116**: 349–56.

16. Mellon P. L., Windle J. J., Goldsmith P. C., Padula C. A., Roberts J. L., Weiner R. I. Immortalization of hypothalamic GnRH neurons by genetically targeted tumorigenesis. *Neuron*, 1990, **5**: 1–10.

17. Pearson D., Shainberg A., Sachs H. The hypothalamo–neurohypophysial complex in organ culture: morphologic and biochemical characteristics. *Endocrinology*, 1975, **96**: 982–93.

18. Davidson K., Gillies G. E. Neuronal vs glial somatostatin in the hypothalamus: a cell culture study of the ontogenesis of cellular location, content and release. *Brain Res*, 1993, **624**: 75–84.

19. Herbison A. E., Theodosis D. T. Absence of estrogen receptor immunoreactivity in somatostatin (SRIF) neurons of the periventricular nucleus but sexually dimorphic colocalization of estrogen receptor and SRIF immunoreactivities in neurons of the bed nucleus of the stria terminalis. *Endocrinology*, 1993, **132**: 1707–14.

20. Murray H., Gillies G. E. Investigations of the ontogenic patterns of rat hypothalamic dopaminergic neurone morphology and function *in vitro*. *J Endocrinol*, 1993, **139**: 403–14.

21. Buckingham J. C., Hodges R. J. The use of corticotrophin production by adenohypo-

physial tissue *in vitro* for the detection and estimation of potential corticotrophin releasing factors. *J Endocrinol*, 1977, **72**: 187–93.

22. Negro-Vilar A., Lapetina E. G. 1,2-didecanoylglycerol and phorbol 12,13-dibutyrate enhance anterior pituitary hormone secretion *in vitro*. *Endocrinology*, 1985, **117**: 1559–64.

23. Cowell A. M., Flower R. J., Buckingham J. C. Studies on the roles of phospholipase A$_2$ and eicosanoids in the regulation of corticotrophin secretion by rat pituitary cells *in vitro*. *J Endocrinol*, 1991, **130**: 21–32.

24. Busbridge N. J., Chamberlain G. V. P., Griffiths A., Whitehead S. A. Non-steroidal follicular factors attenuate the self-priming action of gonadotrophin releasing hormone on the pituitary gonadotroph. *Neuroendocrinology*, 1990, **51**: 493–9.

25. Gillies G., Lowry P. J. Perfused rat isolated anterior pituitary cell column as bioassay for factor(s) controlling release of adrenocorticotropin: validation of a technique. *Endocrinology*, 1978, **103**: 521–7.

26. Cover P. O., Buckingham J. C. Changes in the responsiveness of perifused rat adenohypophyseal cells to luteinizing hormone releasing hormone. *Acta Endocrinol*, 1986, **113**: 479–86.

27. Childs G. V. The use of counterflow centrifugation to enrich pituitary corticotropes: The method and its perils and pitfalls. In Greenstein B. (ed), *Neuroendocrine Research Methods*. Chur, Harwood Academic Publishers, 1991, pp 39–56.

28. Vanderschueren B., Denef C., Cassiman J. J. Ultrastructural and functional character-istics of rat pituitary cell aggregates. *Endocrinology*, 1982, **110**: 513–23.

29. Hogan B., Constanti R., Lacy E. (eds) *Manipulating the mouse embryo*. New York, Cold Harbor Springs Laboratory Press, 1986.

30. Galli-Taliadoros L. A., Sedgewick J. D., Wood S. A., Korner H. Gene knock-out technology: a methodological overview for the interested novice. *J Immunol Methods*, 1995, **181**: 1–15.

31. Landgraf R. Antisense targeting in behavioural neuroendocrinology. *J Endocrinol*, 1996, **151**: 333–40.

32. Morris M., Lucion Q. B. Antisense oligonucleotides in the study of the neuroendocrine system. *J Neuroendocrinology*, 1995, **7**: 493–500.

33. Kaplitt M. G., Rabkin S. D., Pfaff D. W. Molecular alterations in nerve cells: direct manipulation and physiological mediation. In Imura H. (ed), *Current Topics in Neuro-endocrinology*, 1993, **11**: 169–91.

34. Polak J. M., van Noorden S. V. (eds) *An Introduction to Immunocytochemistry: Current Techniques and Problems*. Oxford, Oxford University Press, 1988.

35. Cuello A. C. (ed) *Immunocytochemistry. IBRO Handbook Series: Methods in the Neurosciences. Volume 14.* Chichester, John Wiley & Sons Ltd., 1993.

36. Emson P. C. *In situ* hybridization as a methodical tool for the neuroscientist. *TINS*, 1993, **16**: 9–16.

37. Sambrook J., Fritisch E. F., Maniotis T. (eds) *Molecular cloning. A Laboratory Manual.* 2nd edition, New York, Cold Spring Harbour Laboratory Press. 1989.

38. Kohler T. H., Lassaer D., Rost A. K, Thamm B., Pustowoit B., Ranke H. *Quantification of mRNA by polymerase chain reaction. Nonradioactive PCR methods.* New York, Springer Verlag, 1995.

39. Walker W. H. C. An approach to immunoassay. *Clin Chem*, 1977, **23**: 384–402.

40. Mayer R. J., Walker J. H. *Immunochemical Methods in the Biological Sciences: Enzymes and Proteins.* London, Academic Press, 1980.

41. Miyai K., Ishibashi K., Kumahara Y. Enzyme-linked immunoassay of thyrotropin. *Clin Chim Acta*, 1976, **67**: 263–8.

42. Signorella A. P., Hymer W. C. An enzyme-linked immunosorbent assay for rat prolactin. *Anal Biochem*, 1984, **136**: 372–81.
43. Farrington M. A., Hymer W. C. An enzyme immunoassay for rat growth hormone: applications to the study of growth hormone variants. *Life Sci*, 1987, **40**: 2479–88.
44. Kilpatrick I. C. Rapid, semi-automated HPLC analyses of catecholamines and metabolites in microdissected brain regions and brain slice superfusates using coulometric detection. In Greenstein B. (ed), *Neuroendocrine Research Methods*. Chur, Harwood Academic Publishers, 1991, pp 527–53.
45. Wilson C. A., Hole D. R., Slater D. M. The measurement of biogenic amines and their metabolites in brain tissue and plasma. In Greenstein B. (ed), *Neuroendocrine Research Methods*. Chur, Harwood Academic Publishers, 1991, pp 579–600.
46. Conn P. M., Braden T. D. Methods for studying the gonadotropin releasing hormone receptor. A model for peptide-receptor interactions. In Greenstein B. (ed), *Neuroendocrine Research Methods*. Chur, Harwood Academic Publishers, 1991, pp 673–97.
47. Wilkinson M., MacDonald M. C., Landymore K., Wilkinson D. Opioid receptors in micropunches of fresh hypothalamic tissue. A binding assay for everyman. In Greenstein B. (ed), *Neuroendocrine Research Methods*. Chur, Harwood Academic Publishers, 1991, pp 723–46.

Chapter 6

Assessment of the Autonomic and Behavioural Effects of Stress

Sandra V. Vellucci

The Babraham Institute, Cambridge, UK

6.1 INTRODUCTION

As detailed in Chapter 2, stress causes marked changes in the activity of the autonomic nervous system and in behaviour, the characteristics of which depend on the nature, the intensity and the duration of the insult as well as on the individual subjects. Meaningful evaluation of these responses requires a detailed knowledge of the normal physiological and behavioural patterns of the species under study. It also requires the exploitation of methods which themselves do not impose further stress on the subject; thus, techniques involving minimal handling and restraint and painless sampling procedures have obvious advantages. This chapter describes:

(a) established methods for the assessment of various parameters of autonomic function, and
(b) procedures used commonly to determine the effects of stress on behaviour.

Stress, Stress Hormones and the Immune System. Edited by J. C. Buckingham, G. E. Gillies and A.-M. Cowell
© 1997 John Wiley & Sons, Ltd.

The latter section includes brief descriptions of several specific behavioural tests which are used as experimental models of fearfulness and anxiety; it also describes a number of animal models which are considered to be analogues of human psychiatric conditions (e.g. anxiety and depression) in which certain types of stress may play a permissive role. A comprehensive reference list has been included as precise details of the experimental techniques involved are beyond the scope of this chapter.

6.2 MEASUREMENT OF AUTONOMIC ACTIVITY

The predominant autonomic response to stress is a pronounced increase in sympathetic outflow although in some instances parasympathetic activation may also occur (see Chapter 2). These responses may be evaluated in freely-moving or restrained conscious animals by the assessment of target organ activity and catecholamine output by invasive or non-invasive procedures. Further measurements may also be carried out *post mortem* (e.g. determination of catecholamine synthetic enzyme activity or histological examination of tissue).

6.2.1 Cardiovascular Function

Stress normally elicits significant increases in heart rate, cardiac output and blood pressure which are associated with specific changes in regional blood flow.

Measurement of Heart Rate

The simplest method of measuring heart rate is via electrocardiograph (ECG) leads connected directly to a recording machine. This is easily accomplished in man and in anaesthetised or restrained laboratory animals. However, although not invasive, the leads make this direct method unsuitable for studies in conscious, freely-moving animals and telemetric procedures are therefore advised. These involve transmitting information from ECG electrodes attached to the surface of the skin to a radio receiver via a small device which may be either fastened externally to the animal (e.g. attached to a collar or velcro strap in cats, dogs and rodents (1), covered by a close-fitting jacket in monkeys (2), fastened to the wrist in human) or implanted surgically (e.g. subcutaneously or intraperitoneally (3)) in advance of the experiment. Telemetric recording may also be used to monitor other aspects of cardiovascular function including, for example, blood pressure, blood flow, cardiac output and blood pH together with other parameters such as body temperature (4).

Measurement of Blood Pressure

The measurement of arterial blood pressure includes evaluation of systolic, diastolic and mean arterial pressures. The simplest, non-invasive method involves the use of an inflatable cuff to occlude blood flow in a superficial artery either in a limb (5) or, in the case of small rodents (e.g. the rat (6)) the tail. The pressure in the cuff is measured to determine the points at which blood flow is interrupted (systolic pressure) and unimpeded (diastolic pressure) but it does not provide an accurate measure of mean arterial blood pressure. This procedure is used routinely in clinical medicine; it may also be used in experimental animals (e.g. dogs, monkeys, rats) provided that they are first habituated to the procedure. Sustained or repeated measurements of systolic, diastolic and mean arterial pressure may be obtained directly from all major arteries in various species by means of a pressure transducer attached to an indwelling catheter. Alternatively, telemetric devices (outlined above) may be employed, particularly for measurements in freely-moving animals.

Imaging and Histological Measurements

Exposure to chronic or severe stress can also give rise to a range of structural changes in the vasculature and myocardium which can be detected and evaluated *in vivo* by imaging techniques and *post mortem* by routine histological methods. These include focal myocardial necrosis and fibrosis together with smooth muscle thickening, loss of elasticity and plaque formation in the vasculature, notably the coronary arteries. These structural changes occur in a variety of species (e.g. chicken, mice, rats, cats, pigs, monkeys) which provide valuable experimental models as well as in man (7).

6.2.2 Measurement of Catecholamines and Their Metabolites in Body Fluids and Tissues

Measurements of catecholamines and their metabolites in plasma, urine and cerebrospinal fluid are frequently used to assess sympatho-adrenal activity in conditions of stress. In addition, tissue concentrations of these substances and the enzymes responsible for their biosynthesis and degradation may be determined *post mortem*. It is important to note that the ratio of adrenaline to noradrenaline produced varies according to the nature of the stress. For example, in man, exposure to anxiety- or aggression-provoking situations (emotional stress) produces a marked increase in adrenaline release but only a modest rise in noradrenaline. Conversely, stimuli causing increased physical activity without emotional distress cause a preferential increase in noradrenaline secretion.

Hence, evaluation of a catecholamine response to stress requires indices of both adrenaline and noradrenaline output.

Determination of Adrenaline and Noradrenaline in Plasma

Plasma adrenaline and noradrenaline determinations may be carried out accurately by radio-enzymatic assays or high performance liquid chromatography (HPLC) with electrochemical detection (8, 9). The technique of sampling is critical as catecholamine release occurs very rapidly after stress exposure and the plasma half-life of the amines is extremely short (e.g. 70 seconds in rat plasma), with activity being terminated by metabolism in the liver and kidney or, in the case of the sympathetic nerves, by uptake into the nerves or surrounding tissue. Thus, sampling must be carried out very soon after the application of an acute stress and extreme care taken to ensure that the sampling procedure does not cause further catecholamine release. To minimise sampling stress the experimental subjects should be accustomed to handling or restraint and, in situations where repeated sampling is necessary, use may be made of an indwelling arterial or venous catheter.

It is important to note that the validity of measurement of venous plasma noradrenaline as a direct index of sympathetic neuronal discharge has been questioned. Regional or general differences in sympathetic activity may not be reflected accurately by measurements of catecholamines in venous blood samples taken from a single site. Furthermore, the noradrenaline content of venous blood from a given region is influenced by a variety of factors which include the concentration of the amine in arterial blood, its extraction from the blood during passage through the tissues and neurotransmitter overflow from sympathetic nerve terminals in the tissue. There are also problems in interpreting measurements of noradrenaline in arterial blood as these reflect the levels attained in mixed venous blood and the efficacy of catecholamine removal during the passage of blood through the lungs.

Determination of Catecholamine Metabolites in Urine

The estimation of adrenaline and noradrenaline metabolites in urine offers a simple, non-invasive method for the determination of sympatho-adrenomedullary activity (10), although it does not enable the source of the parent substance to be identified. Sampling is straightforward, both in experimental animals (via metabolism cages) and in man and the metabolites, namely 3-methoxy-4-hydroxymandelic acid (vanillylmandelic acid, VMA) and 3-methoxy-4-hydroxyphenylglycol (MHPG, which may be converted to VMA), are readily detected by standard laboratory methods, for example HPLC. Care must be taken to account for alterations in fluid intake and urine output in the design of the study and the calculation of the data. For acute studies in experimental animals or man, urinary metabolites may be compared in samples collected from the same subjects before and after exposure to an acute stimulus. Alternatively, single samples may be taken from different groups of subjects before, during or after stress and the concentrations of catecholamine metabolites compared. Measurements may also be made on urine samples taken over a 24 hour period to give an indication of long-term sympatho-adrenal activation.

Measurements of Catecholamines in Cerebrospinal Fluid

Measurements of the concentrations of catecholamines, their metabolites and other neurotransmitter substances in the cerebrospinal fluid of experimental animals provide a further valuable index of stress-induced activity. Sample collection is inevitably invasive but, by using pre-implanted indwelling intraventricular cannulae, push-pull cannulae (11) or microdialysis (9), small samples sufficient for assay may be taken repeatedly over extended periods (several hours) in conscious animals with the minimum of disturbance. Microdialysis, which involves the accurate (stereotaxic) placement of a microdialysis probe via a guide cannula, is particularly useful as it enables accurate measurements to be made not only in the ventricles but also in specific brain areas which are of relevance to the control of the autonomic, behavioural and neuroendocrine responses to stress (e.g. hypothalamus and brain stem nuclei, amygdala, hippocampus). This technique has been used in the rat as well as in larger species (e.g. sheep) in which the bigger brain minimises the trauma associated with the insertion of the microdialysis probe (9).

Post Mortem Studies

Quantitative biochemical and histological techniques may be used to examine the distribution and expression of catecholamines, their metabolites and the enzymes involved in their biosynthesis and degradation in central and peripheral tissues. For example, enzyme expression in specific tissues may be monitored by molecular techniques (e.g. *in situ* hybridisation, northern or western blotting), immunohistochemistry or enzyme assay methods. Histochemical methods may also be exploited to visualise the catecholamines at the cellular level, while chemical methods will detect and quantify the amines and their metabolites in tissue extracts.

6.2.3   Other Indices of Autonomic Function

Although changes in cardiovascular function and catecholamine output are the most widely used indices of autonomic activity, other parameters may also be measured. These include respiratory function (e.g. respiratory rate, tidal volume,

PO$_2$, oxygen uptake), blood glucose and lactic acid, gastrointestinal function (gastric acid production, gastrointestinal motility) and surface or deep body temperature (4).

6.3 ASSESSMENT OF BEHAVIOURAL ACTIVITY

6.3.1 Measurement of Stress-induced Behaviours

The behavioural responses to stress include alteration in locomotor and exploratory activity, self-grooming, eating, drinking and reproductive behaviour (see Chapter 2 for further details). Assessment or measurement of these behaviours depends largely on observations made by an experimenter. This may involve studying an animal in its natural or normal habitat or environment, for example groups of monkeys in the wild or laboratory rats in their home cages. Alternatively, it may involve placing the animal (or animals) within a carefully controlled novel environment and monitoring specific behavioural changes, during or after exposure to a suitable fear-provoking stimulus such as the sight, smell or sound of a predator, or a loud noise, bright light or electric shock. Both approaches require a thorough knowledge of the normal and stress-evoked behavioural patterns of the species under investigation. Experimental design and control are critical. Care must be taken to avoid bias, to incorporate appropriate control groups and to make repeated observations, using sufficient animals in each group to permit rigorous statistical analyses. It is also essential that the observer does not distract the animal and thereby influence the ongoing behaviour; this may be prevented either by concealing the observers (e.g. behind a one-way mirror) or by using remotely controlled video cameras. In quantifying the behavioural responses, a given behaviour can be scored numerically in terms of its frequency and duration, for example number and duration of grooming episodes. This is generally carried out by a computerised procedure in which observations are recorded via a keyboard. Alternatively, in some paradigms, scoring can be carried out automatically. For example, infra-red detectors are used to record locomotor activity and, in the case of operant procedures, to monitor the rate of responding (e.g. number of lever presses per unit time) and to determine the response latency. Although most of the behavioural tests described in this chapter were designed originally for rodents, many may also be usefully applied to non-rodent species, particularly those based on unconditioned reactions. Indeed, while the majority of laboratory studies on stress-induced behaviours has been performed in rodents, there are many reports of comparable studies in a wide range of mammalian species, including non-human primates, pigs, sheep and cats. The sections which follow describe a number of experimental models which may be used not only to monitor and quantify stress-induced behaviours but also to evaluate the long-term strategies which enable the individual to cope. These tests are used widely to screen potential anxiolytic and anxiogenic drugs and antidepressant agents as well as to investigate basic physiological mechanisms. They thus have an important role in the development of novel therapies for psychological and psychiatric disorders.

6.3.2   Experimental Models of Fear and Anxiety

These models use specific stimuli to evoke behaviours that are characteristic of fear and anxiety. They are used widely to screen potential anxiolytic or anxiogenic drugs and to examine the influence of other experimental manipulations (e.g. lesioning of specific CNS pathways) on behaviour. The tests fall into two broad classes, spontaneous (unconditioned) and conditioned behaviours, the latter incorporating operant conditioning, classical conditioning or drug-discrimination.

Tests Based on Unconditioned Reactions

Tests of exploratory activity.   These are based on the premise that procedures which cause stress or discomfort reduce exploratory behaviour in rodents (rats or mice) placed in a test arena. In order to eliminate trauma associated with a novel environment, the test animals are initially exposed daily to the arena until levels of exploratory activity stabilise, i.e. until the animals become habituated. On the day of the test a stressor (normally a bright light) is introduced to the arena. The impact of the stress (termed the disturbance index) is calculated by comparing the activity on the test-day with that on the preceding control day. It is important to note that many procedures which may be inherent to the experiment (e.g. intraperitoneal or intra-foot pad injections, prior restraint, oral administration of fluids or handling by an inexperienced handler) can produce reductions in activity compared with control levels (i.e. a negative disturbance index). Tight regulation of the experimental conditions is therefore essential, as also is the inclusion of appropriate control groups.

The most commonly used test of exploratory activity is the *open field test* in which the animal is placed in a large, intensely illuminated arena and its locomotor activity monitored. Movements may be recorded readily by automatic devices (infra-red sensors or electronic monitors). Alternatively, an observer may note the number of times that an animal crosses between squares marked on the arena floor during a given period, the location the animal adopts within the arena (e.g. centre or sides) and the number of rears it makes. This test was originally described as a test of emotionality as animals freeze in the test situation and exhibit increased autonomic nervous activity as indexed by increased defecation.

Its value as a model of anxiety or emotionality has since been questioned but, nevertheless, the behaviours observed are typical of stress responses.

Other tests of exploratory behaviour include the *hole-board* and the *elevated plus-maze*. The hole-board consists of an apparatus with a number of holes (frequently four) in the floor through which an animal can poke its head. This test is used to assess direct exploration (number and duration of head dips) and locomotor activity. In the elevated plus maze test (12) animals are placed in the centre of a + shaped maze, which is raised above ground, with two opposing arms having closed sides and the other two being open. Fearful or anxious animals will avoid the open arms. Thus, measurement of the number of entries an animal makes into the open arms of the maze provides an index of fear-induced inhibition of exploratory activity; entries are therefore increased by anxiolytic drugs (e.g. benzodiazepines) and reduced by anxiogenic compounds (e.g. corticotrophin releasing hormone, CRH, and benzodiazepine inverse agonists) and by stresses such as ethanol withdrawal, prior immobilisation and social aggression (defeat).

Light–dark transition test. This test makes use of the natural tendency of rodents to avoid a brightly lit arena (13). Briefly, animals (normally mice) are placed on the brightly lit side of a two compartment chamber and the number of transitions made between the light and dark sides of the chamber is recorded, together with details of locomotor activity. Anxiolytic drugs produce a dose-dependent increase in light–dark crossings and locomotor activity, whereas non-anxiolytic agents do not. On the other hand, anxiogenic compounds decrease the number of transitions between the light and dark sides of the chamber without decreasing the overall level of locomotor activity.

Active social interaction test. This model exploits the capacity of specific test conditions to alter the social behaviour of pairs of male rats (14). When two male rats are placed in a test chamber in which neither has established territory, social interaction is mostly of an investigative nature and aggressive encounters are rarely noted. The time spent in active social interaction is greatest when the animals are tested under non-threatening conditions. Thus, a familiar chamber with low lighting favours interaction whereas an unfamiliar chamber with intense lighting maximises uncertainty and thereby decreases interactions (i.e. active social interaction is reduced in conditions causing fear or "anxiety"). The reductions in active social interaction are parallelled by increases in plasma corticosterone concentration and are exacerbated by anxiogenic substances but reduced by anxiolytic agents. One disadvantage of this test is that it requires the use of pairs of animals. Thus, individual differences in behaviour may not be examined easily as the behaviour of one animal is dependent on that of its test partner.

Tests based on defence behaviours. These tests involve evaluation of the defensive behaviours exhibited by laboratory animals (usually rats) in stressful or anxiety-provoking situations. Useful endpoints include withdrawal, freezing or immobility, tactile stimulation of the vibrissae (facial whiskers), defensive jump attacking in response to a human experimenter and suppression of non-defensive behaviours such as eating, drinking, grooming and sexual behaviour. A further important measure is emission of ultrasound vocalisations which may vary in frequency according to the stress. For example, male rats defeated following an aggressive encounter with a conspecific (i.e. an individual of the same species) emit calls of 22–26 kHz frequency which signal submission and thus prevent further attack; other stressful events (exposure to footshock or a loud noise) give rise to ultrasound calls with a frequency of around 22 kHz. Comparative studies suggest that defensive behaviours exhibited in the absence of a threatening stimulus reflect anxiety, while those observed in the presence of a threat are indicative of fear. Thus, to investigate anxiety, defensive behaviours are assessed in situations where a previous threat has been removed. Conversely, studies on fear require the presence of the threat.

Tests Based on Conditioned Responses

Many animal species may be trained to make conditioned operant responses and may therefore be used as experimental models; these include rats, pigs, cats, birds, goldfish.

Conflict tests. These tests are based on the conditioned emotional response paradigm of Estes and Skinner (1941) which exploits punishment to suppress a conditioned response and thereby create a state of conflict or fear. An important example is the Geller–Seifter test (15). Since its introduction in 1960, this test has been used widely to screen potential anxiolytic or anxiogenic agents and the data accrued show a good correlation between the "anti-conflict" and clinical anxiolytic potencies of drugs. Briefly, hungry animals (normally rats) are trained to press a lever for a food reward which is delivered initially on a variable interval schedule. When the frequency of lever pressing becomes stable, a signal is presented to the animal (e.g. a light or sound) and the schedule is altered so that a food reward follows every lever press (i.e. the schedule is changed from one of variable interval to one of continuous reinforcement). Once the animals are trained, a punishment is introduced; this usually takes the form of a mildly aversive electric shock applied to the feet via the cage floor. Thus, when the animal presses the lever it receives not only food but also a mild shock, i.e. a punishment. This creates a state of "emotional conflict" which is manifested by a reduction in the frequency of lever pressing which is proportional to the level of the shock (i.e. the intensity of punishment) and which is exacerbated by anxiogenic agents but reversed by anxiolytics. This model may be optimized for screening anxiolytics by carefully raising the shock intensity to a level which produces a low but stable frequency of responding. Conversely, if the shock level is adjusted so that it is sufficient to produce only a very small reduction in the response rate, the effects of anxiogenic compounds or prior exposure to anxiety or fear-provoking situations may be investigated. Another model based on punishment of a conditioned response is the Vogel test (16) in which water-deprived rats are subjected to alternate periods of unpunished and punished drinking.

Fear potentiated startle. The animal models of fear or anxiety described above each employ cessation or inhibition of spontaneous or conditioned behaviours as the index of fear. An important criticism of these paradigms is that drugs which merely modulate the neural processes that mediate behavioural inhibition may prove falsely positive. Behavioural measures which do not depend on response-inhibition to assess fear or anxiety do not have this disadvantage. One such measure is fear-potentiated startle (see Chapter 2 and (17)) which exploits the phenomenon that humans and experimental animals startle more when they are afraid. This straightforward test monitors the increase in amplitude of the startle response to a given stress (e.g. loud noise, a strong puff of air) which is triggered by presenting the stress together with a cue (e.g. a light or buzzer) which has previously been paired with an aversive stimulus (e.g. mild footshock). This test is highly sensitive to anxiogenic and anxiolytic compounds and has the added advantage that the end point (skeletal muscle contraction) may be readily quantified (17).

Drug discrimination test. Another operant procedure which may be used in the study of anxiety or fearfulness is the drug discrimination test (18, 19). For this animals are trained in a two lever discrimination paradigm so that, by pressing the appropriate lever, they can reliably distinguish between anxiogenic compounds (e.g. pentylenetetrazole, which is anxiogenic in man) and all other non-anxiogenic agents. The animal's perception of the drug's action provides a cue, the so-called interoceptive discriminable stimulus, for the selection of the appropriate lever. A preference for the lever appropriate for the anxiogenic substance occurs in animals subjected to a potentially fearful situation (20), for example, aggressive defeat of a male rat in its home cage by an intruder; in addition, the animals exhibit a battery of endocrine (e.g. raised serum glucocorticoids) and autonomic responses indicative of stress. These tests are of value not only as screens for potential anxiolytic and anxiogenic drugs but also in basic studies on the physiology or biochemistry of stress for animals can be tested following various manipulations, such as exposure to acute or chronic stress, and pharmacological or surgical manipulation of endocrine or CNS function.

6.3.3   Experimental Models of Anxiety and Depression

While anxiety is generally viewed as an important component of the acute response to the stress, the behavioural responses to more long-term stresses are widely held to be analogous to depressive states. This concept provides the basis for the development of tests that are predictive of mixed anxiety and depression and thus model a frequently observed clinical condition. An important experimental paradigm is "learned helplessness" which refers to the pattern of behavioural deficits (typically immobility and cessation of any attempt to escape the situation) observed when an animal is, for example, either exposed to inescapable shock or forced to swim in a container from which it cannot escape. The ensuing behaviours can be readily monitored using methods based on the principles described in Section 6.3.1. and the latency of the development of the "helpless" response determined.

Further models are based on the evaluation of behaviours due to frustration. These include stereotypies (i.e. repeated pattern of movements with little or no variation and no obvious function, see Chapter 2), apathy or depressed behaviour. Such behaviours are not usually noted in the wild but are exhibited by captive animals, particularly those kept in isolation from their peers, in barren environments or in conditions where space is severely restricted. For example, sows kept in individual stalls are less responsive to external stimuli than those housed in a group. More severe examples of apathy are noted in animals (notably non-human primates) during the despair phase which follows maternal–infant or peer–peer separation (see Section 6.3.4. and Chapter 2). These behavioural paradigms may be readily monitored by recording the incidence and progression of a given response (see Section 6.3.1.) and are regarded as useful models of depressive disease.

6.3.4   Assessment of Behaviours in Social Settings

Many studies on the biology of stress and its physiological and behavioural consequences have been carried out using singly- or pair-tested animals, predominantly rodents. However, this has limitations if the objective is to gain insight into the more subtle aspects of the effects of stress on human physiology and behaviour. Indeed psychiatric disorders such as anxiety and depression are disorders of social behaviour expressed in social settings. This problem may be overcome by utilising techniques that enable the study and quantification of the behaviour of animals, particularly non-human primates, living in social groups. Studies of social behaviour in non-human primates in which the findings have been interpreted as being analogous to those in man have, however, left many questions unanswered. Nevertheless, if one considers the findings in a broad context, for example behaviours with similar functions, then a direct analogy between man and non-human primates may be drawn (21).

Behavioural Patterns Related to Position in the Social Hierarchy

Many group-living animals form social hierarchies in which one animal is dominant and the others are either equally subordinate or they exhibit a linear dominance hierarchy. Potentially stressful situations may arise as a direct consequence of this, for example subordinate members of the group may receive aggression from others higher in the social order. Conversely, the maintenance of a dominant position may also be stressful since it is known that dominant animals (monkeys) are prone to high blood pressure and heart attacks associated with sympatho-adrenal over activity. Although the hierarchies and attachment bonds that are formed within groups remain relatively constant, they can be manipulated by various means and the consequent behavioural responses monitored. Effective stimuli include alteration of the group structure (removing or adding members) or the environmental conditions, pharmacological manipulation of behaviour (treatment with hormones or psychoactive drugs), removal of endocrine organs or placement of lesions in specific regions of the CNS. Various types of non-human primate models have been developed involving observation of the interactions occurring within social groups. Some of these are of relevance to the study of human anxiety and depression (21).

Mother–Infant and Peer–Peer Separation

Other types of primate behaviour that occur in response to specific stressful situations may be utilised in animal models of depression. An important example is maternal separation. This is typified in infant squirrel monkeys which, on separation from their mothers, show a distinct pattern of behaviour which is characterised by agitation and protest followed by a period of despair during which the animal becomes withdrawn and unresponsive. This behavioural profile is accompanied by elevations in plasma cortisol which are of a similar magnitude irrespective of whether the infant is placed in a small cage adjacent to the mother or is completely removed from the room. Early workers suggested that the behavioural and endocrine responses reflect the novel environment rather than the maternal separation. This view was supported by observations that surrogate infant squirrel monkeys removed from their home environment exhibit elevations in plasma cortisol similar to those of infants separated from their mothers. However, other reports that cortisol is unchanged in surrogate-reared infants when the surrogate is removed from the cage but raised in mother-reared infants following removal of the mother strongly favour a response specific to loss of the mother and thereby support the validity of the model. The protest and despair responses made following peer separation are similar to those noted above but the model has the additional advantage that once the relationships are established they are less likely to change drastically with time, enabling repeated observations to be made. Claims that these paradigms are valid models of certain types of human depression, particularly that provoked by separation from an object or individual of affection, are supported by reports that clinically effective antidepressant drugs induce significant improvements in behaviour over a period similar to that observed clinically.

6.4 CONCLUDING REMARKS

An important consideration in quantifying and interpreting the effects of stress on physiology and behaviour is that animals of a given species do not all respond to a given stress in an identical manner. Such variations are important biologically as they allow the individual to develop a strategy which enables it to cope with environmental changes that threaten homeostasis. This is particularly evident in primates, where social rank is a fundamental determinant of the type of response made, and is also applicable to many other species, including the pig (22). There are two different ways of coping with stressful situations:

(a) one in which the individual actively attempts to remove or escape from the stress, and
(b) one in which the individual freezes and gradually withdraws.

The success of these coping strategies is strongly dependent on environmental conditions and an active strategy appears more effective in a stable environment whereas a passive one is better in a changing or unfamiliar environment. Each individual has a preference for one or other type of coping strategy which is determined partly by genetic factors and partly by early life experiences. This preference is established at an early age, for example one to two weeks in the pig (22), and remains constant over time. These two distinct behavioural strategies are highly correlated with different physiological and neural responses to stress and in differential susceptibility to disease. Thus, animals exhibiting the former response have sympatho-adrenal activation whereas those exhibiting the latter behaviour show evidence of parasympathetic activation. These inherent differences must therefore be taken into account when quantifying autonomic and behavioural responses to stress and the data grouped appropriately for statistical analysis.

REFERENCES

1. Nyakas C., Prins A. J. A., Bohus B. Age-related alterations in cardiac response to emotional stress: relations to behavioural reactivity in the rat. *Physiol Behav,* 1990, **21**: 567–72.

2. Manuck S. B., Kaplin J. R., Adams M. R., Clarkson T. B. Behaviourally elicited heart rate reactivity and atherosclerosis in female cynomolgous monkeys (*Macaca fascicularis*). *Psychosom Med*, 1989, **51**: 306–18.
3. Reite M. Implantable biotelemetry and social separation in monkeys. In G. P. Moberg (ed) *Animal Stress*. Maryland, American Physiological Association, 1985, pp 141–60.
4. Amlaner C. J., Macdonald D. W. (eds) *A Handbook on Biotelemetry and Radio Tracking*. Oxford, Pergamon Press, 1979.
5. Turkhan J. S., Ator N. A., Brady J. V., Craven K. A. Beyond chronic catheterization in laboratory primates. In E. F. Segal (ed) *Housing, Care and Psychological Well-Being of Captive and Laboratory Primates*. New Jersey, Noyes Publications, 1989, pp 305–22.
6. Gardiner S. M., Bennett T. The effect of short-term isolation on systolic blood pressure and heart-rate in rats. *Med Biol*, 1977, **55**: 325–9.
7. Manser C. E. Pathological lesions related to stress. In C. E. Manser (ed) *The Assessment of Stress in Laboratory Animals*. UK, RSPCA, 1992, pp 146–8.
8. Houpt K. A., Kendrick K. M., Parrott R. F., de Riva C. F. Catecholamine content of plasma and saliva in sheep exposed to psychological stress. *Horm Metab Res*, 1988, **20**: 189–90.
9. Kendrick K. M. Microdialysis in large unrestrained animals: neuroendocrine and behavioural studies of acetylcholine, amino acid, monoamine and neuropeptide release in sheep. In T. E. Robinson, J. B. Justice (eds) *Microdialysis in the Neurosciences*. New York, Elsevier, 1991, pp 327–48.
10. Baum A., Grunberg N. E., Singer J. E. The use of psychological and neuroendocrinological measurements in the study of stress. *Health Psychol*, 1982, **1**: 217–36.
11. Wuttke W., Denling J., Roosen-Runge G., Siegler R., Fuchs E., Duker E. *In vivo* release of catecholamines and amino acid neurotransmitters. In E. Usdin, R. Kvetansky, J. Axelrod (eds) *Stress: The Role of Catecholamines and Other Neurotransmitters*. *Vol.1*. New York, Gordon & Beach, 1984, pp 93–103.
12. Pellow S., Chopin P., File S. E., Briley M. Validation of open: closed arm entries in an elevated plus maze as a measure of anxiety in the rat. *J Neurosci Meth*, 1985, **14**: 149–67.
13. Crawley J. N., Goodwin F. K. Preliminary report of a simple animal behaviour model for the anxiolytic effect of benzodiazepines. *Pharmac Biochem Behav*, 1985, **13**: 167–70.
14. File S. E. Animal models for predicting clinical efficacy of anxiolytic drugs: social behaviour. *Neuropsychobiology*, 1985, **13**: 55–62.
15. Geller I., Seifter J. The effects of meprobamate, barbiturates, d-amphetamine and promazine on experimentally-induced conflict in the rat. *Psychopharm*, 1960, **1**: 482–92.
16. Vogel J. R., Beer B., Clody D. E. A simple and reliable conflict procedure for testing anti-anxiety agents. *Psychopharm*, 1971, **21**: 1–7.
17. Davis M. Animal models of anxiety based on classical conditioning: the conditioned emotional response and the fear-potentiated startle effect. In S. E. File (ed) *Psychopharmacology of Anxiolytics and Antidepressants*. New York, Pergamon Press, 1991, pp 187–212.
18. Lal H., Emmett-Oglesby M. W. Behavioral analogues of anxiety: animal models. *Neuropharmacology*, 1983, **22**: 1423–1441.
19. Andrews J. S., Stephens D. N. Drug discrimination models in anxiolytic research. In S. E. File (ed) *Psychopharmacology of Anxiolytics and Antidepressants*. New York, Pergamon Press, 1991, pp 107–30.
20. Vellucci S. V., Martin P. J., Everitt B. J. The discriminative stimulus produced by

pentylenetetrazol: effects of systemic anxiolytics and anxiogenics, aggressive defeat and midazolam or muscimol infused into the amygdala. *J Psychopharmac*, 1988, **2**: 80–93.

21. Vellucci S. V. Primate social behaviour—anxiety or depression? In S. E. File (ed) *Psychopharmacology of Anxiolytics and Antidepressants*. New York, Pergamon Press, 1991, pp 83–105.

22. Hessing M. J. C., Hagelso A. M., Schouten W. P. G., Wiepkema P. R., van Beek J. A. M. Individual behavioral and physiological strategies in pigs. *Physiol Behav*, 1994, **55**: 39–46.

Chapter 7

Methods for Monitoring Immune Function

Richard Aspinall

Imperial College School of Medicine, London, UK

7.1   INTRODUCTION

Immunology has benefited from the recent rapid progress wrought by current molecular techniques, by the introduction of more reagents and by more assays to determine immunological phenomena. These have moved rapidly from basic research use to the clinical laboratory, so increasing the means of identifying the immune status of an individual.

In the past, immunologists trying to comprehend some immunological effects took the reductionist view and subdivided the immune system in to compartments. Typically the immune response was subdivided into a humoral arm, mediated by circulating antibodies, and a cellular arm. On the humoral side the term immunoglobulin (Ig) was introduced at the turn of the century and antibodies were classified in terms of their function as, for example, precipitins,

Stress, Stress Hormones and the Immune System. Edited by J. C. Buckingham, G. E. Gillies and A.-M. Cowell
© 1997 John Wiley & Sons, Ltd.

agglutinins, sensitisers and opsonins. More recently antibodies have been purified and reclassified according to their heavy chain structure, namely IgA, IgD, IgE, IgG and IgM (see also Chapter 3). On a cellular basis, only in the past 30 years have we come to understand something of the difference between B and T cells and here the reductionist approach still prevails, with the division and subdivision of each into distinct lymphocyte sub-populations.

We must now begin to view the immune system as an integrated whole. The reductionist approach is useful but can be misleading if considered in isolation. The immune system is a powerful biological war machine whose properties and behaviour one cannot induce from the analysis of one or two of its regiments. In this chapter my aim is to provide a broad outline of the current methods used for monitoring the immune status of an individual. One approach determines whether the products of an immune response are present. The body is constantly under attack and so products of the immune response are present in normal individuals. Measurement of these products in a number of healthy individuals provides us with reference range values. For B cells the product, which is the effector of the immune response, is immunoglobulin and this is relatively simple to measure in serum. Activation of the complement cascade is also a major effector mechanism of the specific immune response (either via the classical pathway after detection of a foreign particle by an immunoglobulin, or via the alternative, antibody independent pathway) and a number of methods are available to assess complement function as a whole or by measurement of its individual components. For T cells the picture is not as simple because although the soluble products of T cells are important in the response, it is the cells that are the active functional entities. Thus measurements of total lymphocyte counts, lymphocyte subset analysis and lymphocyte activation are more informative of the cellular immune status of an individual as, also, are tests of phagocyte cell function. We will consider first the products of the immune system and then the methods for measuring specific cell types and their functional capacity. These methods are widely applied in the clinical situation but may also be used as end-point measurements of immune function in experimental animals where the immune system may have been activated by various substances, such as lipo-polysaccharide (LPS), interleukins or inflammatory mediators, as detailed in later chapters.

7.2   MEASUREMENT OF PRODUCTS OF ACTIVATED B CELLS

The daily confrontation with antigenic molecules derived from the surrounding environment ensures that there is continual activation of antigen specific B cells, with subsequent production of immunoglobulin. We can determine the specificity of some of these antibodies, but it is virtually impossible to determine the specificity for all of them. However it is possible to measure their overall levels and this can be done in samples from several body fluids e.g. blood, saliva. The values found for each immunoglobulin subclass in normal individuals give us reference ranges against which we can compare our test sample.

7.2.1 Detection and Measurement of Immunoglobulin in Serum

Estimation of the levels of immunoglobulin of all classes and subclasses in the serum is based upon the detection of immune complexes resulting from antigen–antibody interactions. In this case, the antigen is the specific class of immuno-globulin and the antibody is directed against this antigen. (The class of an immunoglobulin is determined by the type of heavy chain used in the construc-tion of the molecule. In addition, within each class, variation in the number and type of amino acids in the heavy chain may produce a sub-class. For more information see Chapter 3). Two of the methods used for detecting immune complexes are nephelometry and radial immune diffusion.

Nephelometry

When in suspension as small particles, immune complexes can disperse a beam of light and this dispersion can be measured on a nephelometer. The degree of light scatter is dependent upon the ratio of antigen to antibody and thus is proportional to the amount of antigen, providing the concentration of antibody remains constant. Using a nephelometer, therefore, one can measure quickly the amount of any particular class or sub-class of immunoglobulin in the serum.

Radial Immune Diffusion

This again is based on the principle of detection of immune complexes. Agar containing, for example, antibody against the specific class of immunoglobulin to be measured is poured into a plate and allowed to set. Wells are cut in the agar and dilutions of the test serum are added to the wells. Diffusion is allowed to proceed and when the antigen and antibody are in optimal proportions (equiva-lence) then immune complexes are formed which precipitate in the agar. The area of the ring of precipitation formed is proportional to the antigen concentra-tion. Graphs of size of circle produced for amount of antigen present can be produced using known concentrations of antigen (i.e. a standard curve may be constructed) and used to calculate the amount of antigen present in the test sample producing the circle of precipitation of that specific size. This process is relatively sensitive but slow, with diffusion sometimes taking 48–72 hours.

Serum Electrophoresis

The above methods can provide an accurate means of assessing the amount of immunoglobulin in a sample. Samples giving values higher than the reference ranges are usually analysed further and the methods used for this are based on electrophoretic separation of the serum proteins. This is carried out either on cellulose acetate membranes or in agar. It is performed at a pH between 8 and 9 (usually pH 8.6) because at this pH serum proteins have varying overall charges which, combined with their different molecular sizes, allows effective separation in an electric field. The gel or membrane is then stained with an appropriate protein dye and the intensity of staining of the protein bands measured with a densitometer. This passes a beam of light through the electrophoresed strip and measures the degree of absorbance associated with each band. A typical resulting trace is shown in Fig. 7.1. This initial separation and assessment is semi-quantitative. When there is unregulated proliferation of a single clone of B lymphocytes, the immunoglobulin product (termed a paraprotein) generally

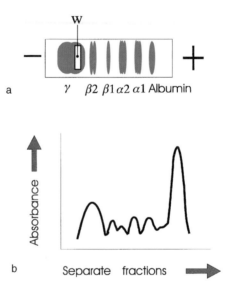

Figure 7.1 Serum electrophoresis. **a** When a serum sample is placed in the well (w) of an agar gel and subjected to an electric field whose polarity is shown, there is separation of the proteins in the serum. After separation the gel can be stained to reveal distinct bands which have been given Greek alphabetical and Arabic numerical notation depending on their distance from the starting well. A typical normal serum sample result is shown here. **b** The relative amount in each peak can be estimated following staining and scanning of the gel with a photometric densitometer, which shines a beam of light through the gel and measures the amount absorbed by the protein bands. An absorbance trace can then be produced for the sample (also see text)

migrates as a compact band which can thus be identified either by immunoelectrophoresis or immunofixation as described below.

Immunoelectrophoresis

In this method the initial electrophoretic separation of serum proteins is carried out in agar gels where several replicates of test sample and normal samples are run in pairs. Troughs are then cut out alongside the separated proteins, between the test and normal samples, and antibodies directed against specific heavy and light chains (typing antibodies) are placed in these troughs. The separated bands and the typing immunoglobulin diffuse through the agar towards each other and, where there is interaction, a visible precipitate occurs, thus allowing identification of the heavy and light chain type of the immunoglobulin (see Fig. 7.2).

Immunofixation

Here the initial electrophoretic separation of sera can be done on cellulose acetate membranes. Various typing antibodies against the different heavy and light chain types are applied over different replica lanes, using a soft camel hair brush. The plates are again electrophoresed, this time for 5 min and then the membranes are washed and stained with an appropriate dye (e.g. amido black, Ponceau S). The washing step removes all proteins except those that have formed an insoluble precipitate of immune complexes following interaction between the typing immunoglobulin and the test sera. These appear as bands after staining, allowing identification of the heavy and light chain of the class of immunoglobulin of interest (see Fig. 7.3).

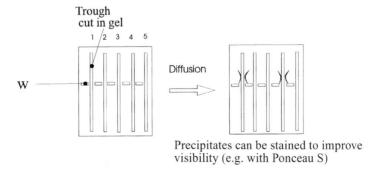

Precipitates can be stained to improve visibility (e.g. with Ponceau S)

Figure 7.2 Immunoelectrophoresis. Proteins in serum samples (placed in wells, w) are separated by electrophoresis and then allowed to interact with typing antibodies. For example, troughs 1, 2 and 3 contain antibodies to the γ, α and μ heavy chains respectively and troughs 4 and 5 contain antibodies to the κ and λ light chains respectively. Samples 1 and 2 are IgGs and samples 4 and 5 have the κ light chain

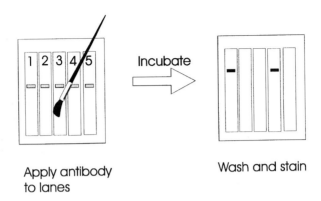

Figure 7.3 Immunofixation. Following electrophoretic separation of serum proteins (e.g. on cellulose acetate) antibody to the light and heavy chains is painted onto the lanes. Here for example anti-γ heavy chain antibody is painted onto lane 1, anti-α on lane 2, anti-μ on lane 3 and anti-κ and anti-λ light chain antibody on lanes 4 and 5. Running the sample again for a short time followed by staining allows visualisation. (See text for further details)

7.2.2 Detection of Specific Immunoglobulin in Serum

There are occasions, for example following a vaccination, when it is important to know whether a specific immune response has been made to an antigen. In addition, when there is a diagnosis of autoimmune disease, there is a need to know whether there is a detectable immunoglobulin response to a specific tissue antigen and, if so, at what level. For these reasons a series of protocols have been devised to detect and quantify the specific immunoglobulin response and the following are some of the tests used.

Diffusion Through Agar

This assay is based on the principle that both antigen and immunoglobulin can diffuse through agar and form a solid, visible precipitate when at equivalence. Precipitating antibodies in serum are usually IgG or IgM. Fig. 7.4 is a diagrammatic representation of the test and shows wells cut in agar around a central well. The test, T, (or the control) serum is placed in the central well with either a range of different antigens or a single antigen at different concentrations placed in the outside wells (A–F). The plates are then left to allow diffusion of antigen and immunoglobulin. If the specific immunoglobulin is present, a visible precipitate will form when antigen and immunoglobulin meet at equimolar concentrations. This method is cheap but takes a relatively long time to produce a result.

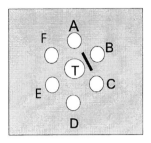

A-F Different Antigens
T   Test serum

Figure 7.4 Detection of specific immunoglobulins by diffusion through agar. A visible precipitation has occurred between the test serum and antigen B. (See text for further details)

Counter Current Electrophoresis

Counter current electrophoresis is also based on the principle of diffusion of antigen and immunoglobulin through agar towards each other until equivalence is reached and a visible precipitate is formed but the process is speeded up by placing an electric field across the agar. Counter current electrophoresis is usually run at a pH between 8 and 9 (usually 8.6). At this pH, precipitating antibodies have a net positive charge and will thus move towards the cathode, while some antigens at this pH have a negative charge and will move towards the anode. The result is a line of precipitation at the point of equivalence in significantly less time than would be needed for normal diffusion (see Fig. 7.5a).

Crossed Electrophoresis

This further refinement to counter current electrophoresis allows simultaneous detection of both antigen and immunoglobulin in the serum. In the example shown in Fig. 7.5b the test serum is positive for both hepatitis B antigen and immunoglobulin to hepatitis B.

Immunoblotting

Here the specific antigen for detection is separated from other antigens by running a solution containing the antigens and the detergent sodium dodecyl sulphate (SDS) on an SDS polyacrylamide gel. SDS is negatively charged and binds to hydrophobic regions of protein molecules, causing them to unfold and become long polypeptide chains. SDS frees the proteins from their association with other protein or lipid molecules and also confers a charge on them which is proportional to their size. Separation by electrophoresis in agar can then occur in a charge:size ratio. After separation the proteins are transferred ("blotted") onto

(a) Counter Current Electrophoresis

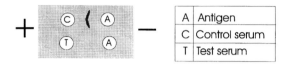

A	Antigen
C	Control serum
T	Test serum

A visible precipitation has occurred between
the control serum and the antigen which is
not apparent in the test serum

(b) Crossed Electrophoresis

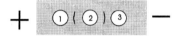

1	Anti-Hepatitis B surface antigen
2	Test serum
3	Hepatitis B surface antigen

Visible precipitation shows that the test sample contains
both anti-Hepatitis B antibody and Hepatitis B surface antigen

Figure 7.5 Demonstration of (a) the absence of a specific antigen in the test serum
using counter current electrophoresis and (b) the presence of both hepatitis B antigen and
specific antibody in a test sample using crossed electrophoresis

nitrocellulose paper which has a positive charge. The presence of a specific
antibody may then be determined by incubating the nitrocellulose with the serum
under test. Any antibody that binds to the antigen attached to the nitrocellulose
paper may then be visualised with a second antibody (an anti-Ig antibody)
labelled either with an enzyme (see below) or a radioactive marker. One
disadvantage of this technique is that the antigen site of the protein may be lost
by this treatment.

Agglutination

This is a very simple method of detecting the presence of an antibody to a
specific antigen in a serum sample. The antigen in question has to be available in

a pure form so that it can be attached to a particle, such as a latex bead or a red cell, and a suspension of these antigen-coated particles is then incubated with the test serum (neat or diluted). As each antibody molecule can bind more than one antigen molecule, any specific antibody present in the serum will effectively link separate particles and agglutination will become visible.

Enzyme-linked Immunosorbent Assays (ELISA)

The general principles of ELISA are explained in Chapter 5.

Sandwich antigen capture ELISA. This form of the ELISA is dependent upon having two antibodies to non-overlapping determinants on the antigen. The antibodies may either both be monoclonal or one may be monoclonal and the other polyclonal. The monoclonal immunoglobulin is attached to the base in the wells of a 96 well plastic plate and this is often referred to as the first layer. Attachment can often be improved by carrying out this part of the procedure at a pH between 9 and 10. The aim is for this antibody to capture the specific antigen in the test sample which will, however, also contain a number of other proteins which could bind non-specifically to the plastic via fairly strong hydrophobic bonds. It is important, therefore, to block the non-specific binding sites by a pre-incubation step with a protein solution. A mild detergent (e.g. Tween 20) may also be used to reduce the strength of these hydrophobic bonds. The sample for analysis is then added to the wells. Any antigen present is captured by the plastic-bound antibody and forms the "second" layer. After incubation, the wells are washed to remove the unbound components and the "sandwich" is then completed by addition of the third layer which is the antibody (monoclonal or polyclonal) against the non-overlapping determinant. Attached to the latter antibody is an enzyme which is usually either horseradish peroxidase or alkaline phosphatase. The plates are again washed and the enzyme substrate added. The product of the enzyme–substrate reaction is coloured and may be quantified by reading the plates at the appropriate wavelength. The absorbance is proportional to the amount of bound, enzyme-linked antibody which in turn is proportional to the amount of antigen captured. A set of wells containing the antigen at a range of known concentrations permits the construction of a standard curve against which the concentration of the unknown samples may be calculated, thus rendering this assay quantitative.

Solid phase single layer ELISA. The object of this assay is to determine whether the test sample contains antibody against this antigen. The antigen must be available in a pure form. It is attached to the plastic base of the multi-well plates and a blocking agent used to block the non-specific binding sites. Diluted serum is then placed in the wells and any antibody specific for the bound antigen will be captured. The plates are washed and bound antibody molecules are visualised with a species specific labelled antibody. Typically, a horseradish peroxidase or alkaline phosphatase label is used and, assuming the test sample derives from human body fluid, the second antibody would be directed against the species specific portion of human immunoglobulin. The plate is then washed, the enzyme substrate added and the reaction allowed to proceed until a colour develops which can be quantified as described above.

Other Markers

As an alternative to enzyme linked immunoglobulins, radioactive, fluorescent or chemiluminescent markers may also be used.

Immunofluorescence. The essentials of this technique are described in Chapter 5. It is commonly used for the detection of autoantibodies in the serum. In the clinical situation, the tissue used to test for the presence of autoantibodies may be human tissue or human cell lines or, alternatively, animal tissue, when there is a known cross-reactivity. The tissue is snap frozen and sections are cut on a cryostat. These sections are placed on slides that have usually been precoated with an agent such as poly-L-lysine or gelatin which improves the adherence of the section to the slide. For the assay, the test serum is placed on the section and incubated for a defined period; the sections are then washed and incubated with a fluorescently labelled second immunoglobulin such as anti-human IgG (see Fig. 7.6). The slides are then viewed under a microscope adapted for the detection of fluorescence. The trained eye can determine something of the characteristics of the autoantibody from the intensity and pattern of staining. For example, serum from patients with pernicious anaemia will stain the gastric parietal cells on a section from mouse stomach. Another example occurs in chronic active hepatitis

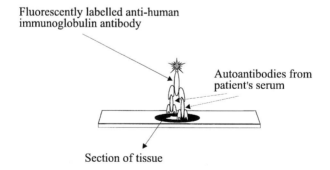

Figure 7.6 Detection of autoantibodies from patients serum can be made by visualising the antibody staining tissue sections using antibody conjugated to a fluorescent molecule which is scanned under a microscope. (See text for more details)

where the patient's serum will stain the smooth muscle found in sections of rat stomach, liver and kidney.

7.3 MEASUREMENT OF COMPLEMENT COMPONENTS

Complement is a collection of heat labile proteins which, when activated, initiates a reaction cascade culminating in osmotic cell lysis and death as a result of immune activation. Individual components of the complement system can be measured immunochemically or the whole system can be assayed functionally. The classical pathway for complement activation is the major effector mechanism for antibody-mediated responses.

7.3.1 Immunochemical Analysis of Individual Complement Components

The availability of antibodies to complement components allows their detection using methodology which has already been described (nephelometry, immuno-diffusion or ELISA) as well as rocket electrophoresis.

Rocket Electrophoresis

In this method antibody against the specific complement component to be assayed is present in the agar used to make the gel. The serum is placed in the well and then the sample is electrophoresed at pH 8.6. The sample components migrate towards the anode and the immunoglobulin in the agar migrates towards the cathode. As electrophoresis proceeds, the antigen at the moving sample front becomes more dilute as it interacts with immunoglobulin and forms insoluble complexes. Eventually all of the antigen is complexed, forming a visible precipitate shaped like a rocket. The area under the rocket is proportional to the concentration of antigen. The use of control sera with known concentrations of the different components allows quantification of complement components in the test serum.

7.3.2 Functional Assay of Complement

The Classical Pathway Haemolytic Complement (CH$_{50}$) Assay

In the classical pathway the complement cascade is triggered by the initial components attaching to an antibody bound to its antigen. In the assay the antigen is a cell surface antigen on red blood cells and sheep red blood cells are often used. Anti-sheep immunoglobulin is then added which will bind to the red blood cells and "sensitise" them. On addition of complement, in the form of the test serum, the red blood cells will lyse. The CH_{50} value is defined as the amount of serum needed to lyse 50% of a standard quantity of sensitised red blood cells. Standard curves of the amount of red cell lysis produced by a specific dilution of complement are constructed using a standard serum (often guinea pig serum) as a source of complement. Sensitised red cells are also mixed with a range of dilutions of the test serum to induce lysis (see Fig. 7.7). After centrifugation, the amount of lysis is determined by the amount of haemoglobin in the supernatant as measured by absorbance of the supernatant at a wavelength of 541 nm. The CH_{50} value can then be calculated. This value is an arbitrary unit and many test variables can influence the result such as the concentration of red cells, their age (which alters their fragility), the amount of immunoglobulin used to sensitise them, the nature of the immunoglobulin, the ionic strength of the buffers and the temperature at which the assay was performed. Probably the commonest cause of a decreased CH_{50} value is an improperly stored sample. For these assays it is important to store the samples at $-70°C$ to preserve the activity of the complement components.

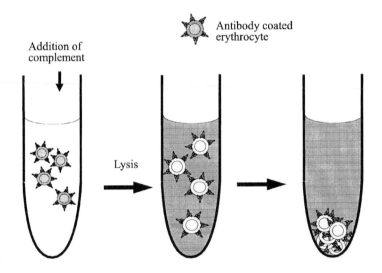

Figure 7.7 Functional measurement of complement using the classical pathway haemolytic complement (CH_{50}) assay

The Alternative Pathway Haemolytic Complement (APCH$_{50}$) Assay

The complement cascade may also be activated by a pathway that does not involve the antigen–antibody interaction but is triggered directly by the surfaces of certain micro-organisms. This is called the alternative pathway. In human serum it can be initiated by the addition of rabbit erythrocytes. These rabbit erthrocytes do not need sensitising with antibody for them to lyse. The APCH$_{50}$ unit is defined in the same way as the CH$_{50}$ unit (see above).

7.4 MEASUREMENT OF T CELL PRODUCTS

The soluble products of T cells play a critical role in mediating the immune response (see Chapter 3 for more details). In some cases they provide the additional signals required to generate effector cells. Many of the original assays for these T cell-derived cytokines were biological tests measuring, for example, the ability of the cytokines to maintain the growth of cytokine-dependent cell lines. Advances in this field have resulted in the production of monoclonal antibodies to many of the cytokines, allowing them to be measured by standard immunoassay methods (ELISA etc.). In addition many of the cytokine genes have been cloned and sequenced. From these sequences, primers have been constructed so that the expression of cytokine genes can be detected by the polymerase chain reaction (PCR). Providing the appropriate stringent controls are used, the polymerase chain reaction is one of the most powerful tools in distinguishing the presence of a transcript of RNA for a specific gene in the tissues under analysis. Firstly, the RNA (total or mRNA) has to be isolated from the cells or tissues of interest and single stranded DNA, complementary to the RNA, is synthesised using a reverse transcriptase enzyme. Then, using a 3′ and a 5′ oligonucleotide primer to define a specific region of the cDNA of interest, this specific signal may be amplified millions of times so that it can be distinguished easily from the surrounding "noise".

7.5 MEASUREMENT OF THE CELLULAR EFFECTORS OF THE IMMUNE SYSTEM BY PHENOTYPE

Leukocytes are the cellular effectors of the immune system and they are categorised as mononuclear cells (lymphocytes, monocytes) and polymorpho-nuclear cells or granulocytes (neutrophils, eosinophils and basophils) described in more detail in Chapter 3. Each of these cell types may be separated by fluorescence-activated cell sorting (FACS) as described below, which may also be used for further subclassifications of lymphocytes. The peripheral lymphoid pool in an individual is in a constant state of flux. Factors such as nutritional status, age, sex, health, the presence of infections or cancers, can all alter the constitution of this pool of cells. Cell-mediated immunodeficiencies are often characterised by recurrent infections which may be due to either a reduction in the number of lymphocytes, or the absence of a specific sub-population, or the presence of lymphocytes that are unable to function properly. In the clinical situation, tests that need to be done to determine the cellular immune status of an individual are total lymphocyte counts, lymphocyte subset analysis and then lymphocyte function tests.

Fluorescent analysis of cell populations is a powerful technique by which one can determine the relative proportions of each sub-population of leuko-cytes within a sample as well as the number of cells in each sub-population. In principle, cells are incubated with a fluorescently labelled antibody directed against a specific cell surface antigen. Although analysis can be done manually using a microscope adapted for the detection of fluorescence, the method of choice is to use a fluorescent cell analyser (cytometer)—see Fig. 7.8.

For most clinical applications the sample most usually analysed is peripheral blood, which at any one time contains approximately 1% of the total body lymphocytes. Analysis must be carried out on fresh blood that has been collected into an anticoagulant, the most preferred of which is EDTA. A typical procedure for analysing samples is as follows:

(a) An aliquot of whole blood is incubated at room temperature with fluores-cently labelled antibodies. For example, a typical analysis may include staining with an anti-CD4 conjugated to FITC (the fluorescent tag) and an anti-CD8 conjugated to R-Phycoerythrin. Both labelled antibodies are avail-able from a number of commercial suppliers. The development of high affinity antibodies has reduced this incubation period to as little as 10 minutes in some cases.

(b) After incubation, red cells within the sample are lysed and the leukocytes fixed. (This part of the process has been automated by some manufacturers).

(c) The fixed sample may be stored at 4°C for a few days, or can be run immediately in the analyser.

The results can then be recorded as the percentage lymphocytes in each sub-group or the total number of cells per microlitre of blood.

Fig. 7.8 represents two typical screens on the fluorescent cell analyser, the first showing separation of leukocytes into their component populations and the second shows the subsequent analysis of the gated population stained with two different antibodies (in this case anti-CD4 and anti-CD8). Reference ranges for some of these sub-populations are given in Table 7.1.

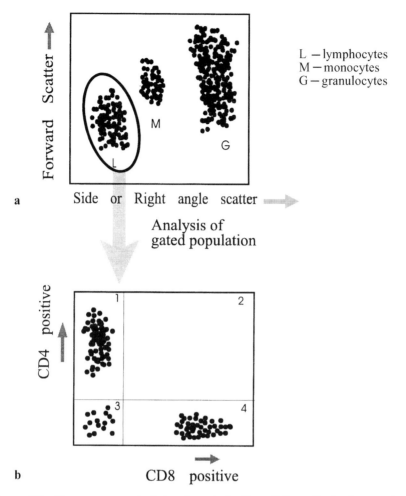

Figure 7.8 Fluorescence activated cell analysis. Essentially, cells in the sample are moved in single file through the path of a laser beam. The deflections produced by each cell are picked up by sensors around the beam which detect the degree of forward scatter (directly proportional to the size of the cell), right angle or side scatter (proportional to the granularity of the cell) and the fluorescence of the cell at different wavelengths. **Screen a** shows the leukocytes in a peripheral blood sample separated on the basis of size versus granularity. Specific populations can be selected (known as gating) by drawing an ellipse around them. This population can then be analysed for their fluorescent staining. For example, **Screen b** shows the expected distribution of blood lymphocytes seen on the screen following staining with anti-CD4 conjugated to FITC and anti-CD8 conjugated to R-Phycoerythrin. Screen b is divided into four regions. Regions 1 and 4 would display cells that were positively stained with one antibody alone. Any cells stained with both antibodies would appear in region 2 whilst cells that were not stained with either would appear in region 3. Here we see that the CD4 positive and CD8 positive cells are in non-overlapping populations

Table 7.1 Reference ranges used by the Department of Immunology at the Chelsea and Westminster Hospital for some sub-populations in normal healthy adults. (From Hobbs *et al.*, 1984), with permission

Population	Normal adult range (number/μl of blood)
Lymphocytes	1382–3712
CD3$^+$ T cells	815–3330
CD4$^+$ T cells	375–2480
CD8$^+$ T cells	280–1350
CD19$^+$ B cells	89–691

7.6 MEASUREMENT OF IMMUNE CELL FUNCTION

Functional analysis is necessary to determine whether a patient can respond to a specific antigen or group of antigens. Phenotypic assays of lymphocytes will only show the quantity of each population or sub-population present, but not its functional status. Although there have been attempts to relate phenotype to function (for example, CD4$^+$ cells are often called "helper" or "regulatory" cells and CD8$^+$ cells are often termed "cytotoxic" or "suppressor" T cells), these are generalisations for which there are exceptions. For example, a patient may have a normal CD4$^+$ count but may be deficient in cells capable of functioning against a specific antigen or group of antigens. Functional assays can be carried out both *in vivo* and *in vitro* and the advantage of *in vitro* assays is the capacity to test how the subject's cells respond to antigens or antigen equivalents which may be potentially hazardous if used as a challenge *in vivo*.

7.6.1 Proliferation Assays

Normal mammalian lymphocytes placed in culture will die within days unless they are provided with a stimulus. In unimmunised subjects only a very small proportion of lymphocytes will recognise a particular antigen-MHC (major histocompatibility complex) complex so that it is extremely difficult to measure antigen-specific responses. In practice, polyclonal activators may be used as non-specific stimulators.

The Stimulus

The stimulus can be a specific antigen, or can be an antigen mimic. The recognition of antigen by T cells (requiring the T cell receptor-CD3 complex which recognises the MHC-associated antigen on the surface of antigen-presenting cells) leads to activation, proliferation and the generation of both effector and memory T cells. The peripheral T cell pool can be subdivided functionally and phenotypically into naive and memory cells, on the basis of whether they have met antigen. Careful selection of the antigenic stimulus can provide a means of discriminating between these populations. Recall antigens may be found, for example, in extracts from *Candida albicans* (a common organism that induces a T cell response which most of us cope with every day) or in purified protein derivative (PPD) extracted from mycobacteria (to which many of us respond since we have been vaccinated with bacille Calmette-Guèrin, a bovine strain of *Mycobacterium tuberculosis*). In normal healthy adults these provide a powerful stimulus to cells in the memory population. The antigenically naive population can be stimulated by alloantigen, which also invokes a response in the memory T cell population. The commonest source of alloantigens are leukocytes derived from a different individual but first these cells require treatment with mitomycin C or irradiation to prevent them from proliferating. Thus they act only as stimulators and do not interfere with the end-point of the reaction described below.

Antigen mimics include antibodies against the antigen receptor, as they will cross-link the receptor and induce activation in the cells that bear the receptor. Generally, antibodies specific for the invariant framework epitopes of the T cell receptor or CD3 proteins are used. Polymeric plant proteins called lectins also act as antigen mimics because they bind to specific sugar residues on T cell surface glycoproteins, including the T cell receptor–CD3 complex, leading to their cross-linkage and hence activation of the T cell. Lectins that stimulate T cells and which are used routinely for the assessment of T cell function are phytohaemagglutinin (PHA), which is derived from *Phaseolus vulgaris* (red kidney bean), and concanavalin A (ConA), derived from *Canavalia ensiformis* (jack bean). For B cells the major mitogenic lectins are LPS, derived from the walls of Gram-negative bacteria e.g. *E. coli*, *S. enteritidis*, *S. typhimurium*, *S. marescens*, and staphylococcal protein A, derived from *S. aureus* (Cowan I strain). Pokeweed mitogen (PWM), derived from the rhizome of *Phytolacca americana* also stimulates B cells, but not without T cell help.

The Assay

The assay is outlined in Fig. 7.9. Briefly, mononuclear cells separated from peripheral blood are cultured in the presence of the stimulus for a defined number of days. The stimulus activates the cells which results in DNA synthesis. The stimulation of DNA synthesis can be determined by the addition of tritiated thymidine, which becomes incorporated into the newly synthesised DNA. The degree of incorporation is used as a measure of the number of responding cells. When interpreting the results of these assays, it should be borne in mind that the

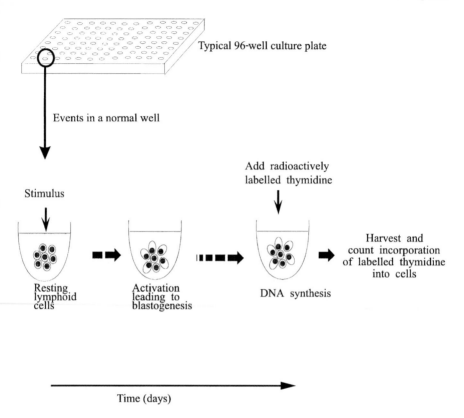

Figure 7.9   Schematic representation of a T cell function assay. Proliferation *in vitro* is only induced by the presence of an appropriate stimulus (see text for details). The degree of proliferation induced is then measured by the amount of radioactively-labelled thymidine incorporated into the DNA of dividing cells

signals required for mitogenesis may be different from those responsible for the development of effector function, depending on the type of T cell population involved. Therefore, the results of T cell activation experiments should ideally be qualified by definition of the T cell type under study.

7.6.2   Cytotoxicity Assays

Classically, this is a measure of the ability of effector cells to lyse target cells over a 4 h incubation period. The effectors of this assay may be either natural killer (NK) cells which show unrestricted killing of target cells or cytotoxic T cells whose killing of target cells is restricted according to MHC type and the presence of the specific antigen on the target and is therefore highly specific. Both NK cells and the precursors of cytotoxic T cells can be found in the blood of normal healthy individuals, although levels may vary. Prior to the assay the target cells are incubated in radioactive chromium, which crosses the cell membrane and binds irreversibly with intracellular proteins. The targets are then washed and used in the assay. Killing of the target cells by the effectors leads to the leakage of these proteins from the cytoplasm into the surrounding media. The surrounding media can be harvested and the amount of radioactive chromium present determined using a gamma counter.

7.6.3 Tests of Phagocyte Function

Neutrophils are produced by the bone marrow and have a finite life span in the periphery (the half-life of a neutrophil in the peripheral blood is 6–8 h). They are central to the inflammatory process because they act both as dispatchers (killing micro-organisms against which an immune response is active) and clearing agents (removing the debris from a response). Deficiencies in this population could therefore appear as an inability to cope with infections. Fig. 7.10 is a schematic diagram of the pathway taken by neutrophils to an area of inflamma-

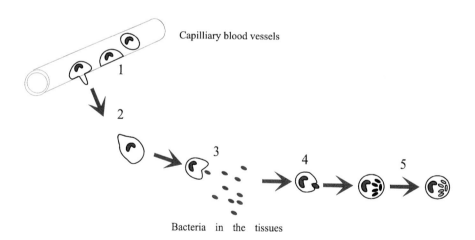

Figure 7.10   Schematic representation of the steps in the interaction of phagocytes with bacteria at the site of inflammation (see text for more details). **1** Phagocytes rolling along the wall of a capillary adhere to the wall through special receptor ligand interactions. **2** Phagocytes push through capillary walls and are drawn by a chemotactic signal to the place of inflammation. **3** Bacteria are opsonised by complement or antibodies. **4** Bacteria are engulfed by phagocytes. **5** Bacteria are killed by the intracellular processes in the phagocyte

tion in the tissues, detailing the steps involved in the response. These steps can be assayed in the laboratory as follows.

Adhesion

Adhesion to glass wool columns, the wells of plastic plates or endothelial cell cultures can be used as a direct measure of adherence. Although both monocytes and neutrophils will perform in these assays, they can be separated using a fluorescent cell analyser (these two populations have differing granular contents of their cytoplasm) or by an indirect measure (the quantity of the CD11 and CD18 family of molecules on these cells). Comparisons are often made between pre and post activation.

Chemotaxis

Chemotaxis is the directed migration of cells towards a stimulus (a chemoattractant), and this can be tested *in vitro* using a simple assay system (Fig. 7.11). Phagocytes are placed in an upper chamber separated from a lower chamber by the presence of a filter of pore size 3–8 μm. The key point about this pore size is that it is smaller than the size of the cell, so cells have to squeeze through the membrane actively. The lower chamber contains a chemoattractant such as zymosan activated plasma, casein or f-met-leu-phe. The apparatus is incubated at 37 °C for a defined period of time (from 1 to 2 h) and the number of cells attracted through the filter and into the lower chamber is then counted. In some laboratories the filters are stained and the number of polymorphonuclear cells attached to the underside of the filters is determined.

Opsonisation

The presence of specific immunoglobulin or complement-derived fragments fixed to the surface of a bacterium allows both more efficient recognition and subsequent phagocytosis of that bacterium. This is termed opsonisation and is

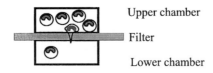

Upper chamber

Filter

Lower chamber

Figure 7.11 A diagrammatic representation of the chemotaxis assay. Cells are placed in the upper chamber and migrate through a filter, the pore size of which is less than the diameter of the cells, to the lower chamber in response to a chemotactic signal placed in the lower chamber

derived from the Greek meaning "to prepare for the table". The presence of opsonins in a sample is determined by the number of bacteria ingested by phagocytes following incubation in the test sera and comparing the results obtained with control sera as the source of the opsonins.

Phagocytosis

Phagocytosis is the ingestion of foreign material and can be assayed by incubation of the phagocytic cells with particles such as latex beads, bacteria or fungi such as *Candida albicans* followed by examination of the cells either microscopically or using the fluorescent analyser, if the particles or bacteria are labelled with a fluorescent dye.

Intracellular Killing

Direct measurement. A method of showing intracellular killing is to incubate the phagocytes with a test organism (e.g. *Candida albicans*) for a defined length of time at 37 °C. The cells are then lysed to release the ingested organisms, which are then assessed for their viability. Dyes such as methylene blue are excluded by viable cells and so the number of organisms which are either dead or alive can be counted following staining with such dyes. Viable counts may also be achieved by culturing the organisms at limiting dilutions and counting the number of colonies formed.

Indirect measurement. One of the most widespread assays for intracellular killing is the nitroblue tetrazolium dye (NBT) reduction test. NBT is a yellow dye which on reduction forms formazan which has a deep blue colour. During the killing process in phagocytes, intracellular enzymes generate superoxide radicals (the "respiratory burst"). These are capable of reducing NBT from a yellow to a blue colour which is the basis of this test. Phagocytes are incubated for a defined period of time with inert particles or bacteria in the presence of NBT. The cells can then either be counted to determine how many contain the blue deposits or, alternatively, the cells can be harvested, washed and lysed and the blue colouration determined spectroscopically. This is an indirect test as it only checks the ability of the cell to generate oxygen free radicals.

An alternative method is to use chemiluminescence. Following particle ingestion and during the respiratory burst one of the most unstable intermediates to be formed is singlet oxygen. This combines with bacteria or other intra-lysosomal components to form electronically unstable carboxyl groups. These return to a more stable ground state following emission of a small amount of electromagnetic radiation which can be detected as light by a photomultiplier tube. (Hence the term chemiluminescence). In this assay the phagocytes are incubated with latex particles or bacterial organisms in a colourless balanced salt solution.

Luminol is then added and this amplifies any electromagnetic radiation emission, which is measured using a photomultiplier tube. The amount of radiation emitted is proportional to the microbicidal activity.

7.7 FUTURE DIRECTIONS

The current rate of progress brought about by the increased use of molecular biological techniques will influence the testing and determination of the immune status of the individual in several ways. Development of new tests will be driven by a requirement in the clinical setting, but advantages may also accrue for research scientists, especially those who may not themselves be immunologists but are investigating immunological phenomena.

Obviously, there will be an increase in the number and quality of reagents available for use in immunological assays. Thus more autoantigens will be identified and the genes cloned and sequenced for use either to make more DNA primers to be used in PCR analysis or to make quantities of the antigen in a pure state for use in the search for specific antibodies in serum e.g. in ELISA. There will also obviously be an increase in the degree of automation in the laboratory. These developments will tend to lead from "after the event" testing, i.e. use of the tests to supplement a diagnosis of an illness that has already occurred, towards "before the event" testing where the tests will be used to identify the propensity of the patient to develop the illness. One of the reasons for the rapid spread of molecular biological techniques has been the marketing of the reagents required to carry out these techniques as "user-friendly" kits. Whereas previously a high degree of skill was required to clone an expressed gene from a cell, the process is now less painstaking with all the reagents available in kit form. The level of expertise required has diminished. This approach will also occur in the immunological laboratory. Many companies now have available dry forms of their reagents which do not demand the strict storage conditions needed in the past. This advance, coupled with the improvements in kit formats, means that in the future more tests will move out of the clinical laboratory into the general practioner's surgery or even into the hands of the individuals themselves. In the future the doctor will be able to substantiate his or her diagnosis with an easy to use patient-testing kit which will give a yes or no answer to questions like "Does this patient have detectable anti-nuclear antibodies in their blood?" The answer "Yes!" may then lead to the doctor sending a blood sample to a laboratory for further screening. The future lies not in small groups of people with specialised skills and knowledge of a number of laboratory tests and their significance, but in the widespread dissemination of those skills which become available because the reagent formats can be made simple and the kit contains the information on the significance of the results.

SOURCES OF INFORMATION AND FURTHER READING

Brostoff J., Scadding G. K., Male D., Roitt I. M. *Clinical Immunology.* London, New York, Gower Medical Publishing, 1991.

Chapel H., Haeney M. *Essentials of Clinical Immunology* (3rd Edn). Oxford, Blackwell Scientific Publications, 1993.

Gooi H. C., Chapel H. (Eds) *Clinical Immunology. A Practical Approach.* Oxford, IRL Press at Oxford University Press, 1990.

Hobbs J. R., Byrom N. A., Chambers J. D., Williamson S. A., Nagvekar N. Secondary T cell deficiencies. In N. A. Byrom, J. R. Hobbs (eds) *Thymic Factor Therapy.* New York, Raven Press, 1984, pp 175–187

Johnstone A., Thorpe R. *Immunochemistry in Practice.* Oxford, Blackwell Scientific Publications, 1982.

Stites D. P., Terr A. I., Parslow T.G. *Basic and Clinical Immunology* (8th edn). Connecticut, Appleton and Lange, 1994.

Functional Interplay Between Stress Hormones and the Immune System

Chapter 8

Glucocorticoids and the Immune System

Nicolas J. Goulding and Roderick J. Flower

The William Harvey Research Institute, St. Bartholomew's and the Royal London School of Medicine and Dentistry at Queen Mary and Westfield College, London, UK.

8.1 GLUCOCORTICOIDS: A CASE OF MISTAKEN IDENTITY?

Glucocorticoid biology in general, and the study of the physiological relevance of these compounds in particular, has struggled over the past 40 years to come to terms with a single clinical observation which changed the course of medical practice almost overnight. In 1949, Philip Hench reported the astounding observation that administering an adrenocortical steroid to a patient with progressive, active rheumatoid arthritis stopped the disease dead in its tracks (1). Over the ensuing decade, these hormones gained a remarkable reputation for effectiveness as their

Stress, Stress Hormones and the Immune System. Edited by J. C. Buckingham, G. E. Gillies and A.-M. Cowell
© 1997 John Wiley & Sons, Ltd.

use widened in the treatment of a range of inflammatory and autoimmune disorders. However, it soon became apparent that there was a price to pay for their efficacy in terms of potentially serious side-effects and considerable doubts arose as to their long-term benefits in modifying the course of chronic diseases such as rheumatoid arthritis. It may be a reflection of the lack of safer, equally potent alternatives that glucocorticoids are still widely employed today in the management of many diseases with autoimmune and inflammatory components. Admittedly, since the 1950s there has been an increasing degree of sophistication in the use of the steroids to minimise side-effects but utilisation is still essentially empirical and there remains much contention over dose schedules and routes of administration (2).

One clear consequence of that initial observation on the therapeutic application of glucocorticoids has been promulgation of the dogma that these compounds are solely drugs. The literature prior to the late 1940s tells a different story. As early as the 1850s, Thomas Addison described effects of adrenal insufficiency in a patient who presented with abnormally high levels of white corpuscles in the blood. This was the earliest description of an effect of low endogenous glucocorticoids on the immune system. The function of the adrenal glands came under close scrutiny in the first three decades of the twentieth century. The importance of these glands to normal physiological function was investigated by studying the effect of their removal. Adrenalectomised rats exhibited thymic enlargement and a reduced ability to cope with a wide range of stress stimuli. Several groups working in the USA in the early years of World War II had access to the novel compounds which had been purified from the adrenal cortex of horses. They demonstrated that these adrenal cortical derivatives were able to reverse the effects of adrenalectomy in terms of thymic changes and susceptibility to stress. This was a period of great advance in understanding of stress-related hormones and the mechanisms controlling their secretion, i.e. the function of the hypothalamo–pituitary–adrenal (HPA) axis. Although no one realised it at the time, it was also a landmark in immunology. The study of immune function as a separate discipline was in its infancy but it was partly the availability of purified hormones of the HPA axis to scientists studying the function of lymphoid tissue which led to a greater understanding of the dynamic nature of the immune system in responding to stress stimuli such as infection.

Allan Munck in his memorable review of the role of glucocorticoids in stress in 1984 (3) described the Hench observations as ". . . the most cataclysmic event in the history of glucocorticoid endocrinology." The emerging concept that endogenous glucocorticoids fulfil a major role as regulators of host defence had been swamped by a host of publications reporting their profound pharmacological actions in a wide range of diseases. Munck's paper in 1984 was really the first to redress the balance. It redefined the purpose of the rise in endogenous glucocorticoid levels observed following a stress stimulus, not in terms of enhancing the organism's resistance to the stressor (which had been deduced from the known pharmacological actions of these hormones) but in terms of prevention of over-reaction of the body's own defence mechanisms in combating the threat to homeostasis.

Cells of the immune system and the soluble mediators which they produce are key components of reactivity to stress stimuli. This review will focus on recent advances in our understanding of the mechanisms of action of the glucocorticoid hormones on these pathways. We will discuss these effects in terms of both their physiological and pharmacological relevance to immune function in health and in autoimmune diseases, such as rheumatoid arthritis, where these mechanisms appear to have failed.

8.2   GLUCOCORTICOID EFFECTS ON IMMUNE CELL FUNCTION

Glucocorticoids exert profound effects on mononuclear and polymorphonuclear leukocytes. Table 8.1 summarises a wealth of *in vitro* data on the effects of glucocorticoids on the functions of monocytes, macrophages, neutrophils, T

Table 8.1   Summary of glucocorticoid effects on immune cell functions

Immune function	Cell type			
	Monocyte/ macrophage	Neutrophil	T lymphocyte	B lymphocyte
Adhesion	−	−	−	?
Antibody production	na	na	na	+ld −hd
Antigen presentation	−	?	−	−
Apoptosis	+	−	+	+
Chemotaxis	−	−	−	?
Cytokine production/release	−	−	−	−
Cytotoxicity	−	−	−	na
Degranulation	?	−	na	na
Diapedesis	−	−	−	?
Endocytosis	−	−	?	?
Growth and differentiation	−	−	−	+ld −hd
Lysis (not human cells)	+	?	+	?
Phagocytosis	+ld −hd	+ld −hd	na	na
Proliferation (antigen or mitogen driven)	−	−	−	−
Respiratory burst	−	−	?	?
Spreading	−	na	na	na

Key: +, enhancing effect; −, suppressive effect; ld, low dose; hd, high dose; ?, unknown effect; na, not applicable

lymphocytes and B lymphocytes. It can be seen from Table 8.1 that the major effects of glucocorticoids are inhibitory. In some cases, the net effect on cell function depends on the dose of steroid as in the case of phagocytosis and B lymphocyte activation and antibody production. Glucocorticoids enhance cell death, whether by apoptosis or lysis. Defects of glucocorticoids on immune cell functions will now be considered in more detail.

8.2.1 Cell Recirculation

One of the most profound and easily detectable effects of administering a single bolus dose of glucocorticoid *in vivo* is the transient alteration in peripheral blood leukocyte populations—reviewed in (4), see also Chapter 3. Although first reported in the 1970s, the mechanisms by which cells travel in and out of the circulation are still incompletely understood. Intravenous administration of hydrocortisone to humans results in a rapid loss of lymphocytes from the circulation. This effect is maximal at 4 hours with numbers in the blood returning to initial levels by 24 hours. Subsets of lymphocytes exhibit differing sensitivities to glucocorticoid. The ratio of T cells bearing the CD4 helper–inducer phenotype to those bearing the CD8 cytotoxic–suppressor phenotype decreases, reflecting the higher sensitivity of CD4 positive cells to glucocorticoid effects. It has also been reported that activated T cells are more sensitive to lysis by glucocorticoids than are resting cells. This could have significant implications for perpetuation of an immune response. Lymphocytes which appear to be most sensitive to gluco-corticoids are those which constantly recirculate between blood and lymphoid tissues, maintaining a surveillance for foreign antigens. Thus, margination of these cells would impair the ability of the immune system to respond to subsequent antigenic challenge. B lymphocytes and natural killer (NK) cells also marginate in response to glucocorticoid, but their proportions increase relative to total lymphocyte numbers. The fate of marginating lymphocytes is unknown but studies in animals have suggested that a main site of redistribution is the bone marrow. Cells of the monocyte lineage which bear the CD14 surface antigen are almost totally depleted within 4–6 hours of a bolus dose of glucocorticoid, although they are restored to normal by 24 hours. There appears to be a paradox between this phenomenon and the glucocorticoid-induced reduction in the ability of these cells to migrate into inflamed tissues. While the latter appears to be mediated by alterations in the expression of adhesion molecules, both on the monocytes and on vascular endothelium (5), the nature of the cell signalling events and/or cell surface marker changes which accompany the blood mono-cytopenia are unknown. In contrast to mononuclear cells, neutrophilic granulo-cytes show a diversity in their trafficking patterns. In response to glucocorticoid, neutrophil numbers increase significantly and are maximal by 5–6 hours. This neutrophilia, which lasts for approximately 18–24 hours, is due in the main to increased release of neutrophils from bone marrow and a reduced rate of their extravasation into tissues. Eosinophils and basophils exhibit a pattern of redistribution akin to that of lymphocytes. Levels of these cell types fall by 6 hours and do not return to pre-treatment levels until 48–72 hours. The numbers of platelets in the circulation are not significantly altered by either acute or chronic glucocorticoid treatment.

Physiological changes in cortisol levels also influence leukocyte trafficking patterns. Studies of peripheral blood lymphocyte populations in man have demonstrated a clear circadian rhythm. Peak numbers of cells occur at night when cortisol levels are at their lowest, while lower numbers of cells are detected in blood during the morning when plasma cortisol levels are high. These findings apply to both B and T lymphocytes. Monoclonal antibodies have been employed to identify cyclic effects on T cell subsets. These have shown circadian rhythms for CD3 (pan-T)- and CD4-positive cells which parallel that of total lymphocytes, although CD8-positive cells do not show a distinct periodicity. This may reflect a greater resistance to glucocorticoid effects.

8.2.2 Cell Growth, Proliferation and Differentiation

Glucocorticoids can exert both positive and negative influences on cell growth. At low concentrations, synthetic glucocorticoids are often used as supplements in culture medium to maintain the growth and viability of primary tissues. Conversely, many tumour cell lines are exquisitely sensitive to glucocorticoids, which rapidly retard their growth. As proliferation of lymphocytes, monocytes and epithelial cells is dependent upon the presence of cytokines and numerous growth factors, glucocorticoids have a negative influence upon proliferative events, as they almost invariably cause a reduction in cytokine and growth factor generation. The development and maintenance of an efficient immune response is dependent upon successful co-ordination of growth, proliferation and differentiation of the many participating cell types. Thus, one future direction of glucocorticoid research must focus upon this molecular choreography. Additionally, cell death is an important facet of glucocorticoid biology relating to immune function. The deletion of immature, self-reactive T cell clones within the thymus is a critical event in ensuring that an organism remains "tolerant" to self-antigens. Failure by these cells to generate the necessary intracellular signals to cause apoptosis (a form of programmed cell death) could result in their potentiation and the development of autoimmunity. Glucocorticoids are potent inducers of lymphocyte cytolysis in animals and apoptosis in humans. The intracellular signals culminating in apoptosis are dependent on glucocorticoid receptor (GR) binding and result in the calcium-dependent enzymatic degradation of internucleosomal DNA. Nuclear transcription factors have been implicated in these processes. Repression of the intracellular oncogene c-*myc* by glucocorticoids is one mechanism by which apoptotic events can be induced. Conversely, elevated expression of another oncogene bcl-2 can overcome gluco-corticoid-induced apoptosis in B cell lines. This is by no means the whole story as experiments have demonstrated the induction of 13 genes by glucocorticoids in apoptosis-sensitive murine WEHI thymoma cell lines. This emphasises the complexity associated with glucocorticoid effects on cell function.

8.2.3   Production of Soluble Mediators

Cytokines

During the mid 1970s, it became clear that ongoing immune and inflammatory reactions were not only fuelled by cell–cell contact but also by the release of soluble mediators, termed cytokines, from many of the cell types which partici-pate in the immune response. Since then, with the routine application of sophisticated molecular biological techniques, an ever-increasing number of cytokines and their respective receptors have been characterised and cloned. These cytokines are involved in both the perpetuation and down-regulation of immune responses and form a complex network of synergistic or antagonistic interactions with many having different effects depending on target cell type. With the possible exception of transforming growth factor-beta (TGF-β) and interleukin-10, glucocorticoids exert suppressive effects on the production of cytokines. This is thought to be a primary mechanism by which these hormones exert their anti-inflammatory and immunosuppressive effects. The production of a wide range of cytokines by immunocompetent lymphoid and non-lymphoid cells is known to be suppressed by glucocorticoids. In most cases this is achieved by direct effects on gene transcription or alteration in the rate of mRNA turnover. However in some cases (e.g. the interleukin-1β precursor), glucocorticoids inhibit translation and post-translational processing. Cytokines whose production is inhibited by glucocorticoids include interleukins (IL-1, IL-2, IL-3, IL-6, IL-8 and IL-12), granulocyte- and granulocyte-macrophage colony stimulating factors (G-CSF and GM-CSF), interferon-γ (IFN-γ), tumour necrosis factor-α (TNF-α) and the monocyte chemotactic protein (MCP-1). Recent data suggest that by depressing the synthesis of IL-12 but not IL-10 induced by stimuli such as bacterial lipopolysaccharide (LPS), glucocorticoids may selectively suppress type 1 T-helper cells (T_H1 cells) but not type 2 T-helper cells (T_H2 cells) and thus depress NK-driven cell-mediated immunity while sparing antibody generation effected by T_H2 cell-driven B cell proliferation (see page 210 and Chapter 3). The potential for interaction between cytokines and glucocorticoids provides an additional dimension of complexity. IFN-γ is able to overcome the effects of glucocorticoids on several monocyte functions including phagocytosis. Further data raise the possibility that the cytokines IL-4 and TGF-β may synergise with glucocorticoids to amplify their effects. Such concerted action may indicate important future therapeutic potential.

Enzymes

The products of arachidonic acid metabolism—prostaglandins, thromboxanes and leukotrienes—are of central importance in generating the classical features of inflammation. Two pivotal enzymes within the eicosanoid pathway are susceptible to inactivation by glucocorticoids. Phospholipase A_2 (PLA_2) catalyses the hydrolysis of phospholipid and the formation of arachidonate, substrate for cyclo-oxygenase and lipoxygenase enzymes, and the subsequent production of eicosanoids (Fig. 8.1). It is known that both PLA_2 and the inducible form of cyclo-oxygenase (COX-2) can be inhibited by pharmacological doses of glucocorticoids. In the case of PLA_2 the lipocortin family of glucocorticoid-induced proteins has been implicated as being putative inhibitors of this enzyme (see below). As far as COX-2 is concerned, it appears that inhibition of enzyme activity is due to direct repression of gene transcription.

Glucocorticoids also inhibit the expression and activity of a number of other enzymes which are up-regulated during inflammatory responses. Synthesis of the proteolytic enzymes elastase and collagenase are suppressed by glucocorticoids both *in vivo* and *in vitro*. Direct inhibition of these activities results in a reduction in connective tissue degradation at an inflamed site. Likewise, an enzyme that is responsible for the generation of highly reactive and potentially damaging oxygen intermediates, namely the inducible form of nitric oxide synthase, is also sensitive to inhibition by glucocorticoids although it is not yet clear whether this is due to a direct effect on gene transcription.

Lipocortins

A potential protein mediator of some glucocorticoid actions was identified in the late 1970s. DNA cloning and expression of the recombinant human protein led to its characterisation as a member of a family of Ca^{2+} and phospholipid-binding proteins known as the lipocortins or alternatively as "annexins". At least thirteen members of this family exist, each possessing a characteristic highly homologous core region containing four 70 amino acid subunits possessing a common sequence motif. Diversity of function within the family is conferred by unique N-terminal domains (6).

Lipocortin 1 (annexin I) has a molecular weight of 37 kDa and is found abundantly in mammalian tissues but has a discrete pattern of cellular distribution that includes secretory epithelium, skin, synovium and blood leukocytes (7). Convincing evidence now exists that synthesis of this member of the annexin family can be induced in monocytes and differentiated macrophage-like cell lines by glucocorticoids. However the synthesis of lipocortin 1 does not appear

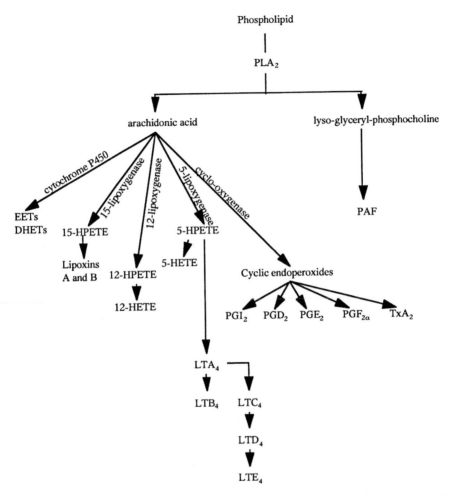

Figure 8.1 Biosynthesis of the products of arachidonic acid. PAF, platelet activating factor; TxA$_2$, thromboxane A$_2$; PGD$_2$, prostaglandin D$_2$; PGE$_2$, prostaglandin E$_2$; PGF$_{2\alpha}$, prostaglandin F$_{2\alpha}$; PGI$_2$, prostacyclin; HPETE, hydroperoxyeicosatetraenoic acid; HETE, hydroxyeicosatetraenoic acid; LT, leukotriene; EET, epoxyeicosatrienoic acid; DHET, dihydroxyeicosatrienoic acid

to be under glucocorticoid control in certain cell lines where its expression appears to be associated with cell differentiation and growth.

A wide range of potential functions has been attributed to members of the annexin family of molecules, some of which could affect the responsiveness of immunocompetent cells. Certain annexins (e.g. annexin VII) have been reported to act as Ca^{2+} channels in reconstituted phospholipid membranes; lipocortin 1 has been implicated in signal transduction pathways through being a substrate for the epidermal growth factor tyrosine kinase. Membrane fusion activities which are potentially important in phagocytosis, including neutrophil granule aggregation and release, have been reported to involve annexins. Also, the ability of lipocortin 1 to be cross-linked by transglutaminases in response to glucocorticoids could be a crucial cytoskeletal event in differentiating cells. Several pharmacological studies have indicated a role for the recombinant human protein and derived peptide fragments as inhibitors of inflammation, cytokine-mediated pyrogenesis and cerebral ischaemia (8).

Extracellular actions of recombinant lipocortin 1 on cells involved in immune responses are significant and parallel some of the effects of glucocorticoids. Exogenous recombinant lipocortin 1 has been shown to mimic glucocorticoid-induced growth arrest in a lung carcinoma-derived epithelial cell line. An indication that the exogenous protein may mediate its effects through specific cell surface receptors comes from the identification of specific lipocortin binding molecules on the surface of peripheral blood monocytes and polymorphonuclear leukocytes. The expression of these surface molecules on leukocytes from patients with rheumatoid arthritis is significantly reduced when compared to healthy individuals or patients with psoriasis or ankylosing spondylitis.

The existence of putative receptors for lipocortin 1 on human leukocytes and their lack in chronic inflammation has lead to the development of a hypothesis regarding the role of lipocortin 1 in glucocorticoid regulation of immune processes (9). The discrete distribution of lipocortin 1 within the basal epidermal keratinocyte layer and its control by even basal levels of glucocorticoids, coupled with our knowledge of receptor-like molecules specific for lipocortin 1 on monocytes and neutrophils, has led to the proposal of lipocortin 1 as a "barrier" to inappropriate inflammatory and autoimmune responses at specific sites around the body, under the tonal control of glucocorticoids via the HPA axis.

The hypothesis, summarised in Fig. 8.2, predicts that following an acute challenge and activation of the local immune response, stress-induced stimulation of the HPA axis (potentially, but not necessarily, by mediators such as IL-1, IL-6 or TNFα) results in the release of cortisol which, in turn, leads to the production of lipocortin 1 at the previously noted discrete sites throughout the body. Neutrophils and monocytes trafficking to tissue sites then have to pass through regions of elevated lipocortin 1 concentration. In peripheral blood, the low plasma lipocortin 1 concentration ($> 5\,ng/ml$) results in low receptor occupancy. However, lipocortin 1 concentrations are much higher within tissues (micromolar concentrations) and either the total or the secreted levels of lipocortin in these tissues are tightly regulated by glucocorticoid. Thus, following sufficient stimulation of the HPA axis, the lipocortin 1 binding molecules on monocytes and neutrophils arriving at tissue sites would become saturated, with resultant moderation of migratory and immunostimulatory activities. The system may be additionally controlled in an autocrine-paracrine fashion with lipocortin

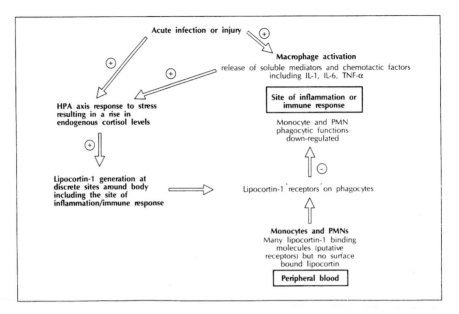

Figure 8.2 Schematic model of the steps involved in regulation of an acute inflamma-tory–immune response by lipocortin 1. HPA, hypothalamo–pituitary–adrenal; IL, inter-leukin; PMN, polymorphonuclear leukocyte; TNF, tumour necrosis factor; +, positive regulation; −, negative regulation. See text for details. (From Goulding N.J. & Guyre P.M. Glucocorticoids, lipocortins and the immune response. *Curr. Opin. Immunol.* 1993; **5**: 108–113. Reproduced with permission)

1 playing a fundamental role in the glucocorticoid feedback loop of HPA axis activity at the level of the anterior pituitary gland and hypothalamus (8).

Possible mechanisms for failure of this system may involve a defective HPA axis response to inflammatory or autoimmune injury—as reported in the Lewis rat (10)—resulting in reduced lipocortin production, permitting chronic influx of activated leukocytes into the inflammatory site. The presence of autoantibodies to lipocortin 1 (which have been described in autoimmune diseases such as rheumatoid arthritis, systemic lupus erythematosus and in MRL autoimmune mice) or a deficiency in the expression of lipocortin receptors (as has recently been demonstrated in active rheumatoid arthritis) could be additional factors conspiring to perpetuate inflammatory and autoimmune activities and their pathological consequences.

It is probably not coincidental that many areas of the body which have high lipocortin 1 concentrations are known to be immunologically privileged sites, including the thymus and skin. Also, cancer in mice has been associated with increased levels of lipocortin 1 *in vivo* and lipocortins have been implicated in the teratogenicity of glucocorticoids. Monocytes and neutrophils contain high intracellular levels of lipocortin 1 as well as expressing high levels of lipocortin 1 receptors. A critical action of glucocorticoids, one which remains poorly understood, is their suppression of phagocyte functions including the inhibition of IgG Fc receptor (Fcγ R) function. Several observations have led to the concept that lipocortin 1, produced by monocytes, epithelial and probably endothelial cells, may be an important mediator of the impaired phagocytic function which is induced by this class of hormones. Recombinant human lipocortin 1 and related peptides inhibit IgG binding to Fcγ receptors without interfering with receptor expression. Few other direct effects of lipocortins on immune receptors have been reported. However, the concept of lipocortin 1 as an immunosuppressive "cytokine", under the control of hormones of the HPA axis, with specific receptor molecules on phagocytic cells is attractive but remains unproven.

8.2.4   Immune Effector Functions

Accessory Functions

The major histocompatibility complex (MHC) class II proteins expressed on cells capable of presenting antigens have a central role in immune recognition. The molecules are involved in the generation of the thymic T cell repertoire and form part of the tripartite class II, antigen, T cell receptor complex which is pivotal in cell-mediated immune responses (see Chapter 3). Glucocorticoid hormones are frequently used in transplantation surgery to prevent allograft rejection. A key marker of graft acceptance is down-regulation of expression of MHC class II antigens on the grafted tissue. In chronic inflammatory diseases such as rheumatoid arthritis, synovial expression of MHC class II antigens is elevated. Intra-articular glucocorticoid administration leads to a reduction in the expression of class II, both in terms of mRNA and protein. These changes parallelled the improvement in clinical measures of joint involvement which often result from intra-articular glucocorticoid use. Elevation of expression of MHC class II antigens at the sites of infection or injury is critical for maintenance of the immune response. Pro-inflammatory cytokines such as IFN-γ or GM-CSF are centrally involved in elevating MHC class II expression. There appear to be essential differences in the ways by which MHC class II antigens are regulated by glucocorticoids in lymphoid and non-lymphoid tissues. On non-lymphoid tissues, it appears that expression is regulated by inhibition of the production of class II-inducing mediators such as IFN-γ and GM-CSF. However, effects of glucocorticoids on the expression of MHC class II on B cells and monocytes appear to be due to direct effects on GR binding to specific areas in the 5′ flanking region of the coding region of the class II gene IAβ. Recent evidence also suggests that certain cytokine-dependent pathways of class II expression on monocytes are relatively glucocorticoid insensitive. While IFN-induced human leukocyte antigen-D-regulated (HLA-DR) expression on monocytes could be suppressed by dexamethasone, the same antigens induced by GM-CSF could not be suppressed by glucocorticoids; in fact there appears to be a synergy between these two agents resulting in a super-induction of class II. Thus, it appears that there are multiple receptor-mediated pathways of up- and down-regulation of class II by glucocorticoids.

T Lymphocyte Activation

In general, immune responses mediated through T lymphocytes are more sensitive to suppression by glucocorticoids than are B cell responses. This is used to great advantage in prevention of allograft rejection by suppressing the activation and proliferation of both cytotoxic and alloreactive T cell populations. These effects are achieved by multiple pathways, including inhibition of production of growth factors and cytokines involved in lymphocyte proliferation and diversion of the cell signalling pathways away from activation and proliferation and towards programmed cell death. Reduced expression of the IL-2 receptor p55 chain appears to play a pivotal role in this process (11).

In vitro experiments have demonstrated that even relatively small doses of hydrocortisone (10^{-8} M), equivalent to physiological levels, are capable of profoundly suppressing allogeneic mixed lymphocyte reactions. This would suggest that adrenal hormones are capable of protecting the body against the generation of self-reactive T cell clones. It has been proposed that autoimmunity results from an impaired HPA axis response to stress with inadequate levels of induced glucocorticoid allowing the potentiation of autoreactive T lymphocyte clones with pathogenic consequences (12).

The identification of subpopulations of human T helper (T_H) cells which differ in their profiles of secreted cytokines has led to a view that T cell activation can be driven down one of two avenues, biasing either towards cell-mediated delayed hypersensitivity responses via T_H1 cells which secrete IL-2 and IFN-γ or humoral responses, such as those to allergens, via T_H2 cells which mainly produce IL-4, IL-5, IL-6 and IL-10. Such a system provides potentially important opportunity for the balance between cell-mediated and humoral responses to be altered by selective modulation of lymphokine production by, for example, stress hormones (glucocorticoids or catecholamines) or other factors (13). Indeed, increasing evidence suggests that, while glucocorticoids may impair cell-mediated responses by suppressing the ability of undifferentiated T_H cells to produce IL-12 (a cytokine which drives the development of mature T_H1 cells) and by inhibiting IL-2 and IFN-γ production by T_H1 cells, the synergistic influence of glucocorticoids and IL-4 on T_H2 cell function coupled with the apparent failure of the steroids to suppress IL-10 production may lead to a net amplification of B lymphocyte-mediated responses. However, the inhibition of lymphokine production by glucocorticoids also has the effect of suppressing lymphocyte cytotoxicity, including both natural killer activity and antibody-dependent cellular cytotoxicity.

B Lymphocyte Activation

Studies on the *in vitro* and *in vivo* effects of glucocorticoids on B lymphocyte activation and antibody generation are conflicting in their conclusions. Patients who receive the potent synthetic glucocorticoid methylprednisolone, intravenously, exhibit a generalised reduction in serum immunoglobulin. Autoimmune diseases such as systemic lupus erythematosus and rheumatoid arthritis are accompanied by the development of specific autoantibodies through the expansion of autoreactive B cell clones. Pulse glucocorticoid therapy usually results in significant reductions in the production of such autoantibodies which parallels its clinical effectiveness. *In vitro* effects of glucocorticoid on B cell function depend on the culture system used, the dose and type of glucocorticoid employed and the aspect of B cell function being monitored. Studies using purified B cells have reported that glucocorticoids work on the early stages of B cell activation by inhibiting signalling pathways leading to activation and blocking entry into the G1 phase of the cell cycle. Events such as differentiation into plasma cells and subsequent immunoglobulin production are relatively resistant to constraint by glucocorticoids. In B cell culture systems which are dependent upon the presence of T cells or T cell-derived factors, glucocorticoids can enhance immunoglobulin production by removing the restraints of T lymphocyte-derived suppressor factors. Thus, while one might predict that even physiological levels of glucocorticoids may suppress cell-mediated autoimmune reactivity, the complexity of factors involved in B cell responsiveness makes it difficult to foresee the net effect of a deficient HPA axis on humoral responses to autoantigens.

Eosinophil, Basophil and Mast Cell Activation

Together with the profound effects on cell redistribution, histamine release by eosinophils and basophils following activation can be inhibited by glucocorticoid. This may be the basis for the effectiveness of these agents in late-phase allergic responses. As far as mast cells are concerned, there is a degree of interspecies variation in response to glucocorticoids. In general, human mast cell activation and mediator release pathways are resistant to glucocorticoid effects, which raises the question of why these compounds are so effective in the treatment of allergic conditions. However, in mouse and rat models, glucocorticoids can suppress the release of IgE, expression of IgE receptors and degranulation by mast cells

Phagocytosis and Antibody-dependent Cellular Cytotoxicity (ADCC)

These end-stage effector functions are crucial for the efficient killing of foreign cells coated with antibody and the elimination of dead cells and immune complexes. Studies on the administration of synthetic glucocorticoids to humans or cattle have reported decreased ADCC and phagocytotic efficiency. Likewise, direct inhibitory effects of glucocorticoids on *in vitro* phagocytic activities of human monocytes and macrophages require culture systems to contain high pharmacological doses of a potent synthetic glucocorticoid for periods of over 18 hours (1 μM dexamethasone for impairment of bacteria or fungi by murine peritoneal macrophages). Where glucocorticoids have been shown to have a negative effect on these functions, the inhibition can be reversed by IFN-γ, suggesting that these compounds act primarily by suppressing the production of immune cytokines. An important paradox exists in that experiments performed on cultured mouse peritoneal macrophages using concentrations of corticosterone comparable to those achieved physiologically in the circulation after stress have demonstrated an enhancement in phagocytosis. This emphasises the caution which must be applied when comparing *in vivo* with *in vitro* studies and also synthetic and natural glucocorticoid effects on immune function. As far as mechanisms are concerned, these effects can be explained by glucocorticoid effects on surface receptors for the Fc portion of IgG. Cells capable of phagocytosis and ADCC, such as monocytes, macrophages and neutrophils, express Fcγ receptors (FcγR) which enable phagocytic cells to recognise invading pathogens to which the body has produced specific antibodies. Complexes of bacteria, virus or tumour cell which have antibody bound through its F(ab) domain can be efficiently bound, internalised and eliminated via receptors recognising the Fc "tail" of the antibody molecule. Interferon-γ increases the expression of Fc receptors on human monocytes; this effect is parallelled by a significant enhancement in phagocytic or cytotoxic activity. Thus, if high dose glucocorticoid suppresses IFN-γ production, ADCC and phagocytosis could be inhibited. Human and murine monocytes and macrophages cultured with relatively low levels of glucocorticoid and IFN-γ demonstrate that the two agents synergise to up-regulate FcγR expression to a level higher than IFN-γ alone, with accompanying increases in ADCC and phagocytic activity (14). This could explain the increased phagocytotic activity in mice receiving corticosterone.

8.3 THE MOLECULAR BASIS FOR GLUCOCORTICOID ACTION

8.3.1 Transport Proteins

Glucocorticoids, being highly lipid soluble molecules, are capable of passing through the phospholipid membranes of cells without the need for any cell surface receptor system. However there is increasing evidence that these hormones can be "targeted" to particular tissues through the existence of glucocorticoid transport proteins present in the blood. In normal circumstances, less than 10% of natural cortisol exists in the unbound form, although up to 40% of synthetic glucocorticoids administered exogenously remain in the free form. The remaining proportions of glucocorticoid are bound either to albumin with relatively low affinity or to the specific corticosteroid binding globulin (CBG) with relatively high affinity. It appears that when bound to carrier proteins, glucocorticoids are pharmacologically inactive. Thus, these transport proteins play an important role in regulating glucocorticoid availability and action. A mechanism which would allow effective targeting of glucocorticoid to areas of inflammation or immune injury has been proposed involving CBG (15). Cleavage of CBG by elastase enzymes released in such areas results in a 10-fold reduction in the affinity of this molecule for glucocorticoid. This conversion of CBG from a "stressed" form to a "relaxed" form could represent an efficient "drug-delivery system" of glucocorticoid to areas where it is particularly required to suppress inflammation or an immune response. There are also hints that the system may be even more specific, with cells from a wide range of tissues expressing a 160 kDa cell surface CBG-binding molecule. One could foresee that, if expression of these receptor-like proteins were to be up-regulated by immune cytokines, it may represent an important feed-back control loop for immune responses.

8.3.2   The Glucocorticoid Receptor

It is now widely accepted that most, if not all, glucocorticoid actions on cells are mediated through interactions with specific intracellular GR (see also Chapter 4). These receptors are distributed in many different mammalian tissues with a common range of expression of the order of 10^3 to 10^4 molecules per cell. As far as the immune cells are concerned, GR are expressed in monocytes, macrophages, granulocytes and all lymphocyte sub-populations. The density and affinity of GR varies between leukocyte types. Receptor numbers also fluctuate depending on the stage in the cell cycle, on whether the cell has been activated and on ambient glucocorticoid levels. Adrenalectomised animals, in which endogenous glucocorticoid levels are minimal, exhibit increased GR expression in most tissues. Conversely, GR levels fall in response to prolonged glucocorticoid administration. The human GR has been isolated and cloned and sequence data have confirmed that it is typical of the steroid receptor superfamily and thus possesses two "zinc-finger" motifs which are critical for DNA binding. Two alternate splice variants of a single gene have been described. The α form consists of 777 amino acids while the β form is expressed as a 742 amino acid protein, being truncated at the C terminus. Unlike the α form, the β form of the receptor is unable to bind ligand although it has the capability to bind DNA. The widespread expression of the β form in cells and tissues has led to speculation that this truncated receptor may function as an endogenous inhibitor of glucocorticoid action and that its expression may be enhanced in some types of steroid resistance (16)—see also Section 8.4.

The glucocorticoid receptors in man and other species comprise three functionally distinct domains. The N-terminal region contains amino acid sequences important for transactivation or transrepression of specific genes. The central "core" of the molecule possesses the motifs which define the gene family and are required for DNA binding, while the C-terminal domain contains the regions responsible for binding to the glucocorticoid ligand and to a 90 kDa chaperone molecule which has been characterised as a heat shock protein (hsp 90) and whose probable function is to stabilise the receptor in the absence of hormone. Two hsp 90 molecules are associated with each GR and are released upon hormone binding, increasing the affinity of the receptor for DNA. Hormone binding also initiates receptor dimerisation which is important for the subsequent binding to DNA. Study of these processes is at a relatively early stage and it is possible that other "regulatory" molecules such as a 59 kDa immunophilin molecule and a 65 kDa hsp are also involved in receptor association and dissociation. Recent studies have implicated an additional regulatory nuclear protein known as calreticulin (17). Association of this molecule to the GR results in inhibition of the transcriptional activities of the receptor. Binding of ligand to receptor also initiates the process by which the resultant complex migrates from the cytoplasm to the nucleus. The mechanism by which this occurs is not known but requires the presence of specific sequences within the central domain of the GR. The major structural and functional relationships of the glucocorticoid receptor and associated proteins are portrayed in Fig. 8.3.

8.3.3 Transcriptional and Post-transcriptional Activities

Hormone binding to the GR, dissociation of the regulatory subunits, nuclear translocation and receptor dimerisation events all culminate in the binding to glucocorticoid responsive elements (GREs). These sequences can be either simple (activating), negative (repressive) or composite (effect depends on binding of other factors). These consensus sequences are summarised in Table 8.2. In the last few years it has become increasingly evident that cross-talk between intracellular transcription factors plays an important role in influencing gene expression. At the transcriptional level this is achieved by factors binding downstream of the coding region of genes to cause transactivation or transrepression. For example, in the monocyte, many genes encoding pro-inflammatory cytokines and enzymes are activated through specific response elements recognised by intracellular oncoproteins. The AP-1 (activator protein 1) family of oncogene products consists of either homodimers of *Jun*-related proteins or heterodimers of *Jun*- and *Fos*-related proteins dimerised by a characteristic leucine zipper coupling. These proto-oncoprotein dimers possess the ability to transactivate genes by binding to specific

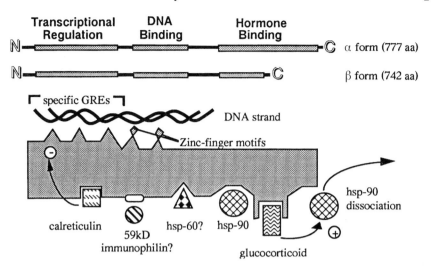

Figure 8.3 Structure and functional representation of the human glucocorticoid receptor. Two splice-variants of the receptor exist, the full length α form and the truncated β form, which is unable to bind ligand. hsp, heat shock protein; GRE, glucocorticoid response element

Table 8.2 Glucocorticoid-related DNA response elements

Consensus element	Binding factors	Type	Effect on transcription	DNA sequence
GRE (Glucocorticoid response element)	glucocorticoid/ receptor complex	simple	enhancing	GGTACAnnn-TGTTCT
		negative	repressing	ATYACnnTnT-GATCn
		composite	enhancing or repressing	GRE adjacent to or overlapping a TRE
TRE (TPA response element)	*Fos*, *Fos*-B, *Fra*-1, *Fra*-2, *Jun*, *Jun*-B, *Jun*-D	simple	enhancing	TGA(C/G)TCA
CRE (cyclic AMP response element)	CREB-1, CREB-2, ATF-1, ATF-2, ATF-3, ATF-4	simple	enhancing	TGACCTCA

regions of DNA known as 12-O-tetradecanoyl phorbol 13-acetate (TPA) response elements (TREs). This consists of the palindromic seven base sequence TGA(C/G)TCA. Cross-talk exists between this activation system and the specific cytoplasmic glucocorticoid receptor which has the ability to alter gene expression through specific GREs downstream of the TATA box transcription start sites of many genes. Some genes such as the mouse proliferin gene contain composite GREs which include TREs. Thus, there is the potential for multiple regulatory activities depending on the relative expression of *Fos* to *Jun* and the presence of GR-hormone complex (18). Recent studies have also indicated that glucocorticoids can suppress immunity by inhibiting the activity of the NF-$_k$B family of transcription factors (19, 20). The NF-$_k$B multiprotein complex has a pivotal role in transducing signals derived from cell surface receptors involved in early host defence reactions. The activation of NF-$_k$B through release of an inhibitory component I$_k$B represents a key stage in inducing nuclear translocation and subsequent activation of the transcription of a wide range of genes whose products are involved in the immune response. Human T lymphocytes and monocytes triggered with TNF-α or phorbol esters exhibit a rapid degradation of I$_k$B and activation of the NF-$_k$B. This process is under feedback control, with NF-$_k$B inducing the *de novo* synthesis of I$_k$B. Glucocorticoids act on at least two levels. Firstly through interaction between the GR-ligand complex and NF-$_k$B, preventing binding of the latter to DNA, and secondly through the induction of I$_k$Bα, thus inhibiting its translocation to the nucleus of the cell and the subsequent increase in cytokine gene activity. Further down the protein synthetic pathway, glucocorticoids can regulate post-transcriptional modification of mRNA, mRNA stability, and as in the case of IL-1 and IL-2 genes polyribosomal activity and post-translational processing of proteins (21). Even if transcriptional and translational activities are unaltered by glucocorticoids, they can still exert profound effects on cell surface expression or release of a protein by affecting intracellular transport and secretory mechanisms.

8.3.4   Mineralocorticoid Receptors and Their Potential Role in the Immune System

Although the regulatory effects of the glucocorticoids on immune function are mediated primarily by the glucocorticoid receptor (sometimes called GR or the type II corticosteroid receptor), it is important to give some consideration to the type I subclass of corticosteroid receptor, namely the mineralocorticoid receptor (often referred to as MR). The distribution of mineralocorticoid and glucocorticoid receptors varies from tissue to tissue but the endogenous glucocorticoids, cortisol and corticosterone, can bind to both receptors and elicit biological responses. Surprisingly, the MR has a much higher affinity for cortisol and corticosterone than the GR (22). From this it may be predicted that the MR should be fully occupied at much lower blood concentrations of cortisol and corticosterone than the GR. Paradoxically, however, in tissues such as the kidney the MR is selectively engaged by aldosterone (the major endogenous mineralocorticoid) rather than the endogenous glucocorticoids. The solution to this enigma lies in an enzyme, type II 11β-hydroxysteroid dehydrogenase, which is expressed in target cells in the kidney and several other tissues where MR abound (23). This enzyme converts cortisol and corticosterone to their respective 11-keto derivatives, cortisone and 11-ketocorticosterone, which have little activity at the MR; it thus permits selective activation of the receptor by aldosterone. Deficiencies in this enzyme lead to over-activation of the MR by endogenous glucocorticoids and through this to pathologies such as excessive sodium conservation and adrenal hyperplasia with associated hypertension.

A further potentially important mechanism of corticosteroid action which may permit a hitherto undiscovered level of fine control of gene transcription has recently been uncovered (24). According to this idea, the genomic actions of these steroids may be effected not only by dimeric pairs of type α GR (see Section 8.3.2.) but also by *heterodimeric* receptor complexes. Such heterodimers may comprise MR and GR or, conceivably, heterodimers of type α and type β GR, or glucocorticoid and other receptors from the same super family (e.g. retinoid acid receptors). Current evidence predicts that heterodimerisation could be important in regulating gene transcription in some target tissues such as those involved in the HPA axis where both MR and GR co-exist. However, in tissues where one or other type of receptor predominates or where the MR is protected by 11β-hydroxysteroid dehydrogenase, the phenomenon would be less important (23).

From the point of immune cell regulation by adrenal steroids, it is important to note that MR are widely expressed by immune cells and tissues, such as lymphocytes and monocytes. Much remains to be learnt about their function and the extent to which they are protected from endogenous glucocorticoids by 11β-hydroxysteroid dehydrogenase. Nonetheless, there is some evidence that activation of these receptors may facilitate responses that oppose those effected by GR, in which case agonists such as cortisol and corticosterone (which have the capacity to stimulate both receptors types) may produce effects which differ subtly from those of the selective GR agonists used clinically, for example, prednisolone, dexamethasone (23). Furthermore, the possibility exists that they may form hetero-dimers with glucocorticoid or other steroid receptors and thereby further refine the control exerted by mixed MR and GR agonists.

8.4   GLUCOCORTICOID RESISTANCE

Glucocorticoid resistance or "steroid resistance" is a fairly common clinical problem and refers to the inability of glucocorticoids to cause an adequate anti-inflammatory response in patients at normal therapeutic doses. In the majority of cases the condition might more accurately be described as "relative steroid resistance" since higher doses bring about the desired beneficial effect, but in others it may be absolute. There are several potential causes of steroid resistance.

In some instances the number of GR may be reduced while in others there may be defects associated with the machinery of steroid-induced protein synthesis (25, 26); as mentioned earlier (Section 8.3.2.), a possible cause of the latter may be increased expression of the type β GR (i.e. the inactive form of the receptor) which may dimerise with the type α species (active) and thus blunt the biological response to the steroid. Another less obvious reason is the occurrence of autoantibodies against lipocortin 1, a protein implicated in certain aspects of glucocorticoid action (see pages 205–9). Such antibodies (both IgG and IgM) have been observed in sera from patients with rheumatoid arthritis or systemic lupus erythematosus although not in subjects with chronic obstructive airways disease or polymyalgia rheumatica (27, 28). Current evidence suggests that the autoantibody titres correlate with the degree of steroid resistance in patients with rheumatoid arthritis and with the severity of the disease in patients with systemic lupus erythematosus, although the relationship evident in the latter appears to be dependent on the way in which the disease was assessed (27, 29). Interestingly in patients with rheumatoid arthritis the occurrence of high titre autoantibodies is often linked with long-term oral use of the synthetic glucocorticoid, predniso-lone, suggesting a role for the exogenous steroid in the pathogenesis of this type of resistance (27).

8.5 ENDOGENOUS ADRENAL STEROIDS AND IMMUNE HOMEOSTASIS

8.5.1 Glucocorticoids

Thus far we have concentrated on "blunderbuss" effects of glucocorticoids on immunity, reviewing data which has derived from *in vivo* or *in vitro* studies generally employing doses of glucocorticoid which would only be achieved pharmacologically. Hormonal actions of natural cortisol are far more subtle since even peak plasma levels achieved following stress-induced stimulation of the adrenal cortex are lower than those obtained by doses of glucocorticoid normally employed during immunosuppressive therapy. Again we must reinforce the point that endogenous glucocorticoids can exert permissive as well as suppressive effects on immune function. We have already described some of the mechanisms of glucocorticoid action on immune cells at the molecular level, which clearly tip the balance towards a down-regulation of immunity. How then do glucocorti-coids exert their permissive effects? A simple mathematical model has been proposed by Munck and co-workers (30) which attempts to explain how fluctuations in levels of endogenous glucocorticoids could result in a significant shift in immune function. This model hinges upon the observation that for a variety of immune cytokines (such as IL-1, IL-6 and IFN-γ) glucocorticoids not only inhibit the production of these cytokines in a number of cell types, but also induce the expression of receptors for these cytokines in a number of cell types. Fig. 8.4a describes a hypothetical example of such a system, where levels of cytokine are suppressed by increasing doses of glucocorticoid while levels of the receptor are induced over the same dose range. Fig. 8.4b shows the mathematical product of these curves, being the effective concentrations of the ligand-receptor

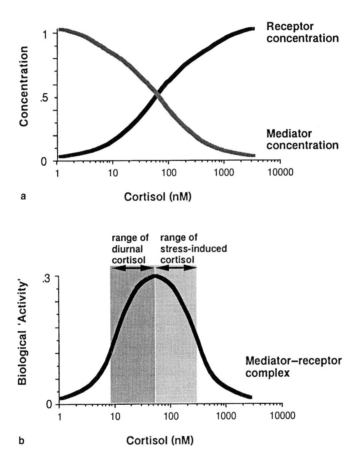

Figure 8.4 Mathematical model for the permissive and suppressive effects of glucocorticoids over a physiological concentration range. **a** dose response curves for a theoretical mediator and its specific receptor; **b** mathematical composite of mediator–receptor complex formation indicating biological activity, suggesting a mechanism by which low cortisol levels could be permissive and stress-induced cortisol surges suppressive in effect. (From Munck A., Naray Fejes-Toth A. *Mol Cell Endocrinol*, 1992, **90**, C1–C4, with kind permission from Elsevier Science Ireland Ltd., Bay 15K, Shannon Industrial Estate, Co. Clare, Ireland)

complex i.e. biological effect of the particular cytokine. It can be seen that at a low glucocorticoid concentration, low expression of receptor leads to an ineffective response, an effect parallelled at high doses of glucocorticoid where cytokine levels are low. It is hypothesised that, at levels of glucocorticoid which occur during the normal circadian cycle, immune function will be primed for activity. However, if the HPA axis is stimulated through stressor pathways to increase circulating glucocorticoid levels, the overall effect is to dampen immune responsiveness i.e. glucocorticoids have their well-described pharmacological effects. The authors themselves recognise the limitations of this model in terms of experimental data. The model is very useful in beginning to explain how glucocorticoids can have paradoxical effects on immune function. It is hoped that studies to test models such as these will reveal new links between endogenous glucocorticoid generation and the development of autoimmunity and cancer. Furthermore, as we unravel the complexity of the mechanisms which accompany glucocorticoid binding to its receptor and the regulatory events leading to alterations in cell function, it is hoped that new therapies based on glucocorticoids and their mediators should increase specificity of action while reducing undesirable side-effects.

8.5.2   Dehydroepiandrosterone

Another potentially important steroid produced by the adrenal cortex is dehydroepiandrosterone (DHEA) which in some species may be secreted in amounts which exceed those of cortisol and corticosterone. Many groups have sought to demonstrate a physiological role for this steroid and increasing evidence suggests that it may exert significant effects in the immune system which oppose the immunosuppressant actions of the endogenous glucocorticoids. Such arguments are supported by evidence that:

(a) the concentration of DHEA in the systemic circulation declines with age and thus parallels the decline in immunocompetence, and
(b) the steroid can antagonise the suppressive actions of dexamethasone on lymphocyte proliferation (31).

The molecular mechanism of DHEA action is unknown. It is transported in the blood as a sulphate and is presumably activated in its target cells by sulphatase enzymes. Reports that DHEA sulphate inhibits TNF production in mice treated with the GR antagonist RU486 suggest its actions are independent of this steroid receptor (32) but a specific DHEA receptor has yet to be identified. Future studies will no doubt clarify the situation and enable us to assign an unambiguous role to this potentially important endogenous steroid hormone.

8.6 OVERVIEW

The glucocorticoids exert considerable influence on the immune system. While the brunt of most research has focused upon their pharmacological actions, it has become clear that they also have important physiological activities in maintaining the organism's "immune tone". These hormones affect cell growth, proliferation and differentiation. They can influence the movement of immune cells around the blood and lymphatics. They can alter the functions of all cells of the immune system with net immunosuppressive consequences. These include effects on the expression of cell surface antigens involved in immune responses, on the production of soluble mediators such as antibodies and cytokines and on the effector functions such as cell killing and phagocytosis.

At the molecular level, most of these activities are mediated through the specific, intracellular GR. On binding hormone, these receptors migrate from cytoplasm to nucleus where they can profoundly alter the transcription and translation of a wide number of proteins. The complexity of the interaction of the glucocorticoid–receptor complex with other transcription factors and DNA regulatory elements has recently become very apparent. Advances in the understanding of the molecular interactions of glucocorticoids, receptors and DNA hold the key to new strategies, both in understanding how the immune system is homeostatically regulated and in the development of new therapeutic modalities where beneficial anti-inflammatory or immunosuppressive effects can be dissected out from those which are potentially harmful.

REFERENCES

1. Hench P., Kendall E. C., Slocumb C. H., Polley H. F. The effects of a hormone of the adrenal cortex and of pituitary adrenocorticotropic hormone on rheumatoid arthritis. *Proc Mayo Clin*, 1949, **24**: 181–97.
2. Kimberly R. P. Mechanisms of action, dosage schedules, and side effects of steroid therapy. *Curr Opin Rheumatol*, 1991, **3**: 373–9.
3. Munck A., Guyre P. M., Holbrook N. J. Physiological functions of glucocorticoids in stress and their relation to pharmacological actions. *Endocr Rev*, 1984, **5**: 25–44.
4. Goldstein R. A., Bowen D. L., Fauci A. S. Adrenal corticosteroids, Inflammation. In J. I. Gallin, I. M. Goldstein, R. Snyderman (eds) *Basic Principles and Clinical Correlates*. New York, Raven Press, 1992, pp 1061–80.
5. Cronstein B. N., Kimmel S. C., Levin R. I., Martiniuk F., Weissmann G. A mechanism for the anti-inflammatory effects of corticosteroids: The glucocorticoid receptor regulates leukocyte adhesion to endothelial cells and expression of endothelial-leukocyte adhesion molecule 1 and intercellular adhesion molecule 1. *Proc Natl Acad Sci USA*, 1992, **89**: 9991–5.
6. Raynal P., Pollard H. B. Annexins: the problem of assessing the biological role for a gene family of multifunctional calcium- and phospholipid-binding proteins. *Biochim Biophys Acta*, 1994, **1197**: 63–93.

7. Fava R. A., McKanna J., Cohen S. Lipocortin I (p35) is abundant in a restricted number of differentiated cell types in adult organs. *J Cell Physiol*, 1989, **141**: 284–93.
8. Flower R. J., Rothwell N. J. Lipocortin-1: cellular mechanisms and clinical relevance. *Trends Pharmacol Sci*, 1994, **15**: 71–6.
9. Goulding N. J., Guyre P. M. Regulation of inflammation by lipocortin I. *Immunol Today*, 1992, **13**: 295–7.
10. Sternberg E. M., Hill J. M., Chrousos G. P., Kamilaris T., Listwak S. J., Gold P. W., Wilder R. L. Inflammatory mediator-induced hypothalamic–pituitary–adrenal axis activation is defective in streptococcal cell wall arthritis-susceptible Lewis rats. *Proc Natl Acad Sci USA*, 1989, **86**: 2374–8.
11. Paliogianni F., Raptis A., Ahuja S. S., Najjar S. M., Boumpas D. T. Negative transcriptional regulation of human interleukin 2 (IL-2) gene by glucocorticoids through interference with nuclear transcription factors AP-1 and NF-AT. *J Clin Invest*, 1993, **91**: 1481–9.
12. Mason D. Genetic variation in the stress response: susceptibility to experimental allergic encephalomyelitis and implications for human inflammatory disease. *Immunol Today*, 1991, **12**: 57–60.
13. Stam W. B., Van Oosterhout A. J., Nijkamp F. P. Pharmacologic modulation of Th1- and Th2-associated lymphokine production. *Life Sci*, 1993, **53**: 1921–34.
14. Munck A., Guyre P. M. Glucocorticoids and immune function. In R. Ader, D.L. Felton, N. Cohen (eds) *Psychoneuroimmunology*. New York, Academic Press Inc, 1991, pp 447–74.
15. Hammond G. L. Molecular properties of corticosteroid binding globulin and the sex-steroid binding proteins. *Endocr Rev*, 1990, **11**: 65–79
16. Bamberger C. M., Bamberger A.-M., de Castro M., Chrousos G.P. Glucocorticoid receptor β, a potential endogenous inhibitor of glucocorticoid action in humans. *J Clin Invest*, 1995, **95**: 2435–41.
17. Burns K., Duggan B., Atkinson E. A, Famulski K. S., Nemer M., Bleackley R. C., Michalak M. Modulation of gene expression by calreticulin binding to the glucocorticoid receptor. *Nature*, 1994, **367**: 476–80.
18. Diamond M. I., Miner J. N., Yoshinaga S. K., Yamamoto K. R. Transcription factor interactions: selectors of positive or negative regulation from a single DNA element. *Science*, 1990, **249**: 1266–72.
19. Scheinman R. I., Cogswell P. C., Lofquist A. K., Baldwin A. S. Jnr. Role of transcriptional activation of IκBα in mediation of immunosuppression by glucocorticoids. *Science*, 1995, **270**: 283–6.
20. Auphan N., DiDonato J. A., Rosette C., Helmberg A., Karin M. Immunosuppression by glucocorticoids: inhibition of NF-κB activity through induction of IκBα synthesis. *Science*, 1995, **270**: 286–90.
21. Boumpas D. T., Paliogianni F., Anastassiou E. D., Balow J. E. Glucocorticosteroid action on the immune system: molecular and cellular aspects. *Clin Exp Rheumatol*, 1991, **9**: 413–23.
22. de Kloet E. R. Brain corticosteroid receptor balance and homoeostatic control. *Frontiers in Neuroendocrinology*, 1991, **12**: 95–164.
23. Funder J. W. Aldosterone action. *Ann Rev Physiol*, 1993, **55**: 115–30.
24. Trap T., Holsbaer F. Heterodimerization between mineralocorticoid and glucocorticoid receptors increases the functional diversity of corticosteroid actions. *Trends Pharmacol Sci*, 1996, **17**: 145–9.
25. Adcock I. M., Lane S. J., Brown C. A., Peters M. J., Lee T. H., Barnes P. J. Differences in binding of glucocorticoid receptor to DNA in steroid resistant asthma. *J Immunol*, 1995, **154**: 3000–5.

26. Adcock I. M., Lane S. J., Brown C. A., Lee T. H., Barnes P. J. Abnormal glucocorticoid receptor/AP-1 interaction in steroid resistant asthma. *J Exp Med*, 1995, **182**: 1951–8.
27. Goulding N. J., Podgorski M. R., Hall N. D., Flower R. J., Browning S. L., Pepinsky R. B., Maddison P. J. Autoantibodies to recombinant lipocortin 1 in rheumatoid arthritis and systemic erythematosus. *Ann Rheum Dis*, 1989, **48**: 843–50.
28. Hirata F., del Carmine R., Nelson C. A., Axelrod J., Schiffmann E., Warabi A., *et al*. Presence of autoantibody for phospholipase inhibitory protein, lipomodulin, in patients with rheumatic diseases. *Proc Natl Acad Sci USA*, 1981, **78**: 3190–4.
29. Podgorski M. R., Goulding N. J., Hall N. D., Flower R. J., Maddisin, P. J. Autoantibodies to lipocortin 1 are associated with impaired glucocorticoid responsiveness in rheumatoid arthritis. *J Rheumatol*, 1992, **9**: 1668–71.
30. Munck A., Naray Fejes-Toth A. The ups and downs of glucocorticoid physiology. Permissive and suppressive effects revisited. *Mol Cell Endocrinol*, 1992, **90**: C1—C4.
31. Blauer K. L., Poth M., Rogers W. M., Bernton E. W. Dehydroepiandrosterone antagonises the suppressive effects of dexamethasone on lymphocyte proliferation. *Endocrinology*, 1991, **129**: 3147–56.
32. Di Sanot E., Sironi M., Mennini T., Zinett M., Savoldi G., Lorenzo D., Ghezzi P. A glucocorticoid receptor-independent mechanism for neurosteroid inhibition of tumour necrosis factor production. *Eur J Pharmacol*, 1996, **299**: 179–86.

Chapter 9

Hypothalamo–Pituitary–Adrenal Activity in Experimental Models of Autoimmune–Inflammatory Disease

Michael S. Harbuz, David S. Jessop and Stafford L. Lightman

Bristol Royal Infirmary, Marlborough Street, Bristol, UK.

9.1 INTRODUCTION

The question as to why one individual is susceptible to an autoimmune or inflammatory condition while another is resistant is intriguing (1). It is apparent from the tendency of particular diseases to cluster within families that there are genetic components which predispose an individual to disease. However, concordance in identical twins falls well short of 100% in common immunologically-mediated inflammatory diseases (e.g. rheumatoid arthritis, systemic lupus erythematosus and multiple sclerosis) suggesting that genetic factors, in themselves, are not necessarily sufficient to initiate the development of such conditions and that other intrinsic or extrinsic factors are required. The nature of these

Stress, Stress Hormones and the Immune System. Edited by J. C. Buckingham, G. E. Gillies and A.-M. Cowell
© 1997 John Wiley & Sons, Ltd.

factors is largely unknown although there is evidence that viruses and other infectious organisms may be important in this regard. Geographical factors are also undoubtedly involved and it is striking, for example, that the incidence of multiple sclerosis is principally confined to the northern and southern latitudes with only a very low incidence in equatorial regions. Relatively little is known also of the factors which determine the severity of the disease and the frequency and duration of remissions and relapses which are characteristic of the inflammatory conditions mentioned above.

Whatever the underlying mechanisms may be, it now seems clear that the interplay between the immune and central nervous systems fulfils a significant role in determining whether an individual develops or resists various autoimmune and inflammatory diseases and in regulating the progress and severity of the disease. An important component of this interaction is the neuroendocrine system, especially the hypothalamo–pituitary–adrenal (HPA) axis. The endpoint of the activation of this axis is the release of glucocorticoids (corticosterone in the rat and cortisol in man) from the adrenal cortex into the general circulation. These steroid hormones, which are released in response to cognitive (e.g. cold) and non-cognitive (e.g. inflammation) stressful insults, exert widespread actions in the body which are required to maintain homeostasis (see Chapter 1); in particular, they are powerful anti-inflammatory and immunosuppressive agents and thereby serve to regulate the body's defence mechanisms and, through this, to limit the inflammatory response and protect the host tissue—for further details see Chapter 8 and (2, 3). Indeed, glucocorticoids and their synthetic analogues, provide an important weapon in the arsenal used to treat acute inflammatory episodes. In the last decade increasing attention has pointed to a role for the HPA axis in the pathogenesis of inflammatory disease and recent observations that a sustained hypersecretion of glucocorticoids ensues in certain conditions of chronic inflammation will form a central theme of this chapter.

Consideration must also be given to the other neuroendocrine axes which are sensitive to stress (see Chapter 1), in particular growth hormone and prolactin which exert pro-inflammatory actions and may counterbalance the anti-inflammatory effects of HPA axis activation. In addition, there are significant gender differences associated with many autoimmune disorders which implicate the neuroendocrine reproductive axis and gonadal steroids in modulating the pathogenesis of a number of diseases (4). The neuroendocrine system may thus exert complex influences on immune function and thereby influence the onset, progress and ultimately the severity of disease (5). This chapter will focus on our current understanding of the role of the HPA axis in relation to autoimmune–inflammatory disease, particularly at the hypothalamic level, with reference also to the influence of gonadal steroids and the expression of "neuroendocrine" peptides in the cells and tissues of the immune system.

9.2 THE HYPOTHALAMO–PITUITARY–ADRENAL (HPA) AXIS AND THE RESPONSE TO ACUTE AND REPEATED STRESS

The HPA axis, also commonly known as the stress axis, responds to a wide variety of stressors and its regulation is described in detail in Chapter 1. For the discussion here it is appropriate to remind ourselves of a few pertinent features concerning the function of this axis (Fig. 9.1). The major corticotrophin releasing

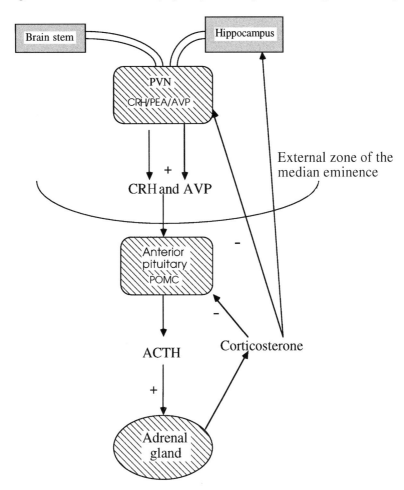

Figure 9.1 The hypothalamo–pituitary–adrenal axis. In response to an acute stress or immune activation (e.g. lipopolysaccharide or cytokines) there is an up-regulation of the components of this axis with increased levels of adrenocorticotrophic hormone (ACTH) and corticosterone, increased pro-opiomelanocortin (POMC) mRNA, and corticotrophic hormone releasing hormone (CRH) and arginine vasopressin (AVP) in the anterior pituitary and PVN respectively. PEA = proenkephalin A. See text for further details

hormone (CRH) is synthesised together with arginine vasopressin (AVP) in the parvocellular cells of the paraventricular nucleus (PVN). In normal animals approximately 50% of the CRH-positive cells are also AVP-positive, the remainder being CRH-positive/AVP-negative. The axons from these neurones terminate in the external zone of the median eminence from whence CRH and AVP are released into the hypophysial portal blood and carried to the anterior pituitary gland where they have a synergistic action to evoke the release of the adrenocorticotrophic hormone (ACTH) into the general circulation. CRH is considered as the principal corticotrophin-releasing factor in many species as it is currently the only factor demonstrated to induce the expression of pro-opiomelanocortin (POMC) mRNA, which encodes the precursor molecule for ACTH. ACTH in turn acts on the adrenal cortex to stimulate the synthesis and the release of the glucocorticoids. The activity of the axis is negatively regulated by the glucocorticoids which act on the anterior pituitary gland, the hypothalamus and elsewhere in the central nervous system to block the release of ACTH and its hypothalamic releasing factors.

Exposure of an individual to acute stress, for example a novel environment or an immune challenge—e.g. injection of lipopolysaccharide (LPS) or cytokines such as interleukin-1 (IL-1) or tumour necrosis factor α—results in increased activity at all levels of the HPA axis (see also Chapters 1 and 13). Thus, there is an increased expression of CRH and AVP mRNAs in the PVN, increased release of CRH and AVP into the hypophysial portal blood, increased POMC mRNA and protein in the anterior pituitary gland and increased circulating levels of ACTH and corticosterone. When the stress is removed the overactivity of the axis abates and the circulating levels of glucocorticoids thus return to the resting level. The HPA response may be further modified by other neuronal populations within the hypothalamus which produce factors such as proenkephalin A and oxytocin and may be differentially activated depending on the nature and intensity of the stimulus. There is thus a complex, multifactorial control mechanism operating at the hypothalamic level to integrate signals transmitted either neurally or hormonally from the periphery to co-ordinate the release of a cocktail of releasing factors into the portal blood.

The HPA responses to chronic stress are less well-defined than those triggered by an acute stress. Most of the experimental chronic stress paradigms employed to date involve the repetition of an acute stress on several successive days. In many, but not all, instances tolerance may develop. Cross-tolerance may also occur with certain types of stress. In other instances, however, exposure to a novel acute stress during a phase of adaptation to the original stress may even result in a supra-normal stress response, suggesting that the system as a whole does not become refractory in these repeated stress paradigms. (For further details see Chapter 1.)

The HPA responses to sustained chronic stress (i.e. where the stressor is not removed) differ markedly from those elicited by daily repeated stress as, in the former condition, the levels of glucocorticoids in the circulation are likely to be elevated continuously. For this reason, experimental protocols involving repeated stresses do not provide accurate models of sustained stress (e.g. inflammatory disease). The mechanisms which allow the HPA axis to continue to respond to an acute stressful stimulus in the face of persistent elevations in circulating glucocorticoid levels are, as yet, unknown but it must be concluded that, in these circumstances, the stress-induced trans-synaptic activation of neurones in the PVN is able to overcome the negative feedback actions exerted by the glucocorticoids (see Chapter 1).

A further paradox lies in the acute and long-term influences of glucocorticoids on the HPA responses to IL-1β. As may be expected, the immediate rise in circulating glucocorticoids (brought about by injection of, e.g., dexamethasone) quells the HPA response to a single intraperitoneal injection of IL-1β; similarly, adrenalectomy augments while dexamethasone depresses the IL-1β-stimulated secretion of CRH and AVP by isolated rat hypothalami *in vitro*. However, the increases in ACTH release and CRH mRNA expression observed *in vivo* following a single injection of IL-1β are abolished by long-term adrenalectomy in rats but restored by steroid replacement, a phenomenon which may reflect the longer term ability of glucocorticoids to upregulate IL-1 receptors.

Clearly much remains to be learnt about the regulation of HPA function in chronic stress. In the following sections we describe evidence from studies performed in man and in animal models of immune-mediated, chronic inflammatory disease which point to alterations in HPA status as a consequence and as a potential causal factor in inflammatory disease.

9.3 THE HPA AXIS IN EXPERIMENTAL INFLAMMATORY CONDITIONS

Inflammatory diseases may be considered as a chronic stress and it is therefore not surprising that animals with experimentally-induced chronic inflammation generally exhibit sustained elevations in circulating glucocorticoids. This section will summarise work which aimed to determine whether dysfunction of the HPA axis contributes to the development and/or to the progression of inflammatory disease.

9.3.1 HPA Responses to Chronic Inflammation

Adjuvant induced arthritis (AA) is a model which has been used extensively for studies on pain, inflammation, arthritis and Reiter's syndrome. It is a T cell-dependent inflammatory disease which is readily induced in susceptible strains of rat by a single intradermal injection of ground, heat-killed *Mycobacterium butyricum* in paraffin oil into the base of the tail. The animals begin to develop hind paw inflammation within 12–14 days of the injection which subsequently spreads to other joints to reach a maximum severity approximately 21 days after injection (6).

The changes which occur at pituitary and adrenal levels on the development of AA are similar to those elicited by an acute or repeated stress paradigm, i.e. increased plasma ACTH and corticosterone concentrations together with raised levels of POMC mRNA in the anterior pituitary gland. It appears, therefore, that in the inflammatory situation, the sustained hypersecretion of glucocorticoids fails to suppress the release of ACTH, i.e. the negative feedback has been overcome. The AA-induced elevation in circulating corticosterone is most pronounced in the morning when levels in the rat would normally be at their circadian nadir. The normal circadian rhythm is thus lost and the animal is continually exposed to raised levels of corticosterone. The loss of the circadian rhythm may have important consequences on immune function as a number of immune parameters mirror the circadian changes in circulating levels of ACTH and glucocorticoids. These include alterations in natural killer cell activity, cytokine expression and lymphocyte counts.

In contrast to the situation in acute stresses, AA does not increase the expression of CRH mRNA in the hypothalamic PVN. Indeed, in the Piebald-Viral-Glaxo (PVG) and Lewis strains of rat the AA-induced increase in hind paw inflammation is associated with a consistent decrease in CRH mRNA in the PVN (6). This paradoxical decrease in CRH mRNA emerges with the first indications of inflammation (around day 11) and reaches a nadir at the time of peak inflammation (day 21). The release of the mature CRH peptide into the hypophysial portal blood is also decreased, suggesting a reduced activity of CRH neurones. In contrast, the expression of AVP mRNA in the parvocellular cells of the PVN is increased in animals with AA, as also is the release of AVP into the portal blood, suggesting that AVP takes over as the major stimulator of the axis. As noted above CRH is the only factor hitherto shown to increase POMC mRNA in the anterior pituitary, so in the chronic immune-mediated disease model of AA the mechanisms controlling the activation of the HPA axis are clearly altered. Whether this represents a fundamental alteration in the regulation of POMC mRNA synthesis by the corticotrophs or whether POMC transcription can be initiated by permissive levels of CRH remains to be determined.

A reduction in CRH mRNA expression in the PVN and concomitant increase in corticotroph POMC mRNA expression has also been reported in the rat model of adoptively transferred experimental allergic encephalomyelitis (EAE) which is used to study features of multiple sclerosis. In this model naive animals are inoculated with activated splenocytes from a donor animal previously injected with myelin basic protein in adjuvant. A similar profile of HPA responses has been reported in rats which develop a condition resembling eosinophilia myalgia syndrome, another T cell-mediated disease which is characterised by muscle pain and oedema followed by muscle and connective tissue inflammation and peripheral neuropathy. These data therefore suggest that, irrespective of the nature of the challenge, the sustained activation of the HPA axis which occurs in T cell-mediated disease is associated with a paradoxical decrease in CRH activity in the PVN. Further work is required to establish the prevalence and implication of this perturbation in HPA function (7).

9.3.2 Correlation of Strain Differences in HPA Activity and Disease Susceptibility

The Lewis strain of rat exhibits marked defects in HPA activity which are characterised by a blunted circadian rhythm and greatly attenuated response to stress (8). Thus, in comparison with the histocompatible Fischer strain, Lewis rats show significant reductions in their corticosteroid, ACTH and CRH responses to a number of inflammatory and other stressful stimuli; in addition, the adrenal and pituitary glands are smaller than those of controls while thymus weight is increased. The impairment of HPA activity in the Lewis rat is associated with a high susceptibility to a number of experimentally-induced autoimmune diseases such as arthritis (AA, collagen-induced and streptococcal cell wall-induced arthritis), EAE and experimental myasthenia gravis (compared to controls). However, the onset or the progression of disease may be halted effectively by administration of glucocorticoids (8). A body of evidence suggests that the HPA defect in the disease-susceptible Lewis strain of rats resides, at least in part, at the pituitary level as evidenced by the paucity of corticotrophs, the reduction in basal POMC mRNA expression, the blunted peak ACTH response to CRH and the enhanced sensitivity of the corticotrophs to the inhibitory actions of the glucocorticoids. Other data suggest that alterations in hypothalamic CRH are also important. Certainly, the expression of CRH mRNA in the PVN is reduced and the ability of hypothalami from Lewis rats to release CRH in response to neurochemical stimuli *in vitro* is impaired. On the other hand, plasma and hypothalamic AVP levels are raised in the Lewis strain, suggesting an attempted compensation for low levels of CRH. These findings have led to suggestions that a hyporesponsive HPA axis may predispose individuals to autoimmune disease (8). This view is supported by the evidence that strains such as the Fischer and PVG strains, which are able to mount a robust HPA response to stress, are resistant to streptococcal cell wall-induced arthritis and EAE respectively. However, the situation is more complicated and depends to some extent on the nature of the inflammatory stimulus. Thus, despite the resistance of the PVG strain to EAE, it is susceptible to AA. Interestingly, the robust response of the PVG rat to an acute stressor is lost when the animals have hind paw inflammation, suggesting that the feedback mechanism is indeed intact. The failure to respond to acute stimulation in such conditions may have profound implications for the ability of the organism to cope with, for example, secondary infections and stresses, which may in turn compromise the individual.

HPA dysfunction has also been noted in strains of several other species that are susceptible to inflammatory disease, indicating a fundamental cross-species role for the HPA axis in the pathogenesis of these conditions. For example, in the obese strain of chicken, which develops an autoimmune thyroiditis, the circulating levels of corticosteroid binding globulin are increased with a consequent decrease in free corticosterone. These animals have a blunted HPA response to IL-1 and other stimulants. Their adrenal glands however respond normally to ACTH, suggesting that the defect resides at the hypothalamo–pituitary level although the precise locus remains to be determined. Attenuated HPA activity is also a feature of inbred mouse strains which develop diseases similar to systemic lupus erythematosus and Sjögren's syndrome. These susceptible strains show an age-related decline in plasma corticosterone, which parallels the development of disease, together with blunted HPA responses to IL-1 and other provocative stimuli.

9.3.3 Importance of HPA Axis Integrity on Disease Activity

The importance of the HPA axis to the integrity of the individual has been demonstrated in many studies (1, 6–11). Removal of the adrenal glands and hence the source of the anti-inflammatory glucocorticoid by adrenalectomy is life-threatening in acute and chronic situations involving immune activation. Injection of cytokines (e.g. IL-1) or LPS, at doses that are sub-lethal in normal animals, can be fatal when given to adrenalectomised rats or mice. Similarly, adrenalectomy results in an earlier onset and greater severity of disease in both AA and EAE in the rat (Fig. 9.2). If left to run its course, the effects of

---

Figure 9.2 Adrenalectomy prevents recovery from experimental allergic encephalomyelitis (EAE). Active EAE was induced by immunization with 50 μg myelin basic protein (MPB) in Freund's complete adjuvant (FCA) on day 0. For passive EAE, spleen cells from MBP/FCA-primed donors were cultured *in vitro* with MBP and 5×10^7 cells were injected intravenously into naive recipients on day 0. Animals were bilaterally adrenalectomised or sham operated 3 d before immunisation or cell transfer, normal basal levels of serum corticosterone being maintained in adrenalectomised rats by subcutaneous steroid implants. For active EAE there were nine control and 10 adrenalectomised animals. For passive EAE there were five control and three adrenalectomised animals. The mean clinical scores apply only to surviving animals. —●— Sham-operated controls; – – ○ – – adrenalectomised; † death. Reproduced from I. A. M. Macphee *et al.*, *The Journal of Experimental Medicine*, 1989, **169**: 437, by copyright permission of The Rockefeller University Press

a Active EAE

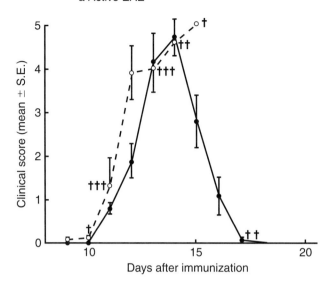

Days after immunization

b Passive EAE

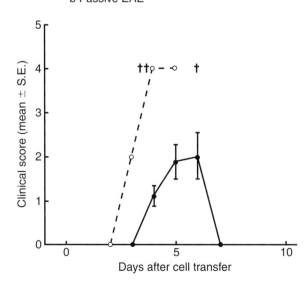

Days after cell transfer

adrenalectomy in these disease models are fatal. Experimental arthritis can also be induced by adrenalectomy or treatment with glucocorticoid antagonists in strains of rat which are normally disease resistant. Conversely, treatment with steroids at physiological doses reduces the severity of disease in susceptible strains and prevents death in adrenalectomised rats. It has been demonstrated in many studies that glucocorticoids are able to suppress a number of host defence mechanisms such as decreasing cytokine production, natural killer cell activity, lymphocyte proliferation and antibody formation (see also Chapter 8). The physiological relevance of these actions were addressed by Munck and colleagues (2) who proposed that "stress-induced increases in glucocorticoid levels protect not against the source of the stress itself but rather against the body's normal reactions to stress, preventing those reactions from overshooting and themselves threatening homeostasis". The available evidence supports the notion that higher organisms have developed defensive immune reactions of such ferocity which, if left unchecked, will run to their natural conclusion resulting in the death of the host organism.

Taken together, the results discussed above provide a body of evidence supporting the view that alterations in HPA function contribute to the development and progression of a wide range of chronic immune-related diseases. The data from animal studies suggest that changes in HPA function may occur as a consequence of the disease process and represent a chronic adaptation. In addition, a congenital perturbation in HPA activity may predispose to disease susceptibility. It is unclear whether such a phenomenon contributes to disease susceptibility in man but considerable evidence, discussed below and in Chapters 18 and 19, suggests that the alterations in HPA activity provoked by various stresses can influence the disease process markedly.

9.4 HPA ACTIVITY IN CLINICAL INFLAMMATORY DISEASE

There are reports of aberrant HPA activity in patients with inflammatory conditions. For example, an inability to mount a cortisol response to the stress of surgery has been described in patients with rheumatoid arthritis. However, when challenged with exogenous CRH, such patients show a normal increase in plasma ACTH as also do those with multiple sclerosis, suggesting that pituitary function is intact in these patients. In accord with findings in animal models, that the role of AVP in regulating ACTH secretion is increased in conditions of T cell mediated disease, the ACTH response to AVP is increased in patients with multiple sclerosis. There are, however, conflicting reports in the literature on HPA activity in patients with rheumatoid arthritis and interpretation of data is inevitably complicated by drug therapy with glucocorticoids or non-steroidal anti-inflammatory drugs which would interfere with prostaglandin synthesis and the HPA responses to cytokines and other stimuli (see Chapters 1 and 13).

Patients suffering from the potentially lethal disease of African sleeping sickness, which is caused by the parasite *Trypanosoma brucei*, are unable to mount appropriate cortisol responses to exogenous CRH or ACTH, suggesting that adrenal function is impaired. However, normal adrenal function is restored on recovery, suggesting that the observed adrenal insufficiency is a consequence of the disease rather than a lesion which predisposed the individual to illness, as suggested for the Lewis strain of rat (see Section 9.3.2).

9.5   STRESS AND THE DISEASE PROCESS

We have seen that the activity of the HPA axis is compromised in a variety of autoimmune disorders. Furthermore we have seen that the ability of an organism to respond to an acute stressful challenge is blunted in these situations. But what effect do stressful stimuli have on the development or the severity of autoimmune diseases? Despite improvements in our ability to control the environment of experimental animals and to reduce the number of variables inherent to investigations on stress, animal studies have produced conflicting results. In the rat various stressful stimuli have been shown to suppress the development of EAE, AA and collagen-induced arthritis. By contrast, some investigators have reported that stress increases severity and advances the onset of both EAE and collagen-induced arthritis. These discrepancies may be due to differences in the strain of rat used and the stress paradigms employed by different research groups. As noted earlier, the activation of central systems is dependent on the type, duration and frequency of the stress (see also Chapter 1). In addition, the ability of the individual to "cope" may be an important factor. Thus, the past history of the experimental animals (feeding, environment, handling, infections etc.) may also be crucial and disease susceptibility may even be dependent on the bacterial flora to which particular strains of rat are exposed. This raises the possibility that exposure to environmental factors at an early age may affect the subsequent resistance or susceptibility balance. In man there is growing evidence that major life events such as the death of a loved one, divorce or separation can result in the onset or increase the severity of a number of diseases such as rheumatoid arthritis, insulin-dependent diabetes, uveitis, Crohn's disease and Grave's disease. The immune consequences of these stressors, whether in animals or man, are not fully understood but it is quite possible that the duration and the timing of glucocorticoid release in response to stress is of fundamental importance in determining the disease outcome.

9.6   INTERACTIONS OF THE STRESS AND REPRODUCTIVE AXES: A FACTOR IN AUTOIMMUNE AND INFLAMMATORY DISEASE?

There is a high degree of communication between the HPA and the hypothalamo–pituitary–gonadal (HPG) axes. Stress inhibits the HPG axis at multiple levels and glucocorticoids also inhibit the effects of sex steroids at many sites. The sex steroids also modulate the activity of the HPA axis. The HPA axis is thus more active in the female than the male, a phenomenon which may relate to the presence of an oestrogen responsive element in the 5' regulatory region of the CRH gene and to the ability of these steroids to augment the neurochemically evoked release of the releasing hormone. Paradoxically, however, in light of the theory that hypo-responsiveness predisposes to autoimmune diseases, females show a greater incidence of disease, shown for example by the female:male ratios for autoimmune thyroiditis (19:1), systemic lupus erythematosus (9:1) and rheumatoid arthritis (4:1). The increase in arthritic flares associated with the post-partum period of pregnancy and changes in disease activity associated with the menstrual cycle strongly implicate gonadal steroids in autoimmune disease. Gonadal competence may be a major factor. Young females are very much more susceptible to rheumatoid arthritis than young males but with increased age the ratio approaches parity. It has been suggested that testosterone has a protective effect in males; there is a decrease in testosterone with age and lowered testosterone levels have been reported in men with rheumatoid arthritis and in experimental animals with adjuvant arthritis. Castration increases the incidence and severity of experimental arthritis in male rats and these effects can be reversed by testosterone treatment. The side-effects associated with testosterone preclude its use clinically, but the increased availability of testosterone analogues with little or no endocrine activity may prove beneficial.

The role of oestrogens is more complex and the effects appear to vary depending on the disease in question. In experimental animals, oestrogen suppresses T cell-dependent conditions such as adjuvant- and collagen-induced arthritis while accelerating the progress of systemic lupus erythematosus. This apparent anomaly may be due to the effects of oestrogen enhancing the B cell (antibody) response, while decreasing T cell-mediated immunity. Testosterone suppresses both B and T cell responses. EAE, AA and collagen-induced arthritis are considered to be T cell mediated disease models. The site of action of the gonadal steroids and the mechanism by which they exert these actions remains to be determined.

Interestingly, female Lewis and Fischer strains of rats have significant differences in their HPG activity, with the former having increased oestrogen and progesterone levels in their circulation. As these steroids are known to enhance both cellular and humoral immunity, their effects on disease susceptibility could be exerted directly. Equally, however, they could affect immune function indirectly via the HPA axis as they have been shown to alter central glucocorticoid and mineralocorticoid receptor expression.

9.7 THE ROLE FOR "NEUROENDOCRINE" PEPTIDES IN THE PERIPHERY

It is now clear that many neuroendocrine peptides, including those which are involved in HPA regulation (namely CRH, AVP and the POMC-derived peptides α-melanocyte stimulating hormone and β-endorphin), along with their receptors, are expressed within the cells and tissues of the immune system (see also Chapters 10, 11, 16, 17) and should therefore be considered as potential local modulators of the inflammatory responses. However, unlike the HPA axis where stress hormones are stored in large amounts in pools for ready release, immune cells normally store only very small amounts of these peptides but synthesise them on demand, for example on stimulation with mitogens such as concanavalin A. This is consistent with the concept that stress hormones expressed in immune tissues may fulfil physiologically relevant roles in the face of an immune challenge (Fig. 9.3); some experimental findings supporting this view will be discussed briefly.

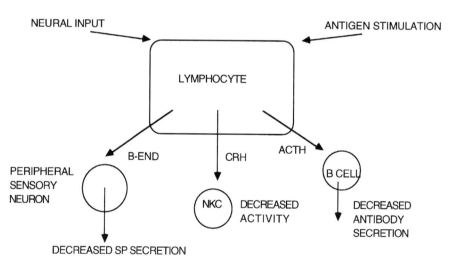

Figure 9.3 Ways in which immunoneuropeptides could control an inflammatory response. Note: both pro- and anti-inflammatory properties have been ascribed to some immunoneuropeptides and thus their actions may be concentration-dependent. B-END, beta-endorphin; SP, substance P; CRH, corticotrophin releasing hormone; ACTH, adrenocorticotrophic hormone; NKC, natural killer cell

CRH immunoreactivity and CRH mRNA are present in synovial tissues taken from rats with experimental arthritis and humans with rheumatoid arthritis. CRH has been shown to stimulate B lymphocyte proliferation, increase cytokine production and increase natural killer cell activity *in vitro*. Immunoneutralisation of the peripheral actions of CRH in experimental models of inflammation results in a decrease in inflammatory exudate volume and cellularity. Together these data support the notion that CRH subserves a pro-inflammatory role in the periphery; however, its site and mechanism of action have yet to be determined. In addition to being produced locally by activated immune cells, CRH may also be delivered to inflamed joints by peripheral nerves. Such a view is supported by evidence that CRH is present in the dorsal sensory and sympathetic interomediolateral columns of the spinal cord and also in the dorsal root and sympathetic ganglia, all of which influence the severity of inflammation in experimental arthritis. Although the bulk of evidence available suggests that the actions of CRH in the periphery are immune-enhancing, there are other data which advocate a direct (i.e. glucocorticoid-independent) immunosuppressive action of the peptide and additional work is now needed to clarify its precise role in the periphery. (For further details see Chapters 10 and 11.)

In rats with adjuvant arthritis the opioid peptides, β-endorphin and met-enkephalin, are abundant in immune cells in inflamed tissue but absent in normal tissue. These opioids exert local anti-nociceptive effects, possibly by inhibiting the release of the inflammatory peptide substance P from nerve terminals in the inflamed tissue (Fig. 9.3) and may therefore fulfil a protective role when released from activated lymphocytes. Rats with adjuvant induced hind paw inflammation exhibit increases in the splenic content of CRH, AVP, ACTH and β-endorphin, demonstrating that "immunoneuropeptide" production is altered by this chronic inflammatory stress. However, while the increases in splenic ACTH are evident as early as day 3 after adjuvant injection, the increases in splenic AVP and CRH do not emerge until day 14, suggesting that the rise in ACTH is independent of a local increase in CRH or AVP. This concept of differential regulation of immune and anterior pituitary POMC-derived products by CRH is further supported by evidence that the stimulation of immune POMC by CRH is not direct, as it is at the pituitary, but mediated through the release of IL-1.

Little is known about the activation of immunoneuropeptides in man. However, in one study an acute stress (insulin-induced hypoglycaemia) caused an increase in leukocyte ACTH content while in a case of ectopic Cushing's syndrome the elevated plasma ACTH concentration was reduced by the removal of a mass of lymphoid tissue which stained positively for ACTH. Thus, some conditions can result in the stimulation of POMC expression in the human immune system.

9.8 CONCLUSIONS

In summary, we are only just beginning to understand the complex interactions between the neuroendocrine and immune systems, particularly in relation to autoimmune and inflammatory disease. In the last decade, the accumulation of evidence that neuropeptides are expressed in immune tissues and may directly influence the progression of a chronic inflammatory response, together with knowledge that cytokines are synthesised in the central nervous system where they exert important regulatory actions, has broken down the rigid boundaries which once existed between neuroendocrinology and immunology. Much of the phenomenology has now been completed. Hence, the increasing numbers of scientists drawn from both disciplines to the new discipline of neuroendocrine-immunology now face the exciting challenges of unravelling the factors and mechanisms that confer susceptibility or resistance to inflammatory disease and those that modulate the progression and severity of the condition.

REFERENCES

1. Olliver W., Symmons D. P. M. *Autoimmunity*. Oxford, BIOS Scientific Publishers Ltd., 1992.
2. Munck A., Guyre P. M., Holbrook N. J. Physiological functions of glucocorticoids in stress and their relation to pharmacological actions. *Endocr Rev*, 1984, **5**: 25.
3. Bateman A., Singh A., Kral T., Solomon S. The immune hypothalamic–pituitary–adrenal axis. *Endocr Rev*, 1989, **10**: 92.
4. Harbuz M. S., Lightman S. L. Stress and the hypothalamic–pituitary–adrenal axis: acute, chronic and immunological activation. *J Endocrinol*, 1992, **134**: 327.
5. Wick G., Hu Y., Schwarz S., Kroemer G. Immunoendocrine communication via the hypothalamo–pituitary–adrenal axis in autoimmune disease. *Endocr Rev*, 1993, **14**: 539.
6. Rook G. A. W., Hernandez-Pando R., Lightman S. L. Hormones, peripherally acting prohormones and regulation of the Th1/Th2 balance. *Immunol Today*, 1994, **15**: 301.
7. Chrousos G. P., Gold P. W. The concepts of stress and stress system disorders:overview of physical and behavioural homeostasis. *JAMA*, 1992, **267**: 1244–52.
8. Derijk R., Sternberg E. M. Corticosteroid action and neuroendocrine-immune interactions. *Ann N Y Acad Sci*, 1994, **746**: 33–41.
9. Wilder R. L. Neuroendocrine-immune system interactions and autoimmunity. *Ann Rev Immunol*, 1995, **13**: 307.
10. Ader R., Cohen N., Felten D. Psychoneuroimmunology: interactions between the nervous system and the immune system. *Lancet*, 1995, **345**: 99.
11. Wilckens T. Glucocorticoids and immune function: physiological relevance and pathogenic potential of hormonal dysfunction. *Trends Pharmacol Sci*, 1995, **16**: 193–7.

Chapter 10

Expression, Biological Actions and Receptors for Stress Peptides within the Immune System

Edward W. Hillhouse and Dimitris Grammatopoulos

The University of Warwick, Coventry, UK

10.1 INTRODUCTION

The central nervous regulation of immune function via the autonomic (principally the sympathetic division) and neuroendocrine systems has been discussed in the preceding chapters. The activation of these systems by stress leads to the manifestation of a series of adaptive responses which are integrated at the hypothalamic level and typically include stimulation of the sympathetic nervous system and the hypothalamo–pituitary–adrenal (HPA) axis together with alterations in behavioural activity and in cellular and humoral immune responses. The precise effects of stress on immune function are complex and depend not only on the nature of the stress and the individual but also on the duration and intensity of the stress. The predominant effect of acute stress on immune function appears to be one of suppression whilst the consequences of chronic stress are relatively poorly understood and may be influenced by the activation of various adaptive mechanisms. Repeated mild stress may, however, enhance immune function and autoimmune diseases may be aggravated by stress.

Although the precise molecular mechanisms whereby stress influences immune function remain uncertain, there is growing evidence that the molecular messengers of the HPA axis can interact with and modulate the immune system.

Stress, Stress Hormones and the Immune System. Edited by J. C. Buckingham, G. E. Gillies and A.-M. Cowell
© 1997 John Wiley & Sons, Ltd.

Similarly the products of activated immune cells profoundly influence the activity of the HPA axis (see Chapters 1, 13). Indeed, the neuroendocrine and immune systems appear to have evolved a common biochemical code based on the exploitation of common chemical messenger and receptor mechanisms. This may have emerged in order to simplify communication between these two highly complex systems and the phylogenetic conservation of vital stress and immune peptides supports the premise that these molecules fulfil fundamental roles in the adaptive responses to stress and, hence, in promoting the survival of the individual. The aim of this chapter is first to review the evidence that peptides associated with the stress axis are also produced by cells of the immune system and secondly to discuss the possible roles of these peptides in host defence processes and in certain disease states where immune cell activity is affected.

10.2 STRESS PEPTIDES AND THEIR RECEPTORS IN IMMUNE CELLS

Numerous studies have suggested that the principal signalling molecules of the hypothalamo–pituitary stress axis are also expressed by cells of the immune system. The quantities of peptides produced by these cells, however, are small suggesting that their predominant role may be autocrine, paracrine or intracrine (i.e. within cells). Evidence in support of this assumption has been provided by the observation that immune cells, in particular lymphocytes and macrophages, express specific, high affinity and saturable binding sites for many of the neuroendocrine peptides. In general immune cells do not store "stress peptides" but synthesise them *de novo* as required via processes which take several hours. The small amounts of peptides synthesised may reach high concentrations locally. However, they are unlikely to be released in sufficient quantities to produce classical "endocrine" effects within the body although it is conceivable that they exploit the mobility of immune cells and may thus be delivered to distant sites when required. Details of the peptides and peptide receptors expressed by immune cells, together with their putative roles in the regulation of immune cell function, are summarised in Tables 10.1 and 10.2 and are discussed in more detail below.

10.2.1 Corticotrophin Releasing Hormone (CRH)

Expression of CRH

Brodish (1) provided the first evidence for the existence of extra hypothalamic corticotrophin releasing factors in the blood of stressed rats. This was followed by studies which showed that monkey thymus extracts contain CRH-like

Table 10.1 Expression of stress peptides within the immune system ir-CRH, immunoreactive corticotrophin releasing hormone; AVP, arginine vasopressin; POMC, pro-opiomelanocortin; ir-ACTH, immunoreactive corticotrophin

Cell type	Hypothalamic peptides	POMC-derived peptides
Macrophages	CRH mRNA	POMC mRNA (spleen)
	ir-CRH-authentic	ir-ACTH, β-endorphin
Fibroblasts	CRH mRNA	
	ir-CRH-authentic	
Endothelial cells	CRH mRNA	
	ir-CRH-authentic	
T-lymphocytes	CRH mRNA	POMC mRNA (spleen)
	ir-CRH-authentic	ir-ACTH, β-endorphin
	ir-CRH-novel form	
B-lymphocyte	ir-CRH	ACTH (1-39)
		Truncated ACTH (1-25)
		α, β, γ endorphin
Leukocytes	CRH mRNA	ACTH
Thymus	CRH mRNA	
	ir-CRH-authentic, ir-AVP	
	ir-CRH-novel form	

bioactivity which is clearly distinguishable from immunoreactive CRH (ir-CRH) of hypothalamic origin. Further *in vivo* and *in vitro* studies provided evidence for a CRH-like substance in immune cells and in inflamed tissues which can activate the HPA axis (2). Since then further studies have confirmed the presence of bioactive and ir-CRH-like material together with CRH mRNA in cells of the immune system. These include splenic macrophages, thymic cells and peripheral blood lymphocytes and monocytes.

Human leukocytes appear to express a form of CRH mRNA which is larger than the hypothalamic CRH mRNA and which is translated into a peptide with a chromatographic profile which differs from that of human hypothalamic CRH (3). In contrast, human T lymphocytes show mitogen-induced expression of a CRH mRNA which is similar in size to rat hypothalamic CRH MRNA and which is translated into material with biochemical and immunological characteristics that closely resemble those of synthetic human hypothalamic CRH. In addition, however, the T lymphocytes secrete at least three other ir-CRH-like molecules which can be separated from the main CRH component by high performance liquid chromatography (HPLC). Careful measurements on subcellular fractions have shown that ir-CRH is distributed in several T cell compartments, with a particular concentration in the cell nucleus. This is interesting in view of recent work which has shown that pro-CRH expressed in stably transfected Chinese hamster ovary cells is translocated to the nucleus where it remains in close association with DNA and chromatin (5). The biological function of this nuclear

Table 10.2 Receptors for stress hormones on cells of the immune system and modulation of immune responses. CRH, corticotrophin releasing hormone; AVP, arginine vasopressin; ACTH, corticotrophin

Hormone receptors	Cell type	Modulating effect
CRH	– murine spleen macrophages – human T helper lymphocytes – human peripheral blood lymphocytes	– enhanced natural killer cell activity – immunosuppressive – interleukin production
AVP (V_1 and V_2)	– human peripheral blood lymphocytes – mouse splenic lymphocytes – thymic lymphoma derived murine T cells	– stimulation of interferon γ
Opioids-Endorphins	– murine spleno- and lymphocytes – human lympho- and leukocytes – thymoma cells – rat splenic T lymphocytes – transformed B lymphocytes	– enhancement of lymphocyte and macrophage cytotoxicity – modulation (stimulation or inhibition) of T cell mitogenesis – enhancement of T cell rosetting – stimulation of human peripheral blood monocyte cells – inhibition of major histocompatability class II antigen expression – enhancement of lymphocyte proliferation
ACTH	– rat B and T lymphocytes – human peripheral blood lymphocytes – mouse spleen cells	– suppression of interferon γ production – modulation of B lymphocyte growth and differentiation – suppression of T cell dependent antibody responses – stimulation of mitogenesis and protein secretion events

pro-CRH is at the moment uncertain although it appears likely that it exerts regulatory effects on gene expression or cell proliferation.

Similar studies have shown that a CRH mRNA similar to the hypothalamic species is expressed by rat thymus and spleen. Furthermore, the rat thymus secretes both authentic and novel immunoreactive and bioactive forms of CRH. The synthesis of the novel form is regulated by interferon (IFN) inducing agents (6) and the active peptide has been shown to stimulate the secretion of adrenocorticotrophic hormone (ACTH), prostaglandin E_2 (PGE_2) and $PGF_{2\alpha}$

both *in vivo* and *in vitro*. In contrast, spleen cells do not secrete CRH when stimulated with IFN-inducing agents but respond to prostaglandin-inducing drugs by secreting a substance, or substances, which initiates the production of both CRH and PGE_2 by the hypothalamus. Thus, a mechanism has evolved which may allow augmentation of HPA activity at multiple sites during an immune response. Studies on the characterisation, purification and *in vitro* translation of the novel CRH produced by rat thymic cells (6) have shown that the secreted form exists as a dimer of a 15 kDa protein which shares important biological and immunological properties with hypothalamic CRH (5 kDa).

Immunoreactive CRH is readily detectable in inflamed tissues. It appears to originate from the immune accessory cells such as macrophages, fibroblasts and endothelial cells, all of which have been shown to express CRH mRNA and ir-CRH during inflammatory reactions. Once again, molecular analysis has revealed multiple CRH isoforms with HPLC profiles similar to those of the ir-CRHs derived from T lymphocytes. The relative contribution of these CRH-like molecules to the inflammatory process is uncertain although there is evidence for a pro-inflammatory action (7) which is discussed in more detail below (see page 247).

Conclusive evidence regarding the nature of immune cell-derived CRH is still awaited. It appears likely, however, that immune cells synthesise and secrete both authentic and novel forms of CRH which may play important roles in the integration of immune and neuroendocrine responses to inflammation. Further evidence for novel CRHs in immune cells is discussed in Chapter 11.

Receptors for CRH

Receptors for CRH have been identified and characterised on murine spleen macrophages (8) and on human T-helper lymphocytes and monocyte/macrophages (9). In the mouse spleen, CRH receptors are localised to the macrophage-rich marginal zones and red pulp regions. These high affinity membrane-bound CRH receptors resemble those in the anterior pituitary gland in that they are functionally linked to adenylyl cyclase via a guanine nucleotide binding protein (see also Chapters 1 and 4) and have an apparent molecular weight of 75 kDa as opposed to 58 kDa for the brain CRH receptor. Although the precise role of the CRH receptors in these cells has not been determined, the presence of CRH immunoreactivity in primary sensory afferent nerves and in human peripheral blood lymphocytes indicates that CRH may be released locally by neurosecretion or by paracrine secretion from leukocytes; it may thus gain access to CRH receptors expressed on peripheral immune cells and thereby play a functional role in modulating immune function.

Recent work (10) has shown that certain tissues express multiple isoforms of the CRH receptor which belongs to the predicted 7-transmembrane G-protein-coupled receptor family (see Chapter 4). It is possible that immune cells also express heterogeneic forms of the receptor which may subserve different physiological functions. Molecular cloning techniques have so far identified two CRH receptor genes (termed CRH-R1 and CRH-R2) which encode for mRNAs that exist in alternatively spliced forms (11, 12). Each of these forms may undergo further, possibly functionally important, post-translational modifications, which are tissue specific and which may vary in different physiological and pathological situations, thus giving rise to a large family of related receptor proteins. Because of the similarities between the third intracellular loops (the major determinant of the coupling of the receptors to G-proteins and adenylyl cyclase) and the C termini of the various CRH receptors, their coupling and signal transduction properties are predicted to be very similar (13). Interestingly, however, studies in which COS-7 cells have been transfected with CRH receptor cDNAs indicate that the CRH-R1 receptor is coupled efficiently to both adenylyl cyclase and phosphoinositol hydrolysis whereas the CRH-R2 receptor is poorly coupled to adenylyl cyclase and not coupled at all to phospholipase C (14). In addition, differences at the N terminus appear to alter the ligand binding properties, suggesting that the major binding determinant probably resides within the N-terminal domain. Thus, the CRH-R2 receptor, which is predominantly expressed in peripheral tissues including immune cells, has a higher affinity for sauvagine than CRH and may therefore preferentially bind novel molecular forms of CRH. Further characterisation of these and other receptor subtypes at a molecular level will undoubtedly help to elucidate the precise and probably complex role of CRH in immune cells (13).

Biological Role of CRH

Current evidence suggests that hypothalamic CRH is involved both directly and indirectly in the pathogenesis of stress-induced immunosuppression (see Chapters 1, 2 and 8). By contrast, CRH produced locally by immune cells appears to augment immune responses. The apparently contradictory roles of central and peripheral CRH may perhaps be explained by visualising two systems providing a counterbalance in the regulation of the inflammatory or immune response. The central CRH-containing neurones receive information from a wide range of stimuli and sensory modalities and serve to co-ordinate the autonomic, behavioural and endocrine responses to stress; these include activation of the sympathetic nervous system and HPA axis, both of which exert predominantly immunosuppressive actions (see Chapters 1, 3, 8 and 15). Immune cells appear to secrete CRH-like substances in response to acute stresses, such as bacterial and viral agents, but not in response to chronic stresses such as adjuvant arthritis. This immune-derived CRH stimulates lymphocyte proliferation, augments the mitogenic response and increases interleukin-2 (IL-2) receptor expression on lymphocytes (7). Furthermore, it can directly stimulate natural killer (NK) cell activity, the production of IL-1 and IL-2 by mononuclear cells *in vitro* and pro-opiomelanocortin (POMC) gene expression in lymphocytes (see also below, page 249). CRH also appears to play a role in local inflammatory reactions. Its precise role in this regard is uncertain but studies on chronic autoimmune inflammatory diseases such as experimental uveitis have provided evidence in favour of a pro-inflammatory role for CRH during the early inflammatory phase. Further evidence in support of such a view has emerged from studies demonstrating the presence of CRH mRNA and immunoreactivity in autoimmune lesions such as rheumatoid arthritis and Hashimoto's thyroiditis. CRH may also play an important role in maintaining pituitary–adrenal activity during inflammatory and infective processes. Other aspects of a role for CRH in inflammatory conditions are discussed in Chapters 9 and 11.

10.2.2 Neurohypophysial Hormones

Expression of Neurohypophysial Hormones

Several lines of evidence suggest that neurohypophysial-like peptides are involved in the regulation of immune function. Immunoreactive arginine vasopressin (ir-AVP) is located in the epithelial cells of the thymus and the plasma cells of the spleen (15). Similarly, bioactive and ir-oxytocin has been identified in the thymic epithelial cells (see also Chapter 17). Moreover, the presence of mRNAs coding for oxytocin and AVP within thymic cells suggests that both peptides are produced locally. However, conclusive evidence for the expression of authentic neurohypophysial peptides has not yet been obtained. Indeed the weight of available evidence suggests that the peptides are related but not identical. For example, ir-AVP has been identified in thymic extracts from Brattleboro rats, a strain of rat that fails to express AVP within the neurohypophysis due to deletion of a single nucleotide in exon-B of the hypothalamic AVP gene. It is possible that the defect in gene expression in the Brattleboro rat is tissue specific and that thymic AVP is thus synthesised normally; on the other hand, the gene encoding the thymic peptide may be distinct from its hypothalamic counterpart. Further studies with oxytocin monoclonal antibodies have also demonstrated clear structural differences between hypothalamic and thymic oxytocin.

Receptors for Neurohypophysial Hormones

Molecular and pharmacological studies have identified three types of AVP receptors, namely V_{1a}, V_{1b} and V_2 receptors, which exhibit 37–50% sequence homology. Binding of AVP to V_1 receptor subtypes stimulates Ca^{2+} mobilisation and breakdown of phosphoinositides whereas binding to the V_2 receptor subtype stimulates adenylyl cyclase activity and production of cyclic adenosine monophosphate (cAMP). Peripheral blood mononuclear cells express both V_1 and V_2

receptor subtypes while a thymic lymphoma derived murine T cell line (RL12-NP) has been reported to express a V_1 receptor subtype, AVP binding to which is inhibited by known V_1 receptor antagonists. In addition, a V_1-like receptor has been identified in mouse splenic lymphocytes which promotes the production of lymphokine IFN-γ via stimulation of phosphoinositides breakdown (16). It appears that the V_{1b} receptor is expressed in both the thymus and spleen, where it may mediate the effects of AVP-like peptides on immune function. Oxytocin receptors are, as yet, less well characterised. Nonetheless, specific oxytocin binding sites have been identified in the rat thymus.

Biological Role of Neurohypophysial Hormones

The biological role of immune-derived neurohypophysial peptides is not certain but they may play a role in enhancing IFN-γ production by spleen cells (16). Such production is regulated by cell to cell interactions involving T-helper and suppressor cells, and IFN-γ producing cells. The role of the helper cells is to provide IL-2 which is a requirement for IFN-γ production by spleen cells. The need for IL-2 can be overcome by either AVP or oxytocin, thus suggesting that both peptides may exhibit lymphokine activity. AVP and oxytocin also play a role in recognising self versus non-self antigens (see Chapter 17).

10.2.3   POMC-derived Peptides

The POMC gene produces a number of biologically active peptides, the most important of which are ACTH and β-endorphin (see Fig 1.2).

Expression of POMC-derived Peptides

The first observation that human leukocytes secrete an ACTH-like substance was made by Blalock and Smith in 1980 (17). This was an extremely important advance which opened up the whole new field of neuroendocrine immunology. The next decade saw an explosion of publications on POMC gene and product expression in immune cells. Much debate has revolved around the central question as to whether immune cells express authentic POMC or a similar protein. Immune cells undoubtedly express POMC gene-related transcripts which are translated into biologically active β-endorphin and ACTH-like peptides. Studies utilising *in situ* hybridisation and immunocytochemistry have detected POMC gene expression and β-endorphin immunoreactivity in a small population of monocyte–macrophage-like cells in the lung and spleen but not in lymphocytes in these tissues (18). These studies have led to the concept that the POMC gene is expressed by discrete populations of immune cells. The biological role of macrophage-derived POMC gene products is unknown but they may mediate local immunoregulatory functions. Interestingly, populations of macrophages within reproductive tissues also express the POMC gene (19), the products of which may play a role in testicular and ovarian function. In these tissues, however, the transcribed POMC mRNA is structurally different from that expressed in the pituitary gland or spleen. Splenic macrophages appear to contain the entire POMC exon-1 sequence, as shown by nuclease protection assay, suggesting that these cell types express a full length POMC RNA transcript which is initiated by the normal pituitary promoter. Reproductive endocrine tissues may contain tissue specific factors which bind to other promoter regions and determine POMC gene activation.

In contrast to splenic macrophages, lymphocytes, like many other extra-pituitary cells, express a smaller transcript which appears to encode for multiple molecular forms of the POMC peptides. Furthermore, endotoxin induces lymphocyte production of a truncated peptide which shows sequence identity to $ACTH_{1-25}$, a POMC gene product which has steroidogenic activity but does not influence antibody production (20, 21). In contrast, stimulation with either CRH or viruses leads to production of $ACTH_{1-39}$ by human peripheral leukocytes. This raises the possibility that different stimuli result in differential processing of various POMC gene products which may fulfil different physiological roles. Interestingly, lymphocyte-derived POMC gene transcripts lack a signal sequence, which is important for packaging of peptides into secretory vesicles, suggesting that the gene products may have intracellular (intracrine) rather than extracellular functions. Some immune cells such as those derived from T cell lines appear to express a POMC mRNA which differs in size from the pituitary species but the functional significance of this is as yet uncertain.

The regulatory elements for the gene-encoding POMC in the B lymphocyte appear to differ from those in the adenohypophysis. The lymphocyte gene can be induced by mitogens and superantigens as well as by conventional stimuli such as CRH and AVP. However, in immune cells, unlike pituitary cells, the effects of CRH are indirect and are mediated via macrophage production of IL-1 which secondarily induces POMC gene expression. Similarly, glucocorticoids, which directly inhibit pituitary POMC gene expression, exert their inhibitory influence on lymphocyte POMC gene by inhibiting macrophage production of IL-1 (22). Recently, *in vivo* studies have confirmed lymphocyte POMC expression in animal models of arthritis and diabetes and following subcutaneous administration of CRH.

Receptors for POMC Hormones

ACTH. In the rat specific high and low affinity membrane-bound receptors for ACTH have been identified on B and T lymphocytes, with the high affinity receptor being expressed in particular abundance on the B cells (23). As in the adrenal cortex, the high affinity receptor appears to be associated with increased

Ca^{2+} influx, possible due to activation of K^+-dependent Ca^{2+} channels, while the low affinity receptor is positively coupled to adenylyl cyclase (24). Collectively, these receptors mediate the various effects of ACTH on immune cell function observed *in vitro*, such as suppression of IFN-γ production by T lymphocytes and modulation of B lymphocyte growth and differentiation (23); they also effect the suppression of T-cell dependent antibody responses in mouse spleen cells *in vivo* while activation of the high affinity receptors on lymphocytes increases mitogenesis and protein synthesis. Specific ACTH binding sites have also been identified on human peripheral blood lymphocytes. Interestingly, the expression of these receptors is reduced in patients with adrenal insufficiency associated with non-functional adrenal ACTH receptors, suggesting that the two receptors are encoded by a common gene.

β-endorphin and other Opioid Peptides

Ligand binding studies have revealed that the four subtypes of opioid receptors (termed μ, δ, κ and σ) which are expressed in the nervous system are also present on immune cells. These high affinity opioid receptors, which have been identified on murine splenocytes and human leukocytes, appear to share many of the unique features of the neural receptors, including molecular size, immunogenicity and intracellular second messenger signalling pathways.

Studies on the roles of opioids within the immune system have placed particular emphasis on β-endorphin. This peptide binds (via its N-terminal sequence) to the δ-receptors, which are expressed on murine splenocytes and lymphocytes and on human lymphocytes and leukocytes (25), as well as to other opioid receptor subtypes. In addition, it recognises a family of atypical receptors, the so called "non-opioid receptors", which are present on transformed B lymphocytes (26) and thymoma cells (27). On the thymoma cells, two distinct atypical protein binding sites have been identified, one of high affinity with a molecular weight of 72 kDa and one of lower affinity with molecular weight of 40 kDa. Activation of the former by β-endorphin results in energy-dependent endocytosis of the ligand, a feature that may allow β-endorphin to modulate events on immune cells via an intracellular mechanism.

Biological Role of POMC-derived Peptides

ACTH appears to exert profound effects on immune function via molecular mechanisms similar to those it employs to stimulates steroidogenesis in adrenal cells. Interestingly, the full length molecule ($ACTH_{1-39}$) has the ability both to stimulate steroidogenesis and to inhibit antibody formation whereas the truncated form ($ACTH_{1-24}$) retains the full steroidogenic activity of the parent molecule but does not affect antibody formation, suggesting that the steroidogenic and immunomodulatory properties reside in separate parts of the molecule (25). The mechanism whereby ACTH interferes with antibody formation appears to involve effects on helper T cell signals. ACTH has other effects on lymphocyte function including stimulation of B cell mitogenesis and differentiation, possibly via a synergistic effect with IL-5. The immunomodulatory effects of ACTH are not confined to lymphocytes and include, for example, stimulation of NK cell activity and suppression of macrophage expression of major histocompatibility (MHC) class II antigens.

The opioid peptides α-, β- and γ-endorphin also exhibit widespread effects on immune function which include modulation of both lymphocyte and monocyte–macrophage function. Examples of the former include: (a) enhancement of the natural cytotoxicity of lymphocytes, (b) modulation (stimulation or inhibition) of T cell mitogenesis, and (c) enhancement of T cell rosetting. Their actions on monocyte–macrophage activity include: (a) stimulation of human peripheral blood mononuclear cells, (b) inhibition of macrophage MHC class II antigen expression, and (c) enhancement of macrophage cytotoxicity towards tumour cells.

In splenocytes β-endorphin has been shown both to inhibit and to stimulate adenylyl cyclase activity, dependent upon the predominant cell type present and the experimental conditions. Similarly, it produces dual effects on lymphocyte proliferation with enhancement being effected via a high-affinity non-opioid receptor and down-regulation via classical opioid receptors.

10.3   SUMMARY

In summary, cells of the immune system express genes for stress peptides which appear to encode both classical and novel forms of stress peptides. These molecules appear to exert profound immunomodulatory activities via classical receptor-mediated mechanisms. Their existence within both the immune and the neuroendocrine systems may allow for a co-ordinated endocrine, behavioural and immune response to stressful situations. It is conceivable that abnormalities in this peptide network could contribute to the pathogenesis of stress-related disease states.

ACKNOWLEDGEMENTS

Dimitris Grammatopoulos is a Sir Jules Thorn Research Fellow. Edward W. Hillhouse is supported by The Wellcome Trust.

REFERENCES

1. Lymangrover J., Brodish A. Tissue CRF: an extra hypothalamic corticotropin releasing factor (CRF) in the peripheral blood of stressed rats. *Neuroendocrinology*, 1973, **12**: 225–35.
2. Hergreaves K., Costello A., Joris J. Release from inflamed tissue of a substance with properties similar to corticotropin-releasing factor. *Neuroendocrinology*, 1989, **49**: 476–82.
3. Stephanou A., Jessop D., Knight R., Lightman S. Corticotrophin-releasing factor-like immunoreactivity and mRNA in human leukocytes. *Brain Behav Immun*, 1990, **37**: 67–73.
4. Ekman R., Servervius B., Castro M., Lowry P., Cederlund A., Bergman O., Sjogren H. Biosynthesis of corticotropin-releasing hormone in human T lymphocytes. *J Neuroimmunol*, 1993, **44**: 7–14.
5. Morrison E., Tomasec P., Linton E., Lowry P., Lowenstein P., Castro M. Expression of a biologically active Procorticotrophin-Releasing Hormone (proCRH) in stably transfected CHO-K1 cells: characterization of nuclear proCRH. *J Neuroendocrinology*, 1995, **7**: 263–72.
6. Milton N., Swanton E., Hillhouse E. Pyrogenic immunomodulator stimulation of a novel thymic corticotrophin-releasing factor. In A. Milton (ed) *Temperature Regulation: Advances in Pharmacological Sciences*. Basel, Birkhauser Verlag, 1994, pp 59–64.
7. Karalis K., Sano H., Listwak S., Chrousos G. Autocrine or paracrine inflammatory actions of corticotrophin-releasing hormone *in vivo*. *Science*, 1991, **254**: 421–3.
8. Webster E. L., Tracey D. E., Jutila M. A., Wolfe S. A., De Souza E. B. Corticotropin-releasing factor in mouse spleen: identification of receptor-bearing cells as resident macrophages. *Endocrinology*, 1990, **127**: 440–52.
9. Audhya T., Jain R., Hollander C. S. Receptor-mediated immunomodulation by corticotropin-releasing factor. *Cell Immunol*, 1991, **134**: 77–84.
10. Grammatopoulos D., Thompson S., Hillhouse E. The human myometrium expresses multiple isoforms of the CRH receptor. *J Clin Endocrinol Metab*, 1995, **80**: 2388–93.
11. Potter E., Sutton S., Donaldson C., Chen R., Perrin M., Lewis P., Sawchenko P., Vale W. Distribution of corticotropin-releasing factor receptor mRNA expression in the rat brain and pituitary. *Proc Natl Acad Sci USA*, 1994, **91**: 8777–81.
12. Perrin M., Donaldson C., Chen R., Blount A., Berggren T., Bilezikjian L., Sawchenko P., Vale W. Identification of a second corticotropin-releasing factor receptor gene and characterization of a cDNA expressed in heart. *Proc Natl Acad Sci USA*, 1995, **92**: 2969–73.
13. Chalmers D. T., Lovenberg T. W., Grigoriadis D. E., Behan D. P., de Souza E. B. Corticotrophin-releasing factor receptors: from molecular biology to drug design. *Trends Pharmacol Sci*, 1996, **17**: 166–72.
14. Xiong Y., Xie L., Abou-Samra A. Signaling properties of mouse and human corticotropin-releasing factor (CRF) receptors: decreased coupling efficiency of human type II CRF receptor. *Endocrinology*, 1995, **136**: 1828–34.
15. Markwick A., Lolait J., Funder J. Immunoreactive arginine vasopressin in the rat thymus. *Endocrinology*, 1986, **119**: 1690–96.
16. Torres B. A., Johnson H. M. Arginine vasopressin (AVP) replacement of helper cell requirement in IFN-γ production: evidence for a novel AVP receptor on mouse lymphocytes. *J Immunol*, 1988, **140**: 2179–83.
17. Smith E., Blalock J. Human leukocyte production of corticotropin and endorphin-like

substances: association with leukocyte interferon. *Proc Natl Acad Sci USA*, 1980, **77**: 5972–4.

18. Mechanick J., Levin N., Roberts J., Autelitano D. Pro-opiomelanocortin gene expression in a distinct population of rat spleen and lung leukocytes. *Endocrinology*, 1992, **131**: 518–25.

19. Li H., Hedger M., Clements J., Risbridger G. Localization of immunoreactive β-endorphin and adrenocorticotrophic and proopiomelanocortin mRNA to rat testicular interstitial macrophages. *Biol Reprod*, 1991, **45**: 282–9.

20. Harbour D., Galin F., Hughes T., Smith M., Blalock J. Role of leukocyte-derived pro-opiomelanocortin peptides in endotoxic shock. *Circ Shock*, 1991, **35**: 181–91.

21. Kavelaars A., Ballieux R., Heijnen C. The role of IL-1 in the corticotropin-releasing factor and arginine vasopressin induced secretion of immunoreactive beta-endorphin by human peripheral blood mononuclear cells. *J Immunol*, 1989, **142**: 2333–42.

22. Johnson H., Downs M., Pontzner C. Neuroendocrine peptide hormone regulation of immunity. In J. Blalock (ed) *Neuroimmunoendocrinology: Chemical Immunology, (2nd edition)*. Basel, Karger, 1992, pp 49–83.

23. Carr D. Neuroendocrine peptide receptors on cells of the immune system. In J. Blalock (ed) *Neuroimmunoendocrinology: Chemical Immunology, (2nd edition)*. Basel, Karger, 1992, pp 84–109.

24. Quinn S. J., Williams G. H. Regulation of aldostrone secretion. In V. H. T. James (ed) *The Adrenal Gland, (2nd edition)*. New York, Raven Press Ltd., 1992, 159–89

25. Carr D. J. J., Kim C.-H., De Costa B., Jacobson A. E., Rice K. C., Blalock J. E. Evidence for a δ-class opioid receptor on cells of the immune system. *Cell Immunol*, 1988, **116**: 44–51.

26. Hazum E., Chang K.-J., Cuatrecasas P. Specific nonopiate receptors for β-endorphin. *Science*, 1979, **205**: 1033–5.

27. Schweigerer L., Schmidt W., Teschemacher H., Gramsch C. β-endorphin: surface binding and internalization in thymoma cells. *Proc Natl Acad Sci USA*, 1985, **82**: 5751–5.

Chapter 11

Corticotrophin Releasing Hormone Binding Protein: A Regulator of the CRH Family of Peptides in Brain and Periphery

P. J. Lowry, S. M. Baigent and R. J. Woods

The University of Reading, Reading, UK

11.1 INTRODUCTION

The 41 amino acid peptide, corticotrophin releasing hormone (CRH) was originally identified as a hypothalamic neuropeptide that regulates the secretion of adrenocorticotrophic hormone (ACTH) by the anterior pituitary gland. The critical role of this peptide, along with arginine vasopressin (AVP), in the control of the hypothalamo–pituitary–adrenocortical (HPA) axis, i.e. the major stress axis, is now well established—see Chapter 1 and (1, 2). It is also well recognised that, in many species, CRH and closely related peptides, which together comprise a growing family, are widely distributed in the brain and periphery. A binding protein for these peptides, termed the corticotrophin

Stress, Stress Hormones and the Immune System. Edited by J. C. Buckingham, G. E. Gillies and A.-M. Cowell
© 1997 John Wiley & Sons, Ltd.

releasing hormone binding protein (CRH-BP), has been characterised recently. This protein is readily detectable in peripheral blood in man and higher apes, although not in rodents, and is also found in the brain of a broader range of species, including rodents and sheep. Growing evidence now supports the view that members of the CRH peptide family, together with their receptors and CRH-BP, are concerned not only with the regulation of HPA function but also with the control of the autonomic nervous and immune systems and with integrating behaviours associated with perturbations of these three systems (see also Chapters 1, 2 and 15). However, our understanding is far from complete and important advances in this area are occurring rapidly. This chapter will identify known and potential players in this field as well as important areas for further investigation.

11.2 EVIDENCE FOR A CORTICOTROPHIN RELEASING HORMONE BINDING PROTEIN (CRH-BP)

11.2.1 Pregnancy

Perhaps surprisingly, a rich extra-hypothalamic source of CRH is the human placenta where both the peptide and its mRNA are readily detected. Placental CRH is secreted into the maternal blood. It is first detected in significant amounts in maternal plasma during the third trimester of pregnancy during which the levels rise to rival those observed in hypophysial portal blood in experimental animals during stress. However, despite the high circulating levels of CRH, plasma ACTH concentrations normally remain within the normal range during this time (3). This apparently discrepant finding may be explained by the existence of a plasma protein (CRH-BP) which binds CRH with high affinity and specificity and which has been shown *in vitro* to abolish the ACTH releasing ability of CRH (4). We have observed that the concentrations of immunoreactive CRH and CRH-BP in human maternal plasma invariably reach molar equivalence at exactly 21 days before parturition, irrespective of whether onset of labour is early, late or normal (5). Thereafter, the circulating levels of CRH-BP decline progressively such that in very late pregnancy levels are lower than those observed in non-pregnant individuals. The physiological significance of these observations remains to be determined but, since the fall in CRH-BP is likely to increase the availability of free CRH, these findings have led to speculation that placental CRH is critical to the events leading up to parturition and that measurement of circulating CRH-related molecules may provide a biochemical index of a placental clock which controls the length of gestation. In this context, it is interesting to note that the plasma CRH concentrations in subjects with pre-term labour and pregnancy-induced hypertension are significantly higher than those observed in a normal pregnancy. Clearly the clinical implications and physiological significance of these findings merit further investigation. A study across species should also prove interesting as the presence of a CRH-BP in the circulation appears to be restricted to higher apes and man. Lower apes (e.g. the gibbon) lack a CRH-BP, despite secreting a placental CRH, but sheep and rats have neither placental CRH nor CRH-BP, although both molecules are found in their central nervous systems (CNS) as is also the case in man.

11.2.2   Non-pregnant Conditions

It seems unlikely that CRH-BP exists solely to subserve events surrounding pregnancy. Although CRH is not detectable in plasma from male and non-pregnant female human subjects, CRH-BP is synthesised in the liver and secreted into the plasma of such individuals. In addition, the binding protein is expressed in many parts of the brain, including the cortex, where CRH is undetectable. Assuming a binding role for this protein, it is possible, therefore, that peptides produced within the brain and periphery (which are closely related to but distinct from the 41 amino acid CRH) may themselves serve as natural ligands for CRH-BP. (See also Section 11.3). CRH itself shows some interesting interactions with the circulating binding protein in non-pregnant individuals. Thus, a bolus injection of CRH, in a dose sufficient to stimulate the HPA axis, produces a rapid fall in the plasma concentration of CRH-BP, which reaches a nadir within 15 minutes. This response appears to be independent of the activation of the HPA axis because ovine-CRH (oCRH) (which differs from the human and rat peptide (r/hCRH) by only seven amino acids and is equipotent with r/hCRH in releasing ACTH) does not reduce the plasma CRH-BP concentration. Other studies have shown that oCRH has only a very low affinity for the hCRH-BP (see Section 11.3.2) thus suggesting a potentially important selectivity for r/hCRH and related peptides.

   The reasons for the rapid disappearance of the CRH-BP from human plasma after a bolus injection of hCRH are intriguing. It is now apparent that CRH binds to CRH-BP on injection and the complex forms a stable dimer, CRH_2/BP_2. We postulate that the formation of this macromolecule constitutes a signal which facilitates the delivery of CRH or CRH-like molecules to appropriate, although as yet unidentified, target sites in the body. Our recent data suggest that the dimer may be taken up or activated by specific tissues (possibly by a receptor-dependent mechanism) and consequently dissociated to yield the active peptide together with CRH-BP in an inactive but stable conformational state; CRH-BP may then be released and reactivated for further use (6). This phenomenon may account, at least in part, for the fall in the levels of circulating CRH-BP seen at the end of pregnancy which may be triggered by a rise in secretion of placental CRH. It is also possible that the binding protein acts as part of a soluble receptor in a manner analogous to that reported for certain cytokines and for growth hormone.

11.2.3   Clinical Conditions

Apart from conditions in which liver and kidney dysfunction may lead to alterations in the synthesis and clearance of the CRH-BP, the only patients we have been able to identify so far with plasma CRH-BP levels which differ significantly from normal are those suffering from rheumatoid arthritis and septicaemia. In these cases plasma CRH-BP is raised (7), a finding which may reflect or contribute to the abnormal HPA responses which have been reported in various cohorts of patients with these conditions (see Chapter 9). The increases in circulating CRH-BP are the direct consequence of increased hepatic synthesis of the protein. Interestingly, the 5′-flanking region of the CRH-BP gene contains enhancer elements implicated in the acute phase response, where a number of genes in the liver are switched on in response to an immune stimulus (see Chapter 3). One element at -305bp binds the nuclear transcription factor NF-κB which also plays a key role in the regulation of production of immunoglobulins and interleukins (which, in turn, trigger other liver-specific genes such as angiotensinogen). Another element, located at -676, binds INF-1, a transcription factor which regulates the interferon gene. The raised levels of CRH-BP in patients with rheumatoid arthritis and septicaemia may thus parallel the associated overactivity of the immune system.

11.2.4   Further Studies on a Role for CRH-BP

Progress in understanding the physiological role of CRH-BP has been severely limited by the lack of a convenient experimental animal with endogenous CRH-BP in the systemic circulation and further strategies are urgently required. A transgenic mouse has recently been produced (8) which, unlike the wild-type strain, secretes significant amounts of CRH-BP into its bloodstream and may thus offer a means whereby the pharmacokinetics of the ligand-binding protein may be studied. Whilst this model may be viewed as "unphysiological", it should serve to enhance our understanding of the effects of exogenous CRH on circulating CRH-BP. Advantage may also be taken of the fact that CRH-BP is expressed in many regions of the rat brain, including higher centres such as the cortex, where it appears to be associated with the cell membrane. The rat may thus provide a valuable model in which to investigate the central roles of CRH-BP and its native ligands; simple experiments involving central injections of the peptide ligands with and without the binding protein are likely to yield interesting data. Further investigations will be assisted also with the cloning of the CRH-BP cDNA (9).

11.3 THE FAMILY OF CRH-RELATED PEPTIDES

11.3.1 Biochemical Evidence for Novel CRH-related Peptides

Some years ago we attempted to isolate the material responsible for giving a positive immunocytochemical signal for CRH in the pituitary gland. Using immunoglobulin isolated from the antiserum we used in our immunocytochemical studies, we isolated a peptide by affinity chromatography which was structurally unrelated to CRH (10). This serves to illustrate the care and caution necessary when interpreting the results from techniques such as immunoassay, immunoneutralisation and immunocytochemistry which depend on antibodies. Such studies may, however, provide evidence for the existence of peptides related to the peptide under investigation and growing evidence suggests that this is the case for CRH (see Fig. 11.1). For some time it has been known that urotensin 1, a peptide found in the urophysis in teleost fish, and sauvagine, a frog skin peptide, are structurally related to CRH. More recently, using a rat cDNA library, the structure of rat urocortin (rUCN) has been predicted to have a 65% homology with fish urotensin 1 (11) and has been located in discrete nuclei of the rat brain. Its mRNA expression seems, however, to be limited to two small nuclei (Edinger-Westphal and lateral superior olive) and such small amounts of peptide appear to be produced that they could not be characterised physiochemically. The restricted distribution of UCN in the rat brain as compared with the wide distribution of CRH-BP suggests that this peptide, like CRH, is unlikely to be the sole ligand for CRH-BP.

The likely existence of other CRH-like molecules is further supported by the recent isolation of a peptide from the sheep brain (12) which has more than ten times the affinity for the CRH-BP than hCRH (see Fig. 11.2). This molecule has been termed the ovine binding protein ligand (oBPLig) and has an ionic mass expected of a 40–41 residue peptide. Its N-terminal sequence shows some

```
oCRH  SQEPPISLDLTFHLLREVLEMTKADQLAQQAHSNRKLLDIA
hCRH  SEEPPISLDLTFHLLREVLEMARAEQLAQQAHSNRKLMEII
UT1   NDDPPISIDLTFHLLRNMIEMARIENEREQAGLNRKYLDEV
Sau   <EGPPISIDLSLELLRKMIEIEKQEKEKQQAANNRLLLDTI
UCN   DDPPLSIDLTFHLLRTLLELARTQSQRERAEQNRIIFDSV
```

Figure 11.1   The corticotrophin releasing hormone (CRH) family of peptides; OCRH = ovine CRH; hCRH = human CRH; UT1 = urotensin 1; Sau = sauvagine; UCN = urocortin

CRH receptor 1

UCN ≥ hCRH = oCRH = UT = Sau

CRH receptor 2$_\alpha$

Sau > UT ≥ hCRH > oCRH

CRH receptor 2$_\beta$

UCN > Sau > UT > hCRH = oCRH

hCRH–BP

oBPLig ≥ UT1 > UCN ≥ hCRH > Sau > oCRH

Figure 11.2   Relative affinities of the corticotrophin releasing hormone (CRH) family of peptides for CRH receptors and binding protein. UCN = urocortin; Sau = sauvagine; oCRH = ovine CRH; hCRH = human CRH; UT = urotensin; BP = binding protein; oBPlig = ovine BP ligand

homology with rUCN but, unlike rUCN (although like CRH-BP itself), it appears to be evenly distributed throughout the sheep brain.

11.3.2   Ligand Interactions with CRH Receptors and CRH-BP

Two classes of CRH receptors, R1 and R2, have now been cloned. These belong to the seven transmembrane G-protein-coupled superfamily (see also Chapter 4) and each may be found as α and β variants which are formed by differential splicing of the initial RNA transcript (13–16). The CRH-R1 variants are found predominantly in the brain and pituitary gland (17) whereas the CRH-R2$_\beta$ is found mainly in tissues such as lung, heart and skeletal muscle. This latter observation would favour the existence of peripheral novel CRH-related peptides as, too, would the differential affinities of the known ligands for the CRH-BP (Fig. 11.2). For example, oCRH has 15-fold lower affinity than hCRH for sheep brain CRH-BP, as well as a low affinity for the murine peripheral receptor (18). Sauvagine, however, has an affinity that is equal to, or even greater than, hCRH for all the CRH receptors cloned to date. Urotensin 1 also has a higher affinity than hCRH for both the peripheral murine CRH receptor (16) and hCRH-BP (18). The recently cloned rUCN has an affinity for the CRH-BP similar to that of hCRH but it has a significantly higher affinity for the cloned receptors (Fig. 11.2). It has also emerged that α-helical CRH_{9-41}, which binds readily to CRH-BP (18), blocks the vascular actions of CRH more readily than it antagonises CRH actions at the pituitary receptors (19). Furthermore, α-helical CRH_{9-41} inhibits the acute phase response to interleukin-1β whereas immunoneutralization of systemic "CRH", with an antibody which blocks the ACTH-releasing activity of synthetic CRH, is without effect (20).

11.3.3   CRH-like Peptides in Human Fluid and Tissues

There is now substantial evidence that CRH or related peptides are produced by leukocytes and that they exert significant effects on immune cell function (see Chapters 9 and 10 for further details). Recent studies, which have shown that CRH immunoreactivity is present in the synovial fluid of patients with rheumatoid arthritis, add further support to the growing evidence that peripheral CRH or related molecules act in concert with other local factors to regulate the inflammatory response. In addition, we have shown that the circulating levels of CRH-BP are elevated in inflammatory disease (Section 11.2.3). Using a two-site immunoradiometric assay which is highly specific for the 41 amino acid hCRH together with an assay which uses CRH-BP to detect ligand (which may or may not be authentic $hCRH_{1-41}$), we have examined the synovial fluid from patients with rheumatoid arthritis. Comparison of the data obtained by the two methods indicates that the bulk of the ligand binding to CRH-BP is distinct from 41 amino acid hCRH and this was further confirmed using high performance liquid chromatography (7). We also have evidence for additional ligands which are chemically distinct from hCRH but which bind CRH-BP in a human liver tumour taken from a patient with Cushing's disease. Further work is needed to characterise these molecules fully.

11.4   CONCLUSION

From what appeared to be a simple neuropeptide with a straightforward, well-defined biological role in controlling ACTH secretion by the pituitary gland, CRH has emerged as a peptide with a complex biology. It now seems likely that it is one of a growing family of peptides whose members interact with a number of different receptors and with a binding protein and are thus likely to fulfil diverse functions at multiple sites within the brain and at the periphery (see also Chapters 1, 2, 9, and 10). The chemical characterisation and validation of the physiological roles of the various CRH-related peptides, CRH receptors and

CRH-BP is, arguably, one of the most exciting and potentially important areas of research in neuroendocrine-immunology which, until recently, has been the subject of some scepticism and controversy. It will be interesting to see just how many new peptides and receptors are characterised in the next few years. There is no doubt that there are still important areas of the brain, such as the locus coeruleus, which are highly responsive to CRH (21) but which appear to be devoid of both type 1 and type 2 CRH-receptors (17). Interestingly, several peptides which appear to belong to an extended family of CRH-like peptides and which exhibit diuretic activity have been identified in insects. Whether there are equivalent peptides in mammals remains to be determined but such peptides could add an important extra dimension to this field.

The impact of the CRH-BP on the varied biological activities of the CRH peptides also requires further investigation and may call for a re-assessment of the effects of the peptide actions. For example, some of the experiments carried out to date on various aspects of immune cell function will have been performed in the presence of varying amounts of liver-derived CRH-BP which could be critical at certain stages of the immune response. In view of the hypotensive and inotropic properties of the CRH-related peptides, intriguing questions are also raised by the expression of the CRH-R2$_\beta$ receptor in the heart. Significantly, perhaps, urotensin 1 and UCN both exhibit a tenfold higher potency than hCRH at this receptor and, along with the oBPLig, these peptides have a high affinity for the hCRH-BP. It is likely, therefore that we are entering a new era of CRH biology with far reaching implications for the interactions between stress, stress hormones and immune function. A greater understanding of how the CRH-BP regulates the CRH family of peptides in the brain and periphery may thus help in the design of novel therapies for a broad range of conditions in a manner similar to that proposed for Alzheimer's disease (22).

REFERENCES

1. Gillies G. E., Lowry P. J. Corticotrophin releasing hormone and its vasopressin component. In W. F. Ganong, L. Martini (eds) *Frontiers in Neuroendocrinology*. New York, Raven Press, 1982, pp 43–75.
2. Antoni F. A. Hypothalamic control of adrenocorticotropin secretion: advances since the discovery of 41-residue corticotropin-releasing factor. *Endocr Rev*, 1986, **7**: 351–78.
3. Campbell E. A., Linton E. A., Wolfe C. D. A., Scraggs C. P., Jones M. T., Lowry P. J. Plasma corticotropin-releasing hormone concentrations during pregnancy and parturition. *J Clin Endocrinol Metab*, 1987, **64**: 1054–9.
4. Linton E. A., Behan D. P., Saphier P. W., Lowry P. J. Corticotropin-releasing hormone binding protein: reduction in the ACTH-releasing activity of placental but not hypothalamic CRF. *J Clin Endocrinol Metab*, 1990, **70**: 1574–80.
5. McLean M., Bisits A., Davies J., Woods R., Lowry P., Smith, R. A placental clock controlling the length of human pregnancy. *Nature Med*, 1995, **1**: 460–3.

6. Woods R. J., Grossman A., Saphier P., Kennedy K., Ur E., Behan D., Potter E., Vale W., Lowry P. J. Association of hCRH to its binding protein in blood may trigger clearance of the complex. *J Clin Endocrinol Metab*, 1994, **78**: 73–6.
7. Woods R. J., David J., Baigent S., Gibbins J., Lowry, P. J. Elevated levels of corticotropin releasing factor binding protein in the blood of patients suffering from arthritis and septicaemia and the presence of novel ligand in synovial fluid. *Brit J Rheumatol*, 1996, **35**: 119–23.
8. Lovejoy D. A., Aubry J. M., Potter E., Matthews L. S., Vale W. W. Analysis of CRF and CRF-binding protein mRNA in transgenic mice over-expressing CRF-binding protein. 77th Meeting of the Endocrine Society, 1995, OR14–2.
9. Behan D. P., Potter E. A., Lewis K. A., Jenkins N. A., Copeland N., Lowry P. J., Vale W. Cloning and structure of the human CRF-binding protein gene. *Genomics*, 1993, **16**: 63–8.
10. Beny J. L., Corder R., Lowry P. J. CRF immunoreactive peptides in the human hypophysis: a cautionary note. *Peptides*, 1985, **6**: 661–7.
11. Vaughan J., Donaldson C., Bittercourt J., Perrin M., Lewis C., Sutton S., Chan R., Turnbill A., Lovejoy D., Rivier C., Rivier J., Sawchencho P., Vale W. Urocortin a neuropeptide related to fish urotensin 1 and corticotropin releasing factor. *Nature*, 1995, **378**: 287– 92.
12. Baigent S., Woods R., Kemp F., Lowry P. Characterization of a novel ligand for hCRH binding protein in sheep brain. *J Physiol*, 1995, **489**: P183.
13. Chen R., Lewis K. A., Perrin M. H., Vale W. W. Expression cloning of a human corticotropin-releasing factor receptor. *Proc Natl Acad Sci USA*, 1993, **90**: 8967–71.
14. Perrin M. H., Donaldson C. J., Chen R., Lewis K. A., Vale W. W. Cloning and expression of a rat brain corticotropin releasing factor (CRF) receptor. *Endocrinology*, 1993, **133**: 3058–61.
15. Lovenberg T. W., Liaw C. W., Grigoriadis D. E., Clevenger W., Chalmers D. T., De Souza E. B., Oltersdorf T. Cloning and characterization of a functionally distinct corticotropin-releasing factor receptor subtype from rat brain. *Proc Natl Acad Sci USA*, 1995, **92**: 836–40.
16. Kishimoto T., Pearse R. V., Lin C. R., Rosenfeld M. G. A sauvagine/corticotropin-releasing factor receptor expressed in heart and skeletal muscle. *Proc Natl Acad Sci USA*, 1995, **92**: 1108–12.
17. Chalmers D. T., Lovenberg T. W., De Souza, E. B. Localization of novel corticotropin-releasing factor receptor (CRF_2) mRNA expression to specific sub-cortical nuclei in rat brain: comparison with CRF_1 receptor mRNA expression. *J Neurosci*, 1995, **15**: 6340–50.
18. Behan D. P., Potter E., Sutton S., Fischer W., Lowry P. J., Vale W. W. Corticotropin-releasing factor binding protein: a putative peripheral and central modulator of the CRF family of neuropeptides. CRF and Cytokines. *Ann NY Acad Sci*, 1993, **697**: 1–8.
19. Corder R., Turnill D., Ling N., Gaillard R. C. Attenuation of corticotropin releasing factor induced hypotension in anaesthetised rats with the CRF antagonist CRF 9-41: Comparison with effect on ACTH release. *Peptides*, 1992, **13**: 1–6.
20. Hagan P. M., Poole S., Bristow A. F. Corticotrophin releasing factor as a mediator of the acute-phase response in rats, mice and rabbits. *J Endocrinol*, 1993, **136**: 207–16.
21. Valentino R. J., Foots S. L., Page M. E. The locus coeruleus as a site for integrating corticotropin-releasing factor and noradrenergic mediation of stress responses. *Ann NY Acad Sci*, 1993, **697**: 173–88.
22. Behan D. P., Heinrichs S. C., Troncoso J. C., Liu X.-J., Kawas C. H., Ling N., De Souza E. B. Displacement of corticotropin releasing factor from its binding protein as a possible treatment for Alzheimer's disease. *Nature*, 1995, **378**: 284–7.

Chapter 12

Interleukin-1 Receptors in the Brain–Endocrine–Immune Axis: Role in the Stress Response and Infection

Toshihiro Takao

Kochi Medical School, Nankoku, Japan and

Errol B. De Souza*

Neurocrine Biosciences, Inc., San Diego, California, USA

12.1 INTRODUCTION

The cytokine interleukin-1 (IL-1) is one of the key mediators of the immunological and pathological responses to stress, infection and antigenic challenge (1).

---

*To whom correspondence should be addressed

Stress, Stress Hormones and the Immune System. Edited by J. C. Buckingham, G. E. Gillies and A.-M. Cowell
© 1997 John Wiley & Sons, Ltd.

Substantial evidence now supports the view that, in addition to its well-documented actions in the immune system (see Chapter 3), IL-1 also serves as a neurotransmitter, neuromodulator and growth factor in the central nervous system (CNS). IL-1 mRNA is present in normal brain (2) and IL-1β-like immunoreactivity has been identified in neurones and glia in the hypothalamus and elsewhere in the human and rat brain (3) as well as in the cerebrospinal fluid (CSF) (4). IL-1β is also produced in abundance by astrocytes and microglia maintained in culture (5) and its expression in the brain is enhanced by cerebral trauma (6) or endotoxin treatment (7).

Administration of IL-1 by central or peripheral routes has potent actions on the CNS; these include significant alterations in neuroendocrine function, the most overt of which are stimulation of the hypothalamo–pituitary–adrenocortical (HPA) axis (8)—see also Chapter 13—and inhibition of the hypothalamo–pituitary–gonadal (HPG) axis (9).

Currently, two forms of IL-1 (termed IL-1α and IL-1β) and one endogenous IL-1 receptor antagonist (IL-1ra) have been characterised (1). IL-1α and IL-1β (collectively referred to as IL-1) and IL-1ra share limited ($<30\%$) sequence homology but elicit many of their biological effects through common receptor molecules on the surface of target cells (see also Chapters 3 and 4). Recent studies have identified at least two types of IL-1 receptor (termed Type I and Type II) that are differentially expressed by certain types of immune cells and by human and murine derived cell lines (10). Recombinant human IL-1α and IL-1β recognise both receptor subtypes. They thus bind to Type I receptors on, for example, T cells, fibroblasts, keratinocytes, endothelial cells, synovial lining cells, chondrocytes and hepatocytes (11) and to the Type II receptors expressed by various B cell lines, including the Raji human B cell lymphoma line (10). IL-1ra was initially reported to be selective for Type I IL-1 receptors and not to recognise Type II receptors (12). However, more recent studies have shown that IL-1ra also competes with IL-1 for the Type II receptors, albeit with only a low affinity (13). Since IL-1 and IL-1ra exhibit differential selectivity for the Type I and Type II IL-1 receptors, they make useful ligands for examining the characteristics of IL-1 receptors in the brain–endocrine–immune axis.

In this chapter, we summarise data from some of our recent studies in which we used a combination of conventional ligand binding techniques on tissue homogenates, receptor autoradiography and *in situ* hybridisation to detect, localise and characterise the IL-1 receptors in the brain–immune system. In addition, we describe factors which modulate the expression of IL-1 receptors *in vitro* and *in vivo*. For the ligand binding and autoradiographic studies ^{125}I-labelled ligands (IL-1 and IL-1ra) were used as probes while for *in situ* hybridisation ^{35}S-labelled antisense cRNA probes derived from a murine T cell IL-1 receptor cDNA were employed to detect and localise type I IL-1 receptor mRNA.

12.2   SPECIES DIFFERENCES IN INTERLEUKIN-1 (IL-1) RECEPTORS

Comparative studies using human recombinant- (hr-) IL-1α and hr-IL-1ra as probes have revealed significant interspecies differences in IL-1 receptor binding in mouse, rabbit, rat and guinea pig (14). In the mouse and rabbit moderate to high levels of ^{125}I-hr-IL-1α and ^{125}I-hr-IL-1ra binding are readily demonstrable in a variety of tissues (hippocampus, testis, spleen); however, the binding of these ligands in comparable tissues from rat or guinea pig is barely within the range of sensitivity of the assay. Representative data from the spleen and testis obtained with ^{125}I-hr-IL-1α are shown in Fig. 12.1. The apparent paucity of IL-1 binding sites in rat tissues is surprising since in the rat, as in many other species, exogenous hr-IL-1 produces diverse functional responses which include altered sleep, anorexia, increased adrenocorticotrophic hormone (ACTH) release (8) and modulation of the acute release of growth hormone-releasing hormone and somatostatin. In addition, IL-1ra reduces the severity of experimental enterocolitis and lipopolysaccharide-induced pulmonary inflammation in the rat (15). It has been suggested that the overt discrepancy between the data from ligand binding and functional studies in the rat may be explained by a multiplicity of IL-1 receptors (10); in this event the radioligands used in the present study

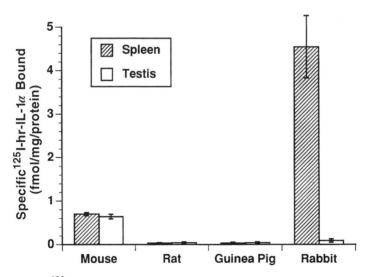

Figure 12.1   ^{125}I-hr-IL-1α binding in mouse, rat, guinea pig and rabbit spleen and testis. Crude membrane preparations from frozen tissues were incubated for 2 h at room temperature with ^{125}I-hr-IL-1α. A saturating concentration of ^{125}I-hr-IL-1α (100 pM) was used in this study primarily to detect changes in receptor density. Nonspecific binding was determined in the presence of 300 nM hIL-1β. Data are expressed as mean specific IL-1 binding $\pm$ SEM, (n = 6)

(^{125}I-hr-IL-1α and ^{125}I-hr-IL-1ra) may only label a subtype of these receptors which is expressed in some species including mouse, rabbit, human and monkey (unpublished data) but not in others such as rat and guinea pig. Some points relevant to this problem are also discussed in Chapter 13.

In subsequent studies we investigated whether the apparent absence of IL-1 binding sites in the rat reflected an inability of the "receptor" to recognise the human recombinant ligands. Various IL-1 receptor ligands (including human, mouse and rat forms of IL-1 and IL-1ra) were used to probe the binding sites in mouse and rat tissues. In the mouse testis, ^{125}I-hr-IL-1α and ^{125}I-hr-IL-1ra showed high specific binding as also did ^{125}I-rat-IL-1β and ^{125}I-rat-IL-1ra while progressively lower binding was observed with ^{125}I-mouse-IL-1β and ^{125}I-hr-IL-1β. By contrast, no specific IL-1 binding was found in rat testis using any of the radioligands described above or in the rat spleen homogenates using ^{125}I-rat-IL-1β or ^{125}I-rat-IL-1ra as probes. Additional studies are necessary not only to resolve these species differences but also to detect and characterise the functional IL-1 receptors in the rat.

12.3 KINETIC AND PHARMACOLOGICAL CHARACTERISTICS OF IL-1 RECEPTORS IN THE MOUSE

Studies performed under equilibrium conditions showed that the binding of ^{125}I-hr-IL-1α and ^{125}I-hr-IL-1ra to mouse tissues is specific, concentration-dependent and saturable (16). Furthermore, Scatchard analysis of the saturation data showed that both ligands have a high affinity for the receptor, with dissociation constants (K_ds) of 60–120 pM for ^{125}I-hr-IL-1α and 20–30 pM for ^{125}I-hr-IL-1ra respectively. Of the tissues studied, the highest density of IL-1 binding sites observed with either ligand was in the testis and the rank order of abundance was testis > spleen (^{125}I-hr-IL-1ra) > hippocampus > kidney (^{125}I-hr-IL-1α). Representative binding curves obtained with ^{125}I-hr-IL-1ra are shown in Fig. 12.2.

The pharmacological specificity of the ^{125}I-hr-IL-1α and ^{125}I-hr-IL-1ra binding sites has been determined by examining the abilities of IL-1-related and IL-1-unrelated peptides to displace specifically bound ^{125}I-hr-IL-1α and ^{125}I-hr-IL-1ra in homogenates of mouse tissues (17). The results are summarised in Table 12.1. IL-1α, IL-1ra and IL-1β readily displaced both radioligands as also did IL-1β^{+} (an analogue of IL-1β with three amino acids added to the carboxy terminal) and IL-1β^{c18} (an analogue of the clone 18 IL-1β with two substitutions at the amino terminus from ala-pro to thr-met); their rank order of potency was IL-1α = IL-1ra > IL-1β > IL-1β^{+} > IL-1β^{c18} which, for the most part, parallelled their bioactivities in a murine thymocyte co-stimulation assay (18). On the other hand, in the concentrations tested (maximum 100 nM) corticotrophin releasing hormone (CRH) and tumour necrosis factor (TNF) had no effect on ^{125}I-hr-IL-1α or ^{125}I-hr-IL-1ra binding.

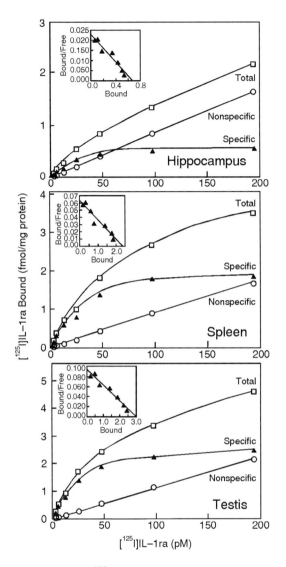

Figure 12.2 The binding of ^{125}I-hr-IL-1ra to mouse hippocampus, spleen and testis as a function of increasing ligand concentration. Direct plot of data shows the total amount of ^{125}I-hr-IL-1ra bound (total), binding in the presence of 300 nM IL-1α or β (nonspecific), and specific (total minus nonspecific) binding. The inserted figures demonstrate Scatchard plots of ^{125}I-hr-IL-1ra specific binding. Crude membrane preparations of mouse tissues were incubated for 120 min at room temperature with increasing concentrations of ^{125}I-hr-IL-1ra. The data shown are from a representative experiment. hr = Human recombinant; ra = receptor antagonist

Table 12.1 Pharmacological specificity of ^{125}I-hr-IL-1α and ^{125}I-hr-IL-1ra binding to mouse tissues. Peptides at between three and 10 concentrations were incubated with approximately 100 pM ^{125}I-hr-IL-1α and 40 pM ^{125}I-hr-IL-1ra for 120 min at room temperature. All assays were conducted in triplicate in three separate experiments. K_i (inhibitory binding-affinity constant) values were obtained from competition curve data analysed using the computer program LIGAND (17). Biological activity data were obtained in a murine thymocyte assay (18). Abbreviations: CRH, rat/human corticotrophin-releasing hormone; IL-1β^+, an analogue of IL-1β with three amino acids added to the carboxy terminal; IL-1β^{c18}, an analogue of the clone 18 IL-1β with two substitutions at the amino terminus from ala-pro to thr-met; TNF, human recombinant tumour necrosis factor-α; ND, not determined.

Peptide	K_i (pM)							Biological activity (units/mg)
	Hippocampus		Spleen	Kidney		Testis		
	^{125}I-hr-IL-1α	^{125}I-hr-IL-1ra	^{125}I-hr-IL-1ra	^{125}I-hr-IL-1α	^{125}I-hr-IL-1ra	^{125}I-hr-IL-1α	^{125}I-hr-IL-1ra	
hr-IL-1α	55 ± 18	70 ± 10	57 ± 9	28 ± 19	ND	14 ± 2	46 ± 8	3.0×10^7
hr-IL-1ra	ND	119 ± 63	104 ± 54	ND	ND	ND	94 ± 49	No activity
hr-IL-1β	76 ± 20	1798 ± 234	3138 ± 1159	53 ± 23	5560 ± 2098	89 ± 6	3672 ± 1317	2.0×10^7*
IL-1β^+	ND	ND	ND	ND	7183 ± 604	ND	ND	1.0×10^6
IL-1β^{c18}	2940 ± 742	2008 ± 350	2780 ± 919	ND	ND	ND	2732 ± 474	ND
TNF	>100 000	>100 000	>100 000	>100 000	>100 000	>100 000	>100 000	8.0×10^2
CRH	>100 000	>100 000	>100 000	>100 000	>100 000	>100 000	>100 000	0.0

*Note, IL-1β used in the ^{125}I-IL-1ra experiments had lower biological activity than IL-1β used in the ^{125}I-IL-α experiments.
hr = Human recombinant; ra = receptor agonist.

12.4   DISTRIBUTION AND ROLE OF IL-1 RECEPTORS IN THE MURINE CENTRAL NERVOUS SYSTEM

12.4.1   Distribution of Type I IL-1 Receptor mRNA and IL-1 Binding Sites

In situ histochemical techniques have been used successfully to investigate the distribution of cells expressing Type I IL-1 receptor mRNA in the murine CNS (19). The strongest autoradiographic signal in the forebrain was found in the hippocampal formation, where an intense signal was observed over the granule cell layer of the dentate gyrus and weak to moderate signals were noted over the pyramidal cell layer of the hilus and the CA3 region. Intense autoradiographic signals were also evident over all aspects of the midline raphe system, over the choroid plexus in the lateral, third and fourth ventricles and over endothelial cells of postcapillary venules throughout the CNS, both in the parenchyma and at the pial surface. Moderate to dense signals were observed over sensory neurones of the mesencephalic trigeminal nucleus, while weak to moderate signals were found over the Purkinje cell layer of the entire cerebellar cortex. In contrast, the signal detected in the hypothalamic paraventricular nucleus and most aspects of the median eminence did not differ significantly from background, suggesting an absence of Type I IL-1 receptor mRNA in this area.

Complementary studies exploited autoradiographic techniques to map the IL-1 binding sites in the murine CNS. The data demonstrated very low densities of IL-1 binding sites throughout the brain using ^{125}I-hr-IL-1α (Figs. 12.3a and 12.3c) or ^{125}I-hr-IL-1ra (Figs. 12.3b and 12.3d) as probes. Discrete areas of high density binding were however evident in the hippocampal formation and in the choroid plexus (Fig. 12.3). Binding sites were also abundant in the molecular and granular layers of the dentate gyrus but were virtually absent in the CA1 to CA3 pyramidal region. No specific binding of either receptor ligand was detected in the hypothalamus, cerebral cortex and other brain areas.

12.4.2   Physiological and Pharmacological Actions of IL-1 in the CNS

IL-1 has been reported to exert a variety of functional effects in the hippocampus; these include enhanced synaptic inhibition in hippocampal neurones *in vitro* and stimulation of nerve growth factor production both *in vitro* and *in vivo* (20). These data suggest that IL-1 may promote neuronal survival or repair in this brain region. Further support for this notion is provided by the demonstration of increased production of IL-1 by hippocampal astrocytes following

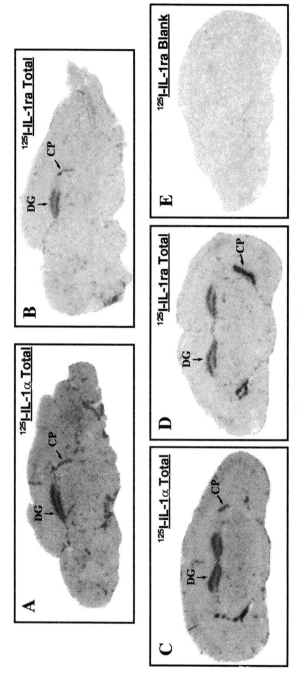

Figure 12.3a–d Autoradiographic localisation of ^{125}I-hr-IL-1α and ^{125}I-hr-IL-1ra binding in mouse brain cut in saggital (top) and coronal (bottom) planes. The tissues were incubated for 120 min with 40 pM of ^{125}I-IL-1ra and 100 pM of ^{125}I-hr-IL-1α. The images were computer generated using autoradiograms on Hyperfilm. The darker areas in autoradiograms correspond to brain regions displaying higher densities of binding. In **Fig. 12.3e** note the absence of specific ^{125}I-hr-IL-1ra binding in an adjacent section (i.e. blank) co-incubated with 100 nM hr-IL-1α. Abbreviations: DG, dentate gyrus; CP, choroid plexus. hr = Human recombinant; ra = receptor agonist

lesions of the entorhinal afferents (i.e. the perforant path) to the dentate gyrus, concurrent with the onset of cholinergic sprouting (21). Since inputs from the hippocampus directly influence thermoresponsive neurones in the preoptic area of the hypothalamus (22) it is possible that the fever-inducing actions of IL-1 are mediated, in part, by the hippocampus (see Chapter 14 for further discussion). Moreover, increasing evidence suggests that at least some of the central effects of IL-1 on the neuroendocrine system and, in particular, on the HPA axis are exerted at the level of the hippocampus—for review see (8). This possibility is particularly appealing given the apparent absence of type I IL-1 receptor mRNA and IL-1 binding sites in the hypothalamus. Nonetheless, it must be recognised that significant quantities of IL-1 are synthesised in the hypothalamus. In addition, IL-1 produces significant functional effects within the hypothalamus; for example, it stimulates the release of CRH from rat hypothalami *in vitro* while *in vivo* it increases the plasma ACTH concentration when injected either into the third ventricle or directly into the median eminence (8)—see also Chapter 13. One possible explanation for the apparent discrepancy between the well-documented hypothalamic effects of IL-1 and the paucity of IL-1 receptors in this brain region (see Chapter 13) is that the endogenous ligand binds avidly to the receptors and thereby prevents the labelled ligand gaining access; such an argument is not however consistent with the reversible IL-1 binding observed in other tissues nor does it explain our failure to detect IL-1 mRNA in this tissue. The possibility that the actions of IL-1 in the hypothalamus are mediated by a subtype of IL-1 receptor that is not labelled by ^{125}I-hr-IL-1α under the conditions used in the present study (see Section 12.2) provides a more attractive hypothesis.

12.5 DISTRIBUTION AND ROLE OF IL-1 RECEPTORS IN THE MURINE PITUITARY GLAND

12.5.1 Distribution of Type I IL-1 Receptor mRNA and IL-1 Binding Sites

Data from experiments using both *in situ* hybridisation and receptor autoradiography suggested that IL-1 receptors are expressed in abundance throughout the mouse anterior pituitary gland. Thus, with both techniques a dense and homogeneously distributed autoradiographic signal was observed over the entire anterior lobe. By contrast, IL-1 mRNA was not detectable in either the intermediate or posterior lobes of the gland. Similarly, no specific ^{125}I-hr-IL-1α or ^{125}I-hr-IL-1ra binding could be detected in these areas. Results from the receptor autoradiography studies using ^{125}I-hr-IL-1α and ^{125}I-hr-IL-1ra as ligands are shown in Fig. 12.4.

^{125}I-IL-1α ^{125}I-IL-1ra

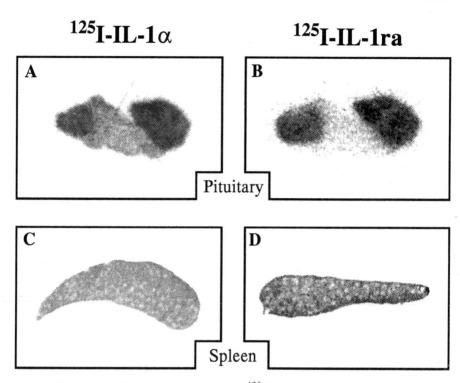

Figure 12.4 Autoradiographic localisation of ^{125}I-hr-IL-1α (**Fig. 12.4a** and **Fig. 12.4c**) and ^{125}I-hr-IL-1ra(**Fig. 12.4b** and **Fig. 12.4d**) binding in mouse pituitary (top) and spleen (bottom). The tissues were incubated for 120 min with 40 pM of ^{125}I-hr-IL-1ra and 100 pM of ^{125}I-hr-IL-1α. The images were computer generated using autoradiogram on Hyperfilm. The darker areas in autoradiograms correspond to regions displaying higher densities of binding

12.5.2 Physiological and Pharmacological Actions

Several studies have demonstrated that IL-1 induces the release of pro-opiomelanocortin (POMC)-derived peptides from cultured anterior pituitary cells (23) and from a pituitary tumour-derived mouse corticotroph cell line, AtT-20 (8). However, the direct actions of IL-1 on the corticotrophs differ from the widely reported stimulatory actions of IL-1 on CRH release from the hypothalamus in that, in most instances, they emerge only after a relatively long contact time (8). These observations have led to the view that the pituitary gland may play a significant role in maintaining and augmenting the HPA response to sustained immune insults. Our finding, that IL-1 mRNA and

[125]I-hr-IL-1 binding sites are distributed homogeneously throughout the anterior lobe, supports this view and further suggests that the cytokine also contributes to the regulation of the secretion of other anterior pituitary hormones. In accord with this premise are widespread reports that IL-1 modulates the release of luteinising hormone, follicle stimulating hormone, thyrotrophin, growth hormone and prolactin.

12.6   DISTRIBUTION AND ROLE OF IL-1 RECEPTORS IN THE MOUSE TESTIS

12.6.1   Distribution of Type I IL-1 Receptor mRNA and IL-1 Binding Sites

In situ hybridisation studies have revealed that IL-1 receptor mRNA is expressed in abundance throughout the interstitial region of the testis proper (i.e. the zone containing mostly Leydig cells) and in the cytoplasm of the epithelial cells lining the epididymal duct, particularly in the head region. By contrast, the hybridisation signals recorded from the seminiferous tubules, the sperm cells within seminiferous tubules and epididymal ducts and the muscular and connective tissue elements throughout the testes were indistinguishable from background. In accord with these data, moderately intense ^{125}I-hr-IL-1α binding has been observed in the interstitial region and in the head, body and tail of the epididymis, while a higher density has been recorded along the luminal borders of the epididymis with a circumferential pattern of distribution. Binding in the luminal centres of the epididymis and the lumen of the seminiferous tubules, by contrast, was weak. These data are illustrated in Fig. 12.5.

12.6.2   Physiological and Pharmacological Actions

The functional nature of the IL-1 binding sites in testis is supported by demonstrations that IL-1 inhibits steroidogenesis by cultured Leydig cells or neonatal testicular cells (24). Further evidence to this effect is provided by a recent study which showed that IL-1 stimulates spermatogonial proliferation *in vivo* (25). The significance of the high density of IL-1 binding sites in the epididymis is, at present, unclear. However, IL-1 activity is readily detectable in extracts of epididymal tissue and epididymal sperm (26) and it has been mooted that the locally produced cytokine may fulfil a role in spermatogenesis (27) or possibly in sperm transit. Although it is outside the scope of this chapter, it should be noted that other studies provide compelling evidence for important roles for cytokines in the reproductive tissues of females, including ovulation

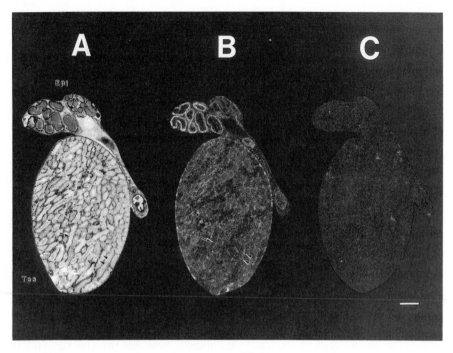

Figure 12.5 Autoradiographic localisation of ^{125}I-hr-IL-1α binding sites in intact mouse testis. **Fig. 12.5a** bright-field photomicrograph showing the histology of a cresyl violet stained section of mouse testis. **Fig. 12.5b** darkfield photomicrograph (using Ultrofilm as a negative) showing the total distribution of ^{125}I-hr-IL-1α binding sites in mouse testis and epididymis. In dark-field illumination, the highest densities of binding sites show up as the lighter areas and the tissue is not visible. Note the high densities of IL-1 binding sites in the epididymis (most notably in the head region) and in the interstitial areas of the testis. The interstitial region of the testis is indicated by the double arrowheads. Note the lower density of ^{125}I-hr-IL-1α binding in the lumen of the seminiferous tubules (arrow). In **Fig. 12.5c**, note the absence of specific ^{125}I-hr-IL-1α binding in an adjacent section (i.e. blank) co-incubated with 100 nM IL-1β. Abbreviations: Tes, testis; Epi, epididymis. Bar = 1 mm

and menstruation which have inherent inflammatory elements and much yet remains to be discovered about these processes.

12.7 DISTRIBUTION AND ROLE OF IL-1 RECEPTORS IN THE SPLEEN

Data from autoradiographic studies using ^{125}I-hr-IL-1α (Fig. 12.4c) and ^{125}I-hr-IL-1ra (Fig. 12.4d) as ligands indicate that IL-1 receptors in mouse spleen are concentrated in the red pulp, which consists of venous sinuses and splenic cord (29), and may be located primarily on macrophages. The white pulp regions (which are enriched with lymphocytes) by contrast are almost completely devoid of IL-1 binding sites. Reports that IL-1 mRNA is expressed in substantial quantities by splenic macrophages located in the marginal zone and red pulp regions suggest that the splenic IL-1 receptors may subserve an autocrine role; this may include internalisation of the cytokine by target cells in a manner analogous to that reported in purified human blood monocytes (30).

12.8 MODULATION OF THE EXPRESSION OF IL-1β AND IL-1 RECEPTORS *IN VIVO*

12.8.1 Effects of Hypophysectomy

Since IL-1 exerts profound effects on the functional activity of the HPA (8) and the HPG (9) axes, experiments were undertaken to elucidate the effects of hypophysectomy (and hence the pituitary hormones) on the expression of IL-1 receptors in the hippocampus and testis (16). Hypophysectomy resulted within 2–3 weeks in atrophy of the hippocampus and a concomitant reduction in the total number of ^{125}I-hr-IL-1α binding sites which was proportional to the decrease in tissue mass. Surgical removal of the pituitary gland also caused atrophy of the testis and a concomitant reduction in IL-1 receptor expression; however, in contrast to the hippocampus, the alterations in receptor expression were not uniform and in some areas of the testis the density of ^{125}I-hr-IL-1α binding sites remained unchanged. These data are difficult to interpret in view of the multiple effects of hypophysectomy in the body. Nonetheless, they support the premise that pituitary hormones contribute to the mechanisms regulating IL-1 receptor expression in both the hippocampus and the testis. In addition, they raise the possibility that specific populations of IL-1 receptors in the testis are regulated by mechanisms which are independent of the pituitary gland.

12.8.2 Effects of Endotoxin Treatment

In an attempt to examine further the mechanisms controlling the expression of IL-1 and IL-1 receptors in the mouse brain–endocrine–immune axis, we examined the effects of an immune insult (intraperitoneal injection of bacterial endotoxin, i.e. lipopolysaccharide, LPS) on these parameters using an enzyme linked immunosorbent assay to determine IL-1β and quantitative autoradiography and conventional ligand binding to evaluate specific ^{125}I-hr-IL-1α binding (31). Low levels of IL-1β were detected in all the tissues taken from control animals, i.e. hippocampus, hypothalamus, pituitary gland, epididymis, testis and spleen. The concentration of IL-1β in the peripheral tissues (pituitary gland, testis and spleen) was dramatically increased at 2–6 h after a single LPS injection but no significant changes were observed in brain (hippocampus and hypothalamus) at this stage. These changes were accompanied by a decrease in ^{125}I-hr-IL-1α binding in the spleen but not in the hippocampus or testis. In order to evaluate whether IL-1 expression in the brain is influenced by more sustained exposure to endotoxin, we examined the effects of two successive injections of LPS given at 12 hour intervals. Significant increases in IL-1β concentration were noted in hippocampus, hypothalamus, spleen, testis and epididymis 12 hours after the second injection; furthermore, ^{125}I-hr-IL-1α binding was significantly decreased in all tissues examined including the pituitary gland (Fig. 12.6). Subsequently, saturation analysis on whole tissue homogenates demonstrated that the LPS-induced decrease in ^{125}I-hr-IL-1α binding was due primarily to a decrease in the density (B_{max}) rather than

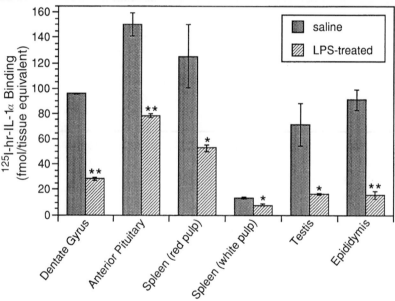

Figure 12.6 Effects of two injections of lipopolysaccharide (LPS) on ^{125}I-hr-IL-1α binding in brain, endocrine and immune tissues using quantitative autoradiography. Mice were injected with LPS (30 μg/mouse) at time 0 and 12 h and sacrificed 12 h after the second LPS injection. Data are expressed as the mean ± SEM of the average sampling values obtained from the autoradiograms. * and **, significant differences at $p < 0.05$ and $p < 0.005$, respectively from saline-injected controls, as determined by Student's t-test

the affinity (K_d) of the receptors. However, in the kidney, LPS treatment caused a significant decrease in the K_d as well as a substantial reduction in the B_{max} value. These data demonstrate that LPS treatment results in a profound increase in IL-1 expression in the brain–endocrine–immune axis and a concomitant down-regulation of IL-1 receptors which may be consequent on the increased IL-1 drive. The dramatic compensatory homologous down-regulation of IL-1 receptors in the tissues further underscores the importance of the cytokine in regulating brain–endocrine–immune function at all levels.

12.9   MODULATION OF IL-1 RECEPTOR EXPRESSION IN THE MOUSE AtT-20 PITUITARY TUMOUR CELL LINE

IL-1 and CRH are considered to be primary candidate mediators involved in co-ordinating the brain–endocrine–immune response to stress. IL-1 is a potent stimulator of hypothalamo–pituitary–adrenocortical hormone secretion through effects both in the brain and at the pituitary level—see Chapters 1, 8 and 13 and (8) for review. We hypothesised that hypothalamic CRH may be integral to the regulation of IL-1 receptors during stress. Accordingly, we used the AtT-20 corticotroph cell line (see Section 12.5.2) as a model in which to examine the influence *in vitro* of rat/human CRH on the binding of ^{125}I-hr-IL-1α and ^{125}I-Tyr[0]-ovine CRH (^{125}I-oCRH, 32). Exposure of the AtT-20 cells to CRH for 24 hours produced a concentration-dependent increase in ^{125}I-IL-1α binding and a parallel concentration-dependent decrease in ^{125}I-oCRH binding. The CRH-induced increase in ^{125}I-hr-IL-1α binding appears to be mediated through specific CRH receptors as it was inhibited by the CRH receptor antagonist, α-helical ovine CRH$_{9-41}$, which itself had no discernible effects. Scatchard analysis of data from saturation studies indicated that the CRH treatment increased the number of IL-1 binding sites (i.e. the B_{max}) without affecting the affinity (K_d). The mechanism underlying the up-regulation of IL-1 receptors is unclear but may include increased synthesis of IL-1 receptors, unmasking of cryptic receptors and a decrease in internalisation of IL-1 receptors. By analogy, if CRH also causes up-regulation of IL-1 receptors in normal anterior pituitary cells, this might provide a mechanism whereby IL-1 (which increases in stressful situations) may act at the pituitary level to maintain the elevated plasma ACTH levels seen following stress (see Sections 12.2 and 12.5.2 and Chapters 1 and 13).

12.10   SUMMARY AND CONCLUSIONS

IL-1 receptors, as defined by ^{125}I-hr-IL-1α and ^{125}I-hr-IL-1ra ligand binding, have been identified, characterised and localised in mouse brain, endocrine and immune tissues. Specific ^{125}I-hr-IL-1 binding in homogenates of the mouse tissues is concentration-dependent, saturable, reversible and of high affinity; in addition it shows a linear relationship with membrane protein concentration. The binding sites for ^{125}I-hr-IL-1 exhibit a pharmacological specificity for IL-1 and its analogues which parallels the relative biological potencies of the compounds in the thymocyte proliferation assay. The kinetic and pharmacological characteristics of the ^{125}I-hr-IL-1 binding sites in brain, endocrine and immune tissues and in AtT-20 cells are similar to those previously observed in EL-4 6.1 mouse thymoma cell membranes, T lymphocytes and fibroblasts (33) and appear to correspond to Type I receptors. Receptor autoradiography and *in situ* hybridisation studies have demonstrated a discrete localisation of IL-1 receptors and Type I IL-1 receptor mRNA in a variety of tissues with high densities occurring in the dentate gyrus of the hippocampus, the choroid plexus, the anterior pituitary gland, the marginal zones and red pulp regions of the spleen, the epididymis and the interstitial area of the testis. Endotoxin administration augments endogenous IL-1 expression, which in turn causes down-regulation of IL-1 receptors in mouse brain and peripheral tissues, suggesting that endotoxin injures host tissues, at least in part, through the action of endogenous IL-1. Studies have demonstrated that IL-1 induces ACTH release directly, by an action on the pituitary, as well as indirectly via hypothalamic CRH secretion. In view of the high density of IL-1 receptors in the anterior pituitary gland and the increase in IL-1 receptor density induced by CRH in AtT-20 cells, we may speculate that IL-1 acts directly at the pituitary level to augment or maintain elevations in plasma ACTH levels seen, for example, in long-term stress. These data provide further support for a role for IL-1 in co-ordinating brain–endocrine–immune responses to stress and infection. Evidence for widespread biological actions of IL-1 in the rat, where IL-1 receptors are largely undetectable, together with the apparent lack of IL-1 receptor expression in the mouse hypothalamus, however, point to the existence of novel receptors or possibly new methods of signalling which are yet to be discovered.

ACKNOWLEDGEMENTS

The data presented in this chapter involved collaborative studies with Steven G. Culp, Emmet T. Cunningham Jr., Robert C. Newton, Daniel E. Tracy, W. Mark Mitchell and Elizabeth L. Webster. We thank them for their contributions.

REFERENCES

1. Dinarello C. A. Interleukin-1 and interleukin-1 antagonism. *Blood*, 1991, **77**: 1627–52.
2. Farrar W. L., Hill J. M., Harel-Bellan A., Vinocour M. The immune logical brain. *Immunol Rev*, 1987, **100**: 361–78.

3. Breder C. D., Dinarello C. A., Saper C. B. Interleukin-1 immunoreactive innervation of the human hypothalamus. *Science*, 1988, **240**: 321–4.
4. Lue F. A., Bail M., Gorczynski R., Moldofsky H. Sleep and interleukin-1-like activity in cat cerebrospinal fluid. *Sleep Research*, 1987, **16**: 51.
5. Fontana A., Kristensen F., Dubs R., Gemsa D., Weber E. Production of prostaglandin E and an interleukin-like factor by cultured astrocytes and C6 glioma cells. *J Immunol*, 1982, **129**: 2413–9.
6. Giulian D., Lachman L. B. Interleukin-1 stimulates astroglial proliferation after brain injury. *Science*, 1985, **228**: 497–9.
7. Fontana A., Weber E., Dayer J. M. Synthesis of interleukin-1/endogenous pyrogen in the brain of endotoxin treated mice: A step in fever induction. *J Immunol*, 1984, **133**: 1696–8.
8. Buckingham J. C., Loxley H. D., Christian H. C., Philip J. G. Activation of the HPA axis by immune insults: roles and interactions of cytokines, eicosanoids and glucocorticoids. *Pharmacol Biochem Behav*, 1996, **54**: 285–98.
9. Rivier C., Vale W. In the rat, interleukin-1α acts at the level of the brain and the gonads to interfere with gonadotropin and sex steroid secretion. *Endocrinology*, 1989, **124**: 2105–9.
10. Bomsztyk K., Sims J. E., Stanton T. H., Slack J., McMahan C. J., Valentine M. A., *et al*. Evidence for different interleukin-1 receptors in murine B- and T-cell lines. *Proc Natl Acad Sci USA*, 1989, **86**: 8034–8.
11. Chizzonite R., Truitt T., Kilian P. L., Stern A. S., Nunes P., Parker K. P., *et al*. Two high-affinity interleukin 1 receptors represent separate gene products. *Proc Natl Acad Sci USA*, 1989, **86**: 8029–33.
12. Carter D. B., Deibel M. R. Jr, Dunn C. J., Tomich C. S., Laborde A. L., Slightom J. L., *et al*. Purification, cloning, expression and biological characterization of an interleukin-1 receptor antagonist protein. *Nature*, 1990, **344**: 633–8.
13. Dripps D. J., Verderber E., Ray K. N., Thompson R. C., Eisenberg S. P. Interleukin-1 receptor antagonist binds to the type II interleukin-1 receptor on B cells and neutrophils. *J Biol Chem*, 1991, **266**: 20311–5.
14. Takao T., Culp S. G., Newton R. C., De Souza E. B. Type I interleukin-1 (IL-1) receptors in the mouse brain–endocrine–immune axis labelled with 125I-recombinant human IL-1 receptor antagonist. *J Neuroimmunol*, 1992, **41**: 51–60.
15. Dinarello C. A., Thompson R. C. Blocking IL-1: interleukin-1 receptor antagonist *in vivo* and *in vitro*. *Immunol Today*, 1991, **12**: 404–10.
16. Takao T., Tracey D. E., Mitchell W. M., De Souza E. B. Interleukin-1 receptors in mouse brain: Characterization and neuronal localization. *Endocrinology*, 1990, **127**: 3070–8.
17. Munson P. J., Rodbard D. LIGAND: a versatile computerized approach for characterization of ligand-binding systems. *Anal Biochem*, 1980, **297**: 220–9.
18. Gery I., Gershon R. K., Waksman B. H. Potentiation of the T-lymphocyte response to mitogens I. The responding cell. *J Exp Med*, 1972, **136**: 128–42.
19. Cunningham E. T. Jr, Wada E., Carter D. B., Tracey D. E., Battey J. F., De Souza E. B. *In situ* histochemical localization of type I interleukin-1 receptor messenger RNA in the central nervous system, pituitary and adrenal gland of the mouse. *J Neurosci*, 1992, **12**: 1101–14.
20. Friedman W. J., Larkfors L., Ayer-LeLievre C., Ebendal T., Olson L., Person H. Regulation of B-nerve growth factor expression by inflammatory mediator in hippocampal cultures. *J Neurosci Res*, 1991, **27**: 347–88.
21. Fagan A. M., Gage F. H. Cholinergic sprouting in the hippocampus: a proposed role for IL-1. *Exp Neurol*, 1990, **110**: 105–20.

22. Hori T., Osaka T., Kiyohara T., Shibata M., Nakashima T. Hippocampal input to preoptic thermosensitive neurons in the rat. *Neurosci Lett*, 1982, **32**: 155–8.
23. Bernton E. W., Beach J. E., Holaday J. W., Smallridge R. C., Fein H. G. Release of multiple hormones by a direct action of interleukin-1 on pituitary cells. *Science*, 1987, **238**: 519–21.
24. Fauser B. C. J. M., Galway A. B., Hsueh A. J. Inhibitory actions of interleukin-1β on steroidogenesis in primary cultures of neonatal rat testicular cells. *Acta Endocrinol (Copenh)*, 1989, **120**: 401–8.
25. Pollanen P., Soder O., Parvinen M. Interleukin-1α stimulation of spermatogonial proliferation *in vivo*. *Reprod Fert Dev*, 1989, **1**: 85–7.
26. Syed V., Soder O., Arver S., Lindh M., Khan S., Ritzen E. M. Ontogeny and cellular origin of an interleukin-1-like factor in the reproductive tract of the male rat. *Int J Androl*, 1988, **11**: 437–47.
27. Werber H. I., Emancipator S. N., Tykocinski M. L., Sedor J.R. The interleukin-1 gene expression by rat glomerular mesangial cells is augmented in immune complex glomerulonephritis. *J Immunol*, 1987, **138**: 3207–12.
28. Antonipillai I., Wang Y., Horton R. Tumor necrosis factor and interleukin-1 may regulate renin secretion. *Endocrinology*, 1990, **126**: 273–8.
29. Fujita T., Kashimura M., Adachi K. Scanning electron microscopy and terminal circulation. *Experientia*, 1985, **41**: 167–79.
30. Uhl J., Newton R. C., Giri J. G., Sandlin G., Horuk R. Identification of IL-1 receptors on human monocytes. *J Immunol*, 1988, **142**: 1576–81.
31. Takao T., Culp S. G., De Souza E. B. Reciprocal modulation of Interleukin-1β (IL-1β) and IL-1 receptors by lipopolysaccharide (endotoxin) treatment in the mouse brain–endocrine–immune axis. *Endocrinology*, 1993, **132**: 1497–1504.
32. Tracey D. E., De Souza E. B. Identification of interleukin-1 receptors in mouse pituitary cell membranes and AtT-20 pituitary tumor cells. *Soc Neurosci Abstr*, 1988, **14**: 1052.
33. Dower S. K., Call S. M., Gillis S., Urdal D. L. Similarity between the interleukin-1 receptors on a murine T-lymphoma cell line and on a murine fibroblast cell line. *Proc Natl Acad Sci USA*, 1986, **83**: 1060–4.

Chapter 13

Responses of the Stress Axis to Immunological Challenge: The Role of Eicosanoids and Cytokines

P. Navarra

Catholic University Medical School, Rome, Italy

G. Schettini

School of Medicine, University of Genoa, Italy and

A. B. Grossman*

St. Bartholomew's Hospital, London, UK

13.1 INTRODUCTION

It was once thought that host defence was performed largely by an autonomous immune system and that the brain was a privileged site, being protected from immune activation. We now appreciate that an effective two-way communication between the immune and brain–neuroendocrine systems exists which is fundamental to bodily homeostatic mechanisms and to host defence in particular, in conditions of health and disease. Co-ordination of these systems in response to a

*To whom correspondence should be addressed

Stress, Stress Hormones and the Immune System. Edited by J. C. Buckingham, G. E. Gillies and A.-M. Cowell
© 1997 John Wiley & Sons, Ltd.

noxious stimulus, whether it be a cognitive stress (e.g. an emotional or physical insult) or a non-cognitive stress (e.g. immunological or inflammatory challenges) relies to a large extent on the rapid activation of the hypothalamo–pituitary–adrenal (HPA) axis, resulting in the secretion of glucocorticoids to restore homeostasis. This process may include metabolic adjustments and behavioural effects as well as modulation of immune and inflammatory processes (see also Chapters 2 and 8).

The regulation of the HPA axis is described in detail in Chapter 1. The major components of this axis are the hypothalamic corticotrophin releasing hormone (CRH) and arginine vasopressin (AVP) which act synergistically to stimulate the secretion of adrenocorticotrophic hormone (ACTH) from the anterior pituitary gland which, in turn, stimulates production of cortisol (in man) or corticosterone (in the rat). These glucocorticoid hormones are the dominant endocrine inhibitors of the immune response and their activities are described in detail in Chapter 8. In the clinical and experimental situation it has now been demonstrated that the immune system equally signals to the neuroendocrine system. While immune challenges may elicit significant changes in the reproductive and growth axes (see also Chapters 9 and 16), the predominant survival need is for up-regulation of glucocorticoid function. Thus, the immune system has access to a pathway whereby it can attenuate its own responses. By analogy to other classical negative feedback pathways, it has been suggested that the purpose of this feedback loop is to prevent immunological processes from "over-shooting" and consequently damaging host tissue. Immunological and inflammatory challenges normally involve the *localised* production of vasoactive mediators (e.g. eicosanoids, cytokines, peptides; see also Chapter 3) which contribute to the manifestation of the local inflammatory response. When such responses become generalised, as in septicaemia, the overriding concern must be the preservation of vascular integrity and blood pressure in order to preserve perfusion and hence function of the brain and other vital organs. The HPA-immune system interaction is critical in all of these processes.

Activated immune cells produce many biologically potent substances, notably interleukin (IL)-1 α and β, IL-2, IL-6, IL-8, interferon-α (IFN-α), lipid metabolites (e.g. eicosanoids, platelet activating factor), amines (e.g. histamine, 5-hydroxytryptamines, 5-HT), peptides (e.g. substance P, bradykinin, angiotensin II, thymic polypeptides) and enzymes (e.g. phospholipase A_2, PLA_2), all of which are released into the general circulation and may potentially influence HPA activity. This chapter will consider the mechanisms through which pro-inflammatory cytokines and eicosanoids activate the HPA axis, either directly within the neuroendocrine organs themselves or indirectly either via the production of intermediates, for example prostaglandins, or via activation of sensory reflexes.

Before discussing how immune signals influence the HPA axis it is important to appreciate the difficulties involved in designing the "perfect" experiment. This issue is addressed in a review elsewhere (1) and a few important points will be summarised here. As discussed in Chapter 5, it is important to be aware that any stresses inherent in the experimental design, including such relatively minor procedures as intraperitoneal (i.p.) injection, could influence results and should be controlled for. The very nature of the immune response, with its chronological, often self-amplifying, cascade of mediators complicates interpretation of experiments. The length of time between the immune challenge and plasma measurements will thus critically affect the spectrum of biological mediators present; measurement of a single component will not provide an overall picture of a very complex, multi-factorial system. Equally, investigations of activities of individual components produced by activated immune cells are limited as these substances act in concert physiologically. Finally, a great many studies utilise injections of bacterial cell wall-derived endotoxin (lipopolysaccharide, LPS) to induce conditions resembling endotoxaemia and septic shock which are, in fact, relatively rare phenomena. The relevance of these experimental findings to day-to-day homeostasis and host defence thus remains to be determined. Indeed, because of their extreme potency and the limitations of assay sensitivities, plasma levels of cytokines in rodent models in conditions of mild infections are not yet being measured reliably (1). However, IL-1β, IL-6 and tumour necrosis factor-α (TNF-α) have been found in the synovial fluid of patients with chronic arthritis, although only IL-6 is detectable in the circulation.

13.2 CYTOKINES AND HYPOTHALAMO–PITUITARY– ADRENAL (HPA) ACTIVATION

Of the cytokines known to activate the HPA axis IL-1, IL-6 and TNF-α have been most studied. The precise spectrum of cytokines released in response to a challenge such as LPS appears to depend to a certain extent on the dose administered. When injected individually, these cytokines, whether purified or recombinant proteins, potently activate the HPA axis. Administration of specific antibodies which immunoneutralise specific cytokines can impair an effective HPA response to a variety of stimuli, including endotoxin. These results, therefore, suggest an involvement of these cytokines in activating the HPA axis in response to immune or inflammatory processes. Fig. 13.1 is a summary of the principal potential sites (at any point within the HPA axis) at which activated immune cell products might exert their actions, *viz.* at any point in the HPA axis, by non-specific stresses due to the pathological effects of infection or inflammation (e.g. pain, hypotension, hypoglycaemia, elevated lactic acid) or via primary nociceptive and other sensory afferents which reflexly activate the HPA axis (2). The third mechanism, possibly mediated by C-fibre and vagal reflexes after activation by local immune or inflammatory mediators, may account for some reports that plasma levels of ACTH may rise in response to LPS injection prior

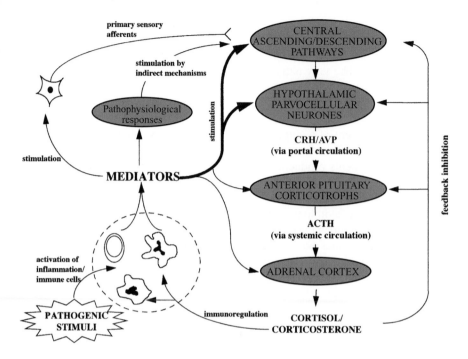

Figure 13.1 Major paths of communication between the immune system and the hypothalamo–pituitary–adrenocortical axis. CRH = corticotrophin releasing hormone; AVP = arginine vasopressin; ACTH = adrenocorticotrophic hormone. From Buckingham J. C. *Brit J Pharmacol*, 1996, **118**: 1–19, reproduced with permission of Macmillan Press Limited.

to the appearance of IL-1β, IL-6 or TNF-α in the circulation. Other cytokines could, however, also be involved or, alternatively, cytokines are such potent substances that they could be active at levels that are below detection. The major emphasis of this chapter will be on the central actions of immune mediators in regulating HPA activity.

13.2.1 Evidence for a Hypothalamic Involvement

In Vivo and In Vitro Studies

On balance, the hypothalamus is the favoured site for mediating cytokine activation of the HPA axis. In the rat, ACTH release in response to IL-1β, IL-6 and TNFα is either reduced or prevented by pre-treatment with CRH antiserum.

Furthermore, peripheral injections of IL-1β increased CRH mRNA expression specifically in the parvocellular division of the hypothalamic paraventricular nucleus (PVN) where the CRH and AVP neurones involved in regulating ACTH secretion are situated (see Chapter 1). Intracerebroventricular administration of IL-1β increases plasma ACTH and serum corticosterone levels in the rat and studies conducted on isolated rat hypothalami demonstrate the ability of IL-1 (α and β) as well as IL-6 and IL-8 to stimulate the release both of CRH and AVP (3). The importance of the AVP response, however, remains controversial. In support of the *in vitro* studies, central (but not peripheral) injections of IL-1β increase AVP mRNA expression in the parvocellular PVN (4) and intra-hypothalamic injections increase AVP release at the median eminence level, as determined by microdialysis (5). However, the immunocytochemical AVP signals and portal AVP blood levels were unchanged in response to cytokines, whereas the CRH signals were increased (6,7). Regarding the *in vitro* results, it must be borne in mind that the preparation employed contains both magnocellular and parvocellular AVP neurones and a component of the AVP response to cytokines may be destined for release from the neurohypophysis to act as an antidiuretic agent and vasoconstrictor.

Some interesting observations from *in vitro* experiments have shown that conditioned media from endotoxin-stimulated peritoneal macrophages produce an increase in CRH and AVP secretion far in excess of the maximum responses to the individual cytokines. Also, low levels of TNF-α, which themselves have no activity, may enhance IL-1β-stimulated AVP release. This raises the possibility of synergism amongst the cytokines which is an aspect of their neuroendocrine actions not yet fully explored. Studies *in vivo* also suggest that the HPA response to LPS is dependent on the synergistic actions of IL-1, IL-6 and TNF-α within the hypothalamus, with IL-6 production being stimulated locally by the other two cytokines (8).

Receptor Location

Receptors for IL-6 and TNF are readily detectable within the hypothalamus, which is consistent with a direct effect of these cytokines at this level of the HPA axis. A hypothalamic site of action for IL-1 is also consistent with early studies showing the presence of IL-1 binding sites in the rat hypothalamus (9,10). However, the precise nature of these binding sites remains controversial, as several workers have failed to detect specific IL-1 receptors in this brain area although they can be detected elsewhere (e.g. hippocampus, see Chapter 12 for further details). The IL-1 receptor antagonist, however, blocks the elevations in circulating ACTH induced by IL-1β (administered peripherally or into the median eminence) and, when centrally administered, the antagonist blocks the HPA response to endotoxin. The apparent paradox of biological actions being exerted by IL-1 at the hypothalamic level while the cytokine's known receptor subtypes (type I and type II) are undetectable is discussed in detail elsewhere (11, 12 and see Chapter 12). Very recently, an IL-1 receptor accessory protein has been described (13). The localisation of this protein in brain tissues raises the possibility that, in the hypothalamus, IL-1 might signal through a novel and as yet uncharacterised receptor complex.

Direct Versus Indirect Activation of the Hypothalamus

Although it seems clear that HPA activation in response to an immune challenge is dependent on CRH and/or AVP release synthesis, it remains to be established whether this response is due to cytokines acting directly at the peptidergic neuronal cell bodies in the PVN. Some studies suggest that cytokines exert their actions at central sites where input pathways to the PVN originate. Of particular interest are the serotonergic pathways from the hippocampus and the adrenergic input from the brain stem, as both of these regions abundantly express receptors for IL-1, IL-6 and TNF and are known to influence HPA function—see (1) for review.

Although evidence points largely to a central site of action for cytokines produced peripherally in response to an immune challenge, it is debatable whether cytokines, which have a molecular mass in the 17–26 kDa region, will cross the blood–brain barrier and to date there is no evidence for their assisted transport. There are certain important areas, however, which are effectively outside the blood–brain barrier. In particular, the median eminence which contains CRH and AVP terminals is thought to be an immediate target for the actions of blood-borne cytokines. Support for this view comes from the ability of IL-1β to release CRH (but not AVP) from a median eminence preparation containing only nerve terminals and from the observation that cytokines injected directly into the median eminence can increase circulating levels of ACTH (2). A further possible site of action is the organum vasculosum of lamina terminalis (OVLT), located in the anterior wall of the third ventricle, which is a region where the barrier is fenestrated and where cytokines could conceivably enter or transmit signals to central nervous system (CNS) structures. In addition, any local inflammation would non-specifically increase the permeability of the cerebral vasculature.

A more complex mechanism whereby cytokines may activate the HPA axis is suggested by the observations that peripheral endotoxin challenge in rodents results in an increase in IL-1 expression in the hypothalamus and other brain areas (14,15) and that either central or i.p. injections of LPS increase mRNA levels for IL-6 in the hypothalamus within two hours (16). In order to explain these effects it has been proposed that the peripherally generated cytokines may act at the level of the endothelium and, via a mechanism involving prostanoids (see also Section 13.3.3), stimulate cytokine expression in the CNS.

13.2.2   Evidence for a Direct Pituitary or Adrenal Involvement

Experiments involving ablation of the PVN prevent the HPA activation produced by peripheral injection of IL-6 and TNF-α, but only partially counteract the response to IL-1β, suggesting that the latter but not the former can act at the level of the anterior pituitary gland. Investigations on anterior pituitary tissue *in vitro* suggest that long term exposure is needed before both IL-1β and IL-6 stimulate ACTH release, whereas a more rapid response is seen with conditioned medium from endotoxin-stimulated macrophages, which presumably contains a cytokine "cocktail" (3). Furthermore, both IL-1β and IL-6 are synthesised in the adenohypophysis and the latter is enhanced by LPS. At the adrenocortical level, several cytokines have weak stimulatory actions on the synthesis and release of glucocorticoids and IL-6 mRNA levels within the cortex appear responsive to LPS administration. Cytokines are thus likely to exert some actions at the pituitary and possibly the adrenal levels, but the biological significance of these actions remains to be determined.

13.3   EICOSANOIDS AND HPA ACTIVATION

Eicosanoids play an important role in effecting in the HPA response to immunological challenge acting at various levels in the axis. These inflammatory mediators are the metabolic products of arachidonic acid, a fatty acid which is liberated either from membrane phospholipids by the action of PLA_2 or from diacylglycerol by the action of diacylglycerol lipase. The major groups of eicosanoids are: (a) the prostanoids (prostaglandins, prostacyclin and thromboxanes), (b) leukotrienes (LTs) and hydroxyeicosatetraenoic acids (HETEs), and (c) the epoxyeicosatrienoic acids (epoxides or EETs) which are produced by the cyclo-oxygenase, lipoxygenase and cytochrome P_{450} (epoxygenase) enzymes respectively (see Chapter 8).

The eicosanoids are rapidly metabolised in the pulmonary and systemic circulations and thus do not normally exert endocrine-like effects but act locally as autocrine, paracrine or intracrine agents.

13.3.1   Prostaglandins

Many studies have been carried out to determine the role of eicosanoids in the control of the HPA axis—for review see (17). It is well established that prostaglandins, administered systemically, are potent stimulators of ACTH secretion. They have actions at hypothalamic, pituitary or adrenal levels. In addition, prostaglandins generated in the periphery may indirectly influence HPA function by, for example, stimulating sensory nerve endings.

Early studies, based on systemic administration of various prostaglandins in rats with median eminence lesions to disrupt hypothalamo–pituitary communication, indicated that prostaglandins can stimulate the HPA axis via an increase in CRH release. Furthermore, local injection of the cyclo-oxygenase inhibitor, indomethacin, into discrete hypothalamic areas, especially in the anterior hypothalamus, inhibited ACTH secretion in response to various stresses, thus supporting a role for prostaglandins produced endogenously within the hypothalamus in regulating CRH release and hence HPA function. Initial reports indicated that the stimulatory actions of the prostaglandins were not specific since prostaglandins of the E, F, A and B series all increased ACTH secretion when injected into the medial basal hypothalamus (18). However, later workers reported that while prostaglandin E_2 (PGE$_2$) and, to a lesser extent, PGE$_1$ stimulated ACTH release following microinjection into the pre-optic area, PGD$_2$ did not (9). Further evidence to support a hypothalamic site of action for prostaglandins comes from an *in vitro* study in which PGF$_{2\alpha}$, although paradoxically not PGE$_2$, stimulated CRH release from the isolated rat hypothalamus (20).

In contrast to their actions at the hypothalamus, prostaglandins exert a significant inhibitory action at the pituitary level. *In vivo* and *in vitro* studies suggest that prostaglandins themselves do not affect basal ACTH secretion (18, 21, 22) but reduce the corticotrophic responses to secretagogues such as CRH and AVP (21, 22). Vlaskovska and colleagues (21) suggested that the inhibitory effect may be specific to PGE$_2$ but other studies have shown that prostanoids such as PGF$_{2\alpha}$ and stable analogues of prostacyclin (PGI$_2$) also attenuate the responses to CRH *in vitro* (22). However, PGE$_2$ synthesis in the pituitary gland is stimulated by CRH or AVP and inhibited by lesions of the hypothalamic PVN (23). Thus, PGE$_2$ may act as a locally produced negative feedback signal within the anterior pituitary gland. This concept is supported by findings *in vivo* that indomethacin, when injected directly into the adenohypophysis, potentiates ACTH release induced by hypothalamic extract (24) and also potentiates the corticotrophic responses of pituitary tissue to CRH and AVP *in vitro* (21). However, one must bear in mind that such responses may not be due necessarily to a reduction in prostanoid tone since, by blocking the cyclo-oxygenase pathway, indomethacin can shunt arachidonic acid metabolism along the lipoxygenase and epoxygenase pathways yielding products which may have prosecretory actions (see later).

Prostaglandins can also act at the adrenal level with most studies suggesting that prostaglandins increase steroidogenesis *in vitro*. Endogenous prostaglandins have also been implicated in the regulation of steroidogenesis, since hypophysectomised rats treated with indomethacin show a reduced corticosterone response to ACTH (25).

13.3.2   Other Eicosanoids

Information about the role of other eicosanoids in the regulation of the HPA axis is limited. The leukotrienes generally fail to influence corticotrophic responses *in vitro* (22, 26, 27) although, in one study, LTA_4 and LTB_4 stimulated the secretion of β-endorphin which is normally co-secreted with ACTH (27). Moreover, the 5-, 12- and 15-HETEs, which are the major lipoxygenase products formed in the adenohypophysis, have been reported to stimulate (27) or to have no effect on (26) β-endorphin release. Investigations into the role of endogenous lipoxygenase products in the control of ACTH secretion have been thwarted by the lack of selectivity and specificity of the lipoxygenase inhibitors available and conflicting data have been produced. Thus, some studies report that corticotrophic activity is reduced by lipoxygenase inhibitors and dual cyclo-oxygenase and lipoxygenase inhibitors (26, 27) while others report that some of these inhibitors have little effect on ACTH secretion (22). Endogenous epoxides have also been implicated in the control of ACTH secretion since inhibitors of cytochrome P_{450} reduce the corticotrophic responses of pituitary tissue (22, 28). However, the identity of the EETs involved is not known. Moreover, the possibility that the high concentrations of the drugs used in some studies may have produced non-specific effects cannot be excluded.

Inhibitors of the lipoxygenase enzymes also reduce ACTH-induced corticosteroid production by rat adrenal cells *in vitro* (29, 30) while 5-hydroperoxy-eicosatetraenoic acid augments the responses to ACTH (29). This raises the possibility that lipoxygenase products play a stimulatory role in the control of steroidogenesis. However, it has been suggested that coupling of ACTH to corticosteroid synthesis may also involve inhibitory influences exerted by lipoxygenase products, in particular LTA_4 (30).

13.3.3   Prostaglandin Mediation of Cytokine Activity

Recently, interest in the involvement of prostaglandins in the control of the HPA axis was rekindled by the observation that prostanoids mediate many biological effects of IL-1 (31). While prostaglandins influence the HPA axis at all levels, there is no evidence to suggest that they modulate the effects of cytokines on the adrenal gland. They also appear not to be involved in the acute IL-1-induced release of ACTH from isolated pituitary cells, although they may be involved in longer term regulation (32). Thus, most of the studies on the interplay between prostaglandins and cytokines in the control of the HPA axis have focused on the actions of these substances within the hypothalamus and on the control of CRH release in particular.

Prostaglandin Mediation of Cytokine-induced CRH Release

A key role for PGE_2 in the control of IL-1-induced ACTH release has been demonstrated in several *in vivo* studies in the rat. Hypothalamic production of prostaglandins is increased after administration of IL-1β or endotoxin (1) and Katsuura *et al.* (33) observed that indomethacin, a cyclo-oxygenase inhibitor, blunts the increase in circulating ACTH induced by intravenous or intracerebroventricular injection of IL-1β. When injected into the anterior hypothalamus, both indomethacin and a PGE_2 receptor antagonist counteract the increase in plasma ACTH induced by intravenous IL-1β, while systemic pre-treatment with indomethacin antagonises the rise in plasma ACTH induced by IL-1α. More recently, evidence has been provided that both IL-6 and TNF also stimulate the HPA axis *in vivo* via mechanisms involving the central activation of prostaglandin biosynthesis.

Both IL-1- and IL-6-induced release of CRH *in vitro* are inhibited by dexamethasone, by inhibitors of cyclo-oxygenase (e.g. indomethacin and naproxen) and by an inhibitor of the epoxygenase pathway (clotrimazol) but not by a selective inhibitor of the lipoxygenase pathway (BW A4C, Burroughs Wellcome). These results further suggest that IL-1 and IL-6 activate, probably in sequence, the PLA_2, cyclo-oxygenase and possibly the epoxygenase pathways to release CRH. This hypothesis has recently been supported by an elegant study by Loxley *et al.* (34) which showed that dexamethasone suppressed CRH release stimulated by IL-1 and IL-6 by mobilising hypothalamic lipocortin 1. Lipocortin 1 is a 37 kDa protein which has been shown to mediate aspects of glucocorticoid action in macrophages by inhibiting PLA_2 and, hence, eicosanoid generation (see Chapter 8). Furthermore, in hypothalamic explants, both IL-1β and IL-6 selectively increase the production and release of PGE_2 without affecting $PGF_{2\alpha}$, thromboxane B_2 and 6-keto-$PGF_{1\alpha}$ (35). Interleukin-1β is also able to stimulate selectively the synthesis and release of PGE_2 from cultures enriched in hypothalamic astrocytes, raising the possibility that a neurone–glial interaction may contribute to the control of CRH release exerted by cytokines.

In all *in vivo* studies where PGE_2 elicited HPA axis activation, injections were placed in the anterior hypothalamus. This led Katsuura *et al.* (19) to hypothesise that PGE_2 is the intra-hypothalamic mediator for IL-1β-induced ACTH secretion and that the OVLT, where the highest density of PGE_2 binding sites is found (36), may be the specific site at which circulating IL-1 increases PGE_2. Subsequent studies confirmed that PGE_2 was markedly increased in the OVLT and, to a lesser extent, in other hypothalamic regions by peripheral (i.v.) injection of IL-1β. The mechanism by which a local increase in PGE_2 in the anterior hypothalamus stimulates neurones within the PVN to release CRH is still unknown. PGE_2 could diffuse across the short distance from the anterior hypothalamus to the PVN or else a PGE_2-activated pathway might communicate between the anterior hypothalamus and the PVN (Fig. 13.2). Alternatively,

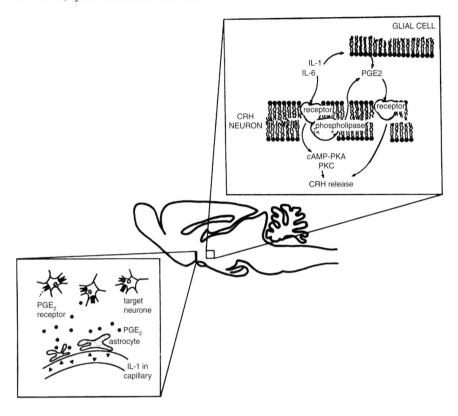

Figure 13.2 Two possible sites in the hypothalamus where prostaglandins (PG) may play a role in mediating the actions of cytokines on the hypothalamo–pituitary–adrenal axis. These are the organun lamina terminalis (OVLT, left panel) and the surface of the corticotrophin releasing hormone (CRH) neurones in the hypothalamic paraventricular nucleus (right panel). In the OVLT, circulating cytokines increase PGE_2 production by glial cells. PGE_2 in turn may stimulate the release of CRH either by diffusing to the PVN or via a specific neuronal pathway connecting the anterior hypothalamus to the PVN. On CRH neurones, PGE_2 synthesised from neuronal and glial cell membranes by cytokine-induced PLA_2 activation may reinforce interleukin-1 (IL-1)- and IL-6-induced CRH release through activation of its own receptor. The median eminence (not marked), which is largely outside the blood–brain barrier, offers a further site where circulating cytokines may stimulate PG to influence CRH release from nerve terminals. cAMP = $3'5'$-cyclic adenosine monophosphate; PKA = protein kinase A; PKC = protein kinase C. (Left panel modified from (19), Katsuura *et al.*, 1990)

prostaglandins may also be involved as mediators of cytokine action in the median eminence to influence CRH and AVP release at the level of the terminals. Whatever the mechanism, elevations in hypothalamic PGE_2 induced by circulating IL-1, or other "pyrogenic" cytokines such as IL-6 (37), are likely to represent a fundamental mechanism subserving various phenomena which take place during the acute phase response; these include activation of the HPA axis as well as febrile and anorectic responses, all of which also require the mediation of CRH (see also Chapter 14).

The foregoing discussion illustrates the powerful effect of prostaglandins on CRH release but it remains unclear whether, in the physiological situation, they act trans-synaptically on specific membrane receptors after release from neurones, whether they are produced locally by glial cells and act in a paracrine fashion or whether they play their role as intracellular modifiers of signal transduction cascades to alter peptide release. The latest studies suggest that prostanoids, produced in the hypothalamus in response to cytokines, trigger the further production of cytokines (3). A self-amplifying cascade may therefore exist whereby peripherally-derived cytokines (e.g. released in response to LPS) stimulate prostanoid production by endothelial cells or adjacent leukocytes which then triggers the hypothalamic production of cytokines which, in turn, stimulate CRH and/or AVP release—see Fig. 13.3 and (33, 35). In this model, PGE_2 should not be thought of as a classical intracellular second messenger of IL-1 and IL-6, but rather as a positive modulator of the cytokines' complex signal transduction mechanisms which trigger CRH release.

Another possible mechanism of action that also should be considered is that the cytokines generated within the periphery may activate sensory neurones, possibly by facilitating the release of PGE_2, and may thereby relay signals to the hypothalamus to augment local cytokine synthesis.

Other Mechanisms Involved in Cytokine Induced CRH Release

The findings that addition of PGE_2 to the incubation medium of hypothalamic explants failed to produce increases in CRH secretion of a magnitude equivalent to those induced by IL-1β or IL-6 (38) suggest that mechanisms other than

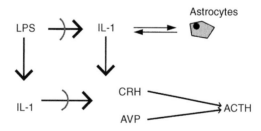

Figure 13.3 Possible schema for the activation of the hypothalamo–pituitary–adrenocortical axis by lipopolysaccharide (LPS). Either LPS or interleukin (IL)-1 must cross the blood–brain barrier to stimulate the release of corticotrophin releasing hormone (CRH) and arginine vasopressin (AVP); it is likely that astrocytes and prostaglandin E_2 mediate this response

activation of PLA_2 may be involved in the responses to the cytokines. Interleukin-1 acutely stimulates PLA_2 through the activation of the sphingomyelin pathway (39) but PLA_2 activation does not appear to be the only IL-1-operated post-receptor event. In fact, evidence suggests that IL-1 can trigger several transduction mechanisms simultaneously in the same cell. This seems to be the case for IL-1 stimulation of CRH release since studies on acutely incubated hypothalami suggest that both protein kinase A and protein kinase C pathways may be involved (40), but inhibition of each of these pathways by specific antagonists inhibits IL-1-induced CRH release completely (40). Some evidence exists also that nitric oxide and catecholamines may be mediators of cytokine activity in stimulating the HPA axis (1).

13.4   CONCLUSIONS

Infective and inflammatory processes communicate with the principal neuroendocrine stress effector, the HPA axis, primarily by modifying the release of hypothalamic CRH and AVP. This may be mediated via an activation of hypothalamic cytokines of neuronal or glial origin which, in turn, stimulate the release of CRH and AVP; alternatively, circulating IL-1 and IL-6 may activate the hypothalamic neurones which produce the releasing hormones. In the latter instance, it is likely that PGE_2 is involved in the transfer of the inflammatory signal to these releasing hormones. There is some evidence that there are self-amplifying positive feedback loops which aid in the amplification of this inflammatory signal which is finally effective in elevating circulating glucocorticoids. Such an increase in glucocorticoids may then serve to feed back at a multitude of sites to switch off the cytokine signal and restore body homeostasis. The feedback sites of the steroids include suppression of cytokine activity in cells of the immune system (see Chapter 8) as well as the classical neuroendocrine negative feedback effects which suppress HPA activation at the hypothalamic and pituitary levels (see Chapter 1). Clinical practice suggests that failure of this complex process is inimical to survival.

REFERENCES

1. Rivier C. Influence of immune signals on the hypothalamic–pituitary axis in the rodent. *Frontiers in Neuroendocrinology*, 1995, **16**: 151–82.
2. Buckingham J. C. Stress and the neuroendocrine–immune axis: the pivitol role of glucocorticoids and Lipocortin 1. *Brit J Pharmacol*, 1996, **118**: 1–19.
3. Buckingham J. C., Loxley H. D., Christian H. C., Philip J. G. Activation of the HPA axis by immune insults: roles and interactions of cytokines, eicosanoids and glucocorticoids. *Pharmacol Biochem and Behav*, 1996, **54**: 285–98.
4. Lee S., Rivier C. Hypophysiotropic role and hypothalamic gene expression of

corticotrophin releasing factor and vasopressin in rats injected with interleukin-1β systemically or into the brain ventricles. *J Neuroendocrinology*, 1994, **6**: 217–24.

5. Watanabe T., Takebe K. Intrahypothalamic perfusion with interleukin-1-beta stimulates the local release of corticotrophin-releasing hormone and arginine vasopressin and plasma corticotrophin in freely moving rat: a comparative perfusion of the paraventricular nucleus and the median eminence. *Neuroendocrinology*, 1993, **57**: 593–9.

6. Sapolsky R., Rivier C., Yamomoto G., Plotsky P., Vale W. Interleukin 1 stimulates the secretion of hypothalamic corticotrophin releasing factor. *Science*, 1987, **238**: 522–4.

7. Berkenbosch F., van Oers J., del Rey A., Tilders F., Besedovsky H. Corticotrophin releasing factor-producing neurones in the rat activated by interleukin 1. *Science*, 1987, **238**: 524–6.

8. Perlstein R. S., Whitnall M. H., Abrams J. S., Moougey E. H. Synergistic roles of interleukin 6, interleukin 1 and tumor necrosis factor in adrenocorticotrophin response to bacterial lipopolysaccharide *in vivo*. *Endocrinology*, 1993, **132**: 946–52.

9. Farrar W. L., Kilian P. L., Ruff M. R., Hill J. M., Pert C. B. Visualization and characterization of interleukin-1 receptors in brain. *J Immunol*, 1987, **139**: 459–63.

10. Katsuura G., Gottshall P. E., Arimura A. Identification of a high-affinity receptor for interleukin-1 beta in rat brain. *Biochem Biophys Res Commun*, 1988, **156**: 61–7.

11. Cunningham E. T. Jr, Wada E., Carter D. B., Tracey D. E., Battey J. F., De Souza E. B. *In situ* histochemical localization of Type I interleukin-1 receptor messenger RNA in the central nervous system, pituitary and adrenal gland of the mouse. *J Neurosci*, 1992, **12**: 1101–14.

12. Mirtella A., Tringali G., Guerriero G., Ghiara P., Parente L., Preziosi P., Navarra P. Evidence that interleukin-1β-induced prostaglandin E$_2$ release from rat hypothalamus is mediated by type I and type II interleukin-1 receptors. *J Neuroimmunol*, 1995, **61**: 171–7.

13. Greenfeder S. A., Nunes P., Kwee L., Labow M., Chizzonite R. A., Ju G. Molecular cloning and characterization of a second subunit of the interleukin 1 receptor complex. *J Biol Chem*, 1995, **270**: 13757–65.

14. De Simoni M. G., del Bo R., de Luigi A., Simard S., Forloni G. Central endotoxin induces different patterns of interleukin 1 (IL)-1β and IL-6 messenger ribonucleic acid expression and IL-6 secretion in the brain and periphery. *Endocrinology*, 1995, **136**: 897–902.

15. Hagan P., Poole S., Bristow A. F. Endotoxin-stimulated production of rat hypothalamic interleukin 1β *in vivo* and *in vitro*, measured by specific immunoradiometric assay. *J Mol Endocrinol*, 1992, **133**: 349–55.

16. Muramani N., Fukata J., Tsukada T., Kobayashi H., Ebisui O., Segawa H., Muro S., Imura H., Nakoa K. Bacterial lipopolysaccharide-induced expression of interleukin 6 messenger ribonucleic acid in the rat hypothalamus, pituitary, adrenal gland and spleen. *Endocrinology*, 1993, **133**: 2574–8.

17. Cowell A.-M., Buckingham J. C. Eicosanoids and the hypothalamo–pituitary axis. *Prostaglandins Leukotrienes and Essential Fatty Acids*, 1989, **36**: 235–50.

18. Hedge G. A. Roles for the prostaglandins in the regulation of anterior pituitary secretion. *Life Sci*, 1977, **20**: 17–34.

19. Katsuura G., Arimura A., Koves K., Gottshall P. E. Involvement of organum vasculosum of lamina terminalis and preoptic area in interleukin-1β-induced ACTH release. *Am J Physiol*, 1990, **258**: E163–71.

20. Bernardini R., Chiarenza A., Calogero A. E., Gold P. W., Chrousos G. P. Arachidonic acid metabolites modulate rat hypothalamic corticotropin-releasing hormone secretion *in vitro*. *Neuroendocrinology*, 1989, **50**: 708–15.

21. Vlaskovska M., Hertting G., Knepel W. Adrenocorticotropin and β-endorphin release from rat adenohypophysis *in vitro*: inhibition by prostaglandin E_2 formed locally in response to vasopressin and corticotropin-releasing factor. *Endocrinology*, 1984, **115**: 895–903.
22. Cowell A.-M., Flower R. J., Buckingham J. C. Studies on the role of phospholipase A_2 and eicosanoids in the regulation of corticotrophin secretion by rat pituitary cells *in vitro*. *J Endocrinol*, 1991, **130**: 21–32.
23. Knepel W., Vlaskovska M., Meyer D. K. Release of prostaglandin E_2 and β-endorphin-like immunoreactivity from rat adenohypophysis *in vitro*: variations after adrenalectomy or lesions of the paraventricular nuclei. *Brain Res*, 1985, **326**: 87–94.
24. Hedge G. A. Stimulation of ACTH secretion by indomethacin and reversal by exogenous prostaglandins. *Prostaglandins*, 1977, **14**: 145–50.
25. Gallant S., Brownie A. C. The *in vivo* effect of indomethacin and prostaglandin E_2 on ACTH and DBCAMP-induced steroidogenesis in hypophysectomized rats. *Biochem Biophys Res Commun*, 1973, **55**: 831–6.
26. Vlaskovska M., Knepel W. Beta-endorphin and adrenocorticotropin release from rat adenohypophysis *in vitro*: Evidence for local modulation by arachidonic acid metabolites of the cyclo-oxygenase and lipoxygenase pathway. *Neuroendocrinology*, 1984, **39**: 334–42.
27. Nishizaki T., Ikegami H., Tasaka K., Hirota K., Miyake A., Tanizawa O. Mechanism of release of beta-endorphin from rat pituitary cells. Role of lipoxygenase products of arachidonic acid. *Neuroendocrinology*, 1989, **49**: 483–8.
28. Okajima T., Hertting G. The possible involvement of cytochrome P-450 monooxygenase in AVP-induced ACTH secretion. *Horm Metabol Res*, 1986, **18**: 281–2.
29. Hirai A., Tahara K., Tamura Y., Saito H., Terano T., Yoshida S. Involvement of 5-lipoxygenase metabolites in ACTH-stimulated corticosteroidogenesis in rat adrenal glands. *Prostaglandins*, 1985, **30**: 749–67.
30. Jones D. B., Marante D., Williams B. C., Edwards C. R. W. Adrenal synthesis of corticosterone in response to ACTH in rat is influenced by leukotriene A_4 and by lipoxygenase intermediates. *J Endocrinol*, 1987, **112**: 253–8.
31. Dinarello C. A., Savage N. Interleukin-1 and its receptor. *Crit Rev Immunol*, 1989, **9**: 1–20.
32. Kehrer P., Turnill D., Dayer J.-M., Muller A. F., Gaillard R. C. Human recombinant interleukin-1 beta and -alpha but not recombinant tumor necrosis factor alpha stimulate ACTH release from rat anterior pituitary cells *in vitro* in a prostaglandin E_2 and cAMP independent manner. *Neuroendocrinology*, 1988, **48**: 160–6.
33. Katsuura G., Gottshall P. E., Dahl R. R., Arimura A. Adrenocorticotropin release induced by intracerebroventricular injection of recombinant human interleukin-1 in rats: possible involvement of prostaglandins. *Endocrinology*, 1988, **122**: 1773–9.
34. Loxley H. D., Cowell A.-M., Flower R. J., Buckingham J. C. Modulation of the hypothalamo–pituitary–adrenocortical response to cytokines in the rat by lipocortin 1 and glucocorticoids: a role for lipocortin in the feed-back inhibition of CRF-41 release? *Neuroendocrinology*, 1993, **57**: 801–14.
35. Navarra P., Pozzoli G., Brunetti L., Ragazzoni E., Besser G. M., Grossman A. Interleukins-1β and -6 specifically increase the release of prostaglandin E_2 from rat hypothalamic explants *in vitro*. *Neuroendocrinology*, 1992, **56**: 61–8.
36. Matsumura K., Watabane Y., Onoe H., Watabane Y., Hayaishi O. High density of prostaglandin E_2 binding sites in the anterior wall or 3rd ventricle: a possible site of its hyperthermic action. *Brain Res*, 1990, **533**: 147–51.
37. Dinarello C. A., Cannon J. G., Mancilla J., Bishai I., Lees J., Coceani F. Interleukin-6

as an endogenous pyrogen: induction of prostaglandin E_2 in brain but not in peripheral blood mononuclear cells. *Brain Res*, 1991, **562**: 199–206.

38. Pozzoli G., Costa A., Grimaldi M., Schettini G., Preziosi P., Grossman A., Navarra P. Bacterial lipopolysaccharide modulation of eicosanoid and corticotrophin releasing hormone release from rat hypothalamic explants and astrocyte cultures *in vitro*: evidence for the involvement of prostaglandin E_2 but not $PGF_{2\alpha}$, and lack of effect of NGF. *J Endocrinol*, 1994, **140**: 103–9.

39. Kolesnick R., Golde D. W. The sphingomyelin pathway in tumor necrosis factor and interleukin-1 signaling. *Cell*, 1994, **77**: 325–8.

40. Hu S. B., Tannahill L. A., Lightman S. L. Interleukin-1β induces corticotropin-releasing factor-41 release from cultured hypothalamic cells through protein kinase C and cAMP-dependent protein kinase pathways. *J Neuroimmunol*, 1992, **40**: 49–56.

Cytokines, Fever and Thermogenesis

Nancy J. Rothwell and Andrew V. Turnbull

University of Manchester, Manchester, UK

14.1 INTRODUCTION AND DEFINITIONS

Fever (also known as pyresis) is one of the commonest symptoms of infectious disease and may also accompany various forms of injury and inflammation. Clinically, fever is defined on the basis of a raised core temperature which is one of the most widely used diagnostic tools for identifying infection. Theoretically, core temperature is the temperature deep within the body (e.g. that of the brain or heart) but in clinical practice it is usually measured as the oral, axillary or rectal temperature, with temperatures above a value of about 37.5 °C indicating fever. However, while these definitions have obvious clinical advantages, not least because of their simplicity, they have a number of disadvantages and are open to considerable misinterpretation. For example, core temperature is usually underestimated. In addition, diurnal variations or other endogenous and exogenous factors such as exposure to low temperatures, age or haemorrhage are rarely taken into account and, most importantly, fever cannot be distinguished from passive hyperthermia simply on the basis of measurement of body temperature in patients or experimental animals. Fever is due to an increase in the set point for body temperature regulation and is therefore defended against external influences. In contrast, hyperthermia is a "passive" increase in temperature which may result from exposure to high environmental temperatures (e.g. saunas), impaired heat loss (e.g. due to excessive clothing) or increased heat production (such as that seen after severe exercise).

Fever may be achieved by activation of mechanisms to reduce heat loss, for

Stress, Stress Hormones and the Immune System. Edited by J. C. Buckingham, G. E. Gillies and A.-M. Cowell
© 1997 John Wiley & Sons, Ltd.

example vasoconstriction, piloerection or postural changes, and/or by increased heat production via shivering or nonshivering thermogenesis. All of these effector mechanisms are controlled by the hypothalamus and are mediated by the autonomic nervous system. Thermogenesis literally means an increase in heat production but is usually applied to changes in energy expenditure which occur independently of muscular contraction and therefore excludes shivering and conscious physical activity. Thermogenesis can be stimulated not only by agents (known as pyrogens) which elicit fever but also by psychological stress, physical injury, exposure to cold or increased energy intake. In all these cases, increases in thermogenesis are dependent on activation of the sympathetic nervous system and in experimental animals have been ascribed to heat production in brown adipose tissue (BAT), although the role of this tissue in adult humans is uncertain (see also Chapter 2).

Fever is undoubtedly a common and important clinical response but much of our understanding of the mechanisms underlying fever, its biological importance and modulation has derived from studies on experimental animals. A variety of experimental models have been established in animals to mimic clinical conditions such as infection and injury and these have proved invaluable in research on fever. Basic research has been undertaken to investigate the synthesis, release and mechanism of action of pyrogens produced within the body (i.e. endogenous pyrogens) and is the subject of a number of reviews (1–4). This research has assumed a much broader relevance since many putative endogenous pyrogens, particularly cytokines (see below), have been shown to control other aspects of

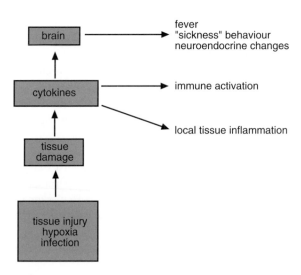

Figure 14.1 Schematic representation of the involvement of cytokines in response to injury or disease

the acute phase response including neuroendocrine, behavioural and immune responses (see Fig. 14.1 and Chapter 13). Indeed, early studies on fever have provided many of the foundations for the emerging and rapidly expanding field of neuroimmunology which addresses important questions on how the nervous, endocrine and immune systems interact and integrate the body's defence responses to disease.

14.2 MEDIATORS OF FEVER AND THERMOGENESIS

Since fever and thermogenesis are under the direct control of the central nervous system (CNS), a fundamental question is how the brain is activated by tissue damage or the presence of foreign material (e.g. pathogens, cancer cells or physical objects) at distant sites in the periphery. This question is in fact also relevant to many of the body's responses to disease described above which are controlled by the CNS.

Very rapid activation of the brain by injury may be achieved by conscious awareness, by the sensation of pain and by other neural afferent signals. Psychological stress not associated with tissue damage can lead to "fever" (raised body temperature) and increased thermogenesis which share many common mechanisms with classical pyrogenic responses (see below). In rodents, the rapid induction of fever and thermogenesis caused by local inflammation can be prevented by blocking C-fibre afferent nerves which provide information to the brain on pain, pressure etc. However, more sustained pyrogenic and thermogenic responses, which may occur without conscious awareness of pain and are present even during deep anaesthesia, appear to depend largely on humoral (circulating) factors which directly or indirectly signal the brain.

A variety of molecules associated with inflammation, including histamine, prostaglandins, bradykinin etc. (see Chapter 8), are released at sites of tissue damage and may enter the circulation and thus influence the brain. However, the most likely candidates for endogenous pyrogens are the molecules known as cytokines. Cytokines are a large and diverse group of polypeptides (molecular weights of 8–40 kDa) of which there are now over 60. The discovery of cytokines has been quite recent, but the study of these molecules has increased exponentially and, largely because of their potential involvement in almost all diseases, has attracted intense interest from scientists and clinicians alike. Cytokines have numerous and varied actions on inflammation, immune function, cell growth and differentiation and on many physiological functions such as temperature regulation, metabolism, neuroendocrine, cardiovascular, gastric and reproductive systems and on behaviour (see also Chapters 12, 13 and 18). They are broadly divided into groups known as interleukins (ILs), tumour necrosis factors (TNFs), interferons (IFNs), growth and cell stimulating factors (GFs, CSFs) and neurotrophins (NTs)—see Chapter 3 for further details. The cytokines most relevant to the study of fever are IL-1, TNF and IL-6, although many others may influence body temperature and thermogenesis (see Table 14.1). In particular IL-1, which was originally known as "endogenous pyrogen" (i.e. the naturally occurring molecule that causes fever), has been considered for many years to be the major circulating factor which influences the brain to cause fever.

A number of cytokines are produced during febrile conditions and elicit fever and thermogenesis when injected at low concentrations into experimental animals. In some cases similar responses have been observed in humans. However, these observations do not necessarily show that a particular cytokine acts as a signal to the brain, nor that it actually causes the pyrogenic response to disease, since fever caused by injection of recombinant cytokines may represent a pharmacological response that merely mimics normal biological events. To assume this role in fever, it is necessary to demonstrate that the cytokine gains access to, or indirectly influences, the CNS and, most importantly, that blocking its action prevents fever. The classical pharmacological approach to blocking the action of biological molecules using receptor antagonists is not readily available because, with the exception of IL-1 (see Chapter 12), no receptor antagonists for cytokines have been identified. Cytokine action can be inhibited *in vivo* and *in vitro* by application of neutralising antibodies which bind to the cytokine and prevent activation of its receptor. Studies in experimental animals have revealed that injection of neutralising antibodies to IL-1 or IL-6 inhibits fever and thermogenesis caused by bacterial endotoxin (a component of bacterial cell walls responsible for many of the responses to infection, including fever). Blocking the actions of other cytokines either has variable effects on fever or has not been tested. These experimental results suggest that both IL-1 and IL-6 are involved in generating fever and probably act in some way to signal to the brain during infection and injury.

Although IL-1 is produced around sites of injury or infection, very little of this cytokine is released into the circulation and in most circumstances its plasma concentrations remain low. However, IL-1 potently stimulates the production of IL-6, the plasma levels of which increase rapidly and dramatically (often by

Table 14.1 Cytokines which stimulate fever and thermogenesis

interleukin 1 (IL-1)	tumour necrosis factor α (TNFα)
interleukin 2 (IL-2)	tumour necrosis factor β (TNFβ)
interleukin 6 (IL-6)	
interleukin 8 (IL-8)	interferon α (IFNα)
	interferon β (IFNβ)
	interferon γ (IFNγ)

granulocyte-macrophage colony stimulating factor (GMCSF)
macrophage inflammatory protein (MIP)

1000-fold) in experimental animals and patients after infection, injury or inflammation. IL-6 concentrations usually correlate closely with fever and thermogenesis and it is therefore likely that IL-6 is the major pyrogen in the circulation but how it actually signals to the brain is uncertain. The brain, unlike other tissues, is protected by the blood–brain barrier which relies primarily on specialised endothelial cells of the cerebral vasculature to prevent access of large molecules, such as cytokines. Cytokines could act at specific sites within the brain where this barrier is poor or absent, such as the organum vasculosum of the lamina terminalis (see Chapter 13) and certain hypothalamic areas, or there may be a specific transport system to allow their entry into the brain. Alternatively, they could cause release of other molecules that more readily enter the CNS (see Fig. 14.2). Very recent studies have demonstrated that cytokines (e.g. IL-1, IL-6 and TNF) are present within the CNS and that brain cytokine synthesis is increased in response to a variety of insults, including direct brain trauma and CNS or peripheral infection. Synthesis of cytokines in the brain can occur in a variety of cell types including glia (microglia and astrocytes), neurones, endothelial cells in blood vessel walls and immune cells such as macrophages and neutrophils which can enter the CNS from blood, particularly after injury (see also Chapter 13).

Since IL-1 and IL-6 elicit fever much more potently when injected directly

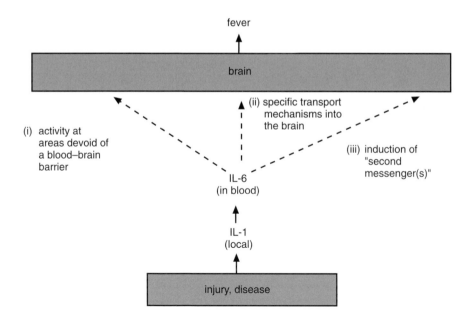

Figure 14.2 Signals to the brain during injury and disease. IL-1 = interleukin-1; IL-6 = interleukin-6

into the CNS (via the cerebral ventricles) than when administered peripherally, it may be that cytokines synthesised within the brain itself play an important role in the development of fever. Indeed this seems a likely mechanism of fever induction following direct brain trauma or infection. However, if the synthesis of cytokines within the brain accounts for fever observed during peripheral injury or infection then there still remains the important question, "How does a damaged tissue communicate with the brain?". Consequently, the hypothesis that a circulating signal (most probably IL-6) stimulates fever either directly or via stimulation of brain cytokine synthesis is currently the most favoured (Fig. 14.2).

14.3   MECHANISMS CONTROLLING FEVER AND THERMOGENESIS IN THE BRAIN

The areas of the brain most involved in the control of fever and thermogenesis are located in the hypothalamus which regulates many autonomic functions (see Chapter 2) including body temperature. Neurones within the pre-optic anterior hypothalamus are particularly sensitive to local changes in temperature and also receive inputs from the periphery via neural and humoral signals (see above) and from other brain regions. The hypothalamus appears to be responsible for integrating these signals, comparing actual body temperature to the "set point" (i.e. the temperature at which the body is regulated) and, if necessary, for activating appropriate mechanisms to raise or lower temperature by adjusting heat loss and heat production. The precise way in which the set point is determined is not known but it may relate to the ratio of concentrations of certain ions or neurotransmitters (particularly noradrenaline, adrenaline and 5-hydroxytryptamine) which alter the rate of firing of specific hypothalamic neurones.

Most forms of fever are due to release of prostaglandins (PGs) within the brain. The synthesis of these compounds is described in Chapter 8. Inhibition of the synthesis of PGs by a group of compounds known as cyclo-oxygenase inhibitors (of which aspirin is one of the most common) reduces fever in patients with infections, inflammation or severe forms of injury and prevents the fevers caused by experimental treatments such as injection of cytokines. There are, however, some exceptions to this. For example, certain forms of injury where raised temperatures and thermogenesis may be resistant to cyclo-oxygenase inhibitors. Interestingly, one group of cytokines, of which IL-8 is an example, causes fever in animals which is not prevented by blocking PG synthesis. Further research is required to determine whether IL-8 is involved in "cyclo-oxygenase resistant" fevers. PGE_2 has been considered the main PG responsible for fever and during infection is released in large amounts in the hypothalamus where it acts on temperature sensitive neurones and may cause an increase in the set point.

As research has progressed, an increasingly complicated pattern of events underlying fever has emerged, indicating the involvement of a number of different brain regions, neurotransmitters and peptides in the CNS. Of these, a neuropeptide known as corticotrophin releasing hormone (CRH, also called corticotrophin releasing factor 41 or CRF-41) has proven particularly interesting. CRH was first defined as a peptide released from the hypothalamus, which acts on the pituitary gland to cause release of adrenocorticotrophic hormone (ACTH) which, in turn, stimulates glucocorticoid production by the adrenal gland. Thus, CRH plays a major role in activating this hypothalamo–pituitary–adrenal (HPA) axis in response to physical and psychological stress (see Chapters 1 and 2). CRH is, however, widely distributed in the CNS and it has a number of actions within the brain which may be relevant to disease and injury. For example, when given centrally it causes increased body temperature and thermogenesis, reduced appetite and changes in cardiovascular, gastric and immune functions—actions which are remarkably similar to those of cytokines in the brain. It has now been shown that the stimulation of fever by certain cytokines and PG is due to release of CRH and can be prevented by injection into the brain of a CRH receptor antagonist, suggesting that CRH is one of the final mediators of fever and

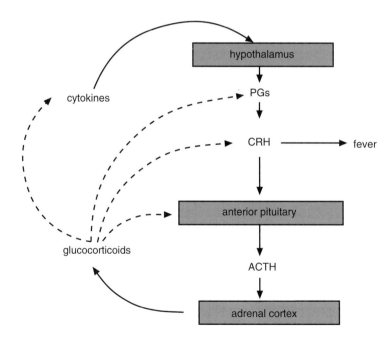

Figure 14.3 Mechanism of action of cytokines on fever and activation of the HPA axis: inhibitory activity of glucocorticoids; CRH, corticotrophin releasing hormone; PGs, prostaglandins; ACTH, adrenocorticotrophin. Intact lines = positive effects; broken lines = negative effects

thermogenesis. Interestingly, the activation of the HPA axis following injury or infection has also been attributed to the action of cytokines on CRH synthesis or release (Fig. 14.3)—see also Chapter 13.

14.4   INHIBITORS OF FEVER AND THERMOGENESIS

Several categories of drugs can inhibit fever and thermogenesis, the most potent and widely used of these being the cyclo-oxygenase inhibitors. However, naturally occurring (endogenous) inhibitors have also been identified which appear to act as modulators of many of the defence responses. Most notably glucocorticoids produced by the adrenal gland (i.e. cortisol in humans or corticosterone in the rat) or their synthetic counterparts, such as dexamethasone, inhibit not only fever and thermogenesis but also immune and inflammatory responses and are widely used clinically for these purposes (see Chapters 8 and 9). Animals in which glucocorticoids have been removed (by surgical removal of the adrenal glands) present greater fevers than their sham-operated counterparts, indicating that the antipyretic activity is not just a pharmacological phenomenon. Glucocorticoids can inhibit fever and thermogenesis in several ways. Firstly, they can reduce the extent of inflammation and damage, therefore inhibiting the actual stimulus itself. They are also potent inhibitors of cytokine synthesis and action, both in peripheral tissues and in the brain, and they also inhibit the synthesis and actions of PG (by inhibiting the enzyme phospholipase A_2 which is responsible for releasing the precursor for PG synthesis, arachidonic acid, from membrane phospholipids, as described in Chapter 8) and CRH (see Fig. 14.3). This inhibitory action of glucocorticoids is thought to play an important role in limiting the severity of host defence mechanisms. However, during chronic stress or disease, where circulating glucocorticoids concentrations may be raised for days or even weeks, some resistance to their inhibitory actions may develop (see Chapter 8).

   Glucocorticoids probably do not influence these processes directly and several of their effects may be due to production of another protein or several proteins known as lipocortins or annexins (see Chapter 8). Lipocortin-1 can also inhibit fever and thermogenesis by reducing PG synthesis (due mainly to inhibition of the release of arachidonic acid by phospholipase A_2 in the brain) or by decreasing the release of CRH or both. Unlike CRH, several other neuroendocrine peptides, for example α-melanocyte stimulating hormone (found in the hypothalamus and in the intermediate lobe of the pituitary gland in species which possess the third lobe) and arginine vasopressin (synthesised in the hypothalamus) can reduce body temperature but the biological significance of these actions remains to be determined.

14.5 BIOLOGICAL AND CLINICAL RELEVANCE OF FEVER AND THERMOGENESIS

Most biological responses have some value or benefit in allowing organisms to survive or maintain normal function since any responses with detrimental effects would impair survival and would be selected against during evolution and eventually lost. Fever appears to be no exception to this. Raised body temperatures help animals to combat infection since many pathogens (bacterial, viral and fungal) do not survive well at temperatures above 38 °C. In addition, fever increases the synthesis of the army of molecules needed to combat illness as most enzymes are highly temperature-dependent. Experimental studies have shown that blocking fever in animals can increase the rate of progression of infection, impair recovery and sometimes lead to death. This has led to questions about the widespread use of drugs (many of which can be purchased over the counter) to prevent fever. Fever is a phenomenon which is not restricted just to mammals or, surprisingly, even to homeotherms. Amphibians show raised body temperatures in response to infection and, since they do not possess homeo-thermic mechanisms such as thermogenesis, the fever is usually achieved by behavioural means. For example, lizards with bacterial infection choose warmer environments than healthy animals and thus raise their body temperature!

Evolutionary benefits and pressures are, of course, most obvious for animals in the wild where severe injury and infection would usually result in rapid death (if not because of the disease itself, then because the animal would be unable to escape predators or search for food). Most humans are not subjected to such hardships and can now survive even severe illness and major injury thanks to medical advances and clinical care. In some of these cases, fever and thermogenesis may have disadvantages, particularly when responses are large or prolonged. For example, high body temperatures in children can lead to fits. Very severe fevers may cause brain damage and even modest increases in body temperature significantly worsen the irreversible brain damage caused by stroke or head injury. Increased thermogenesis can also have harmful effects. In the short term, thermogenesis raises the body's demand for oxygen and increases the production of waste products. During illness oxygen may be limited, for example because of impaired respiratory or cardiovascular func-tion, blood loss or greater oxygen demands for tissue repair and protein synthesis. Prolonged increases in thermogenesis will result in breakdown and use of the body's own energy reserves (fat and protein) and is often accompanied by decreased food intake in illness. Modest weight loss over short periods of time usually poses little problem for adults but in children and the elderly, who may already have nutritional problems, weight loss is likely to seriously worsen their clinical condition and delay recovery. Chronic diseases such as cancer or long term infection (e.g. AIDS) usually lead to severe loss of body weight and general wasting. This condition, known as cachexia, may be a major cause of death.

As our understanding of the mechanisms of fever and thermogenesis improves, new drugs and treatments for inhibiting these processes may arise but it will be important to distinguish situations where fever may be advantageous from those in which blocking fever and thermogenesis will help survival and recovery.

REFERENCES

1. Kluger M. J. Fever: role of pyrogens and cryogens. *Physiol Rev*, 1991, **71**: 93–127.
2. Rothwell N. J. Functions and mechanisms of interleukin-1 in the brain. *Trends Pharmacol Sci*, 1991, **12**: 430–6.
3. Bartfai T., Ottoson D. (eds). *Neuroimmunology of Fever*. Oxford, Pergamon Press, 1992.
4. Busbridge N. J., Rothwell N. J. Thermogenic effects of cytokines: In E. B. De Souza (ed) *Methods and Mechanisms in Neurobiology of Cytokines*. San Diego, Academic Press, 1993, pp 96–110.

Chapter 15

Autonomic Regulation of Immune Function: Anatomical, Biochemical and Functional Studies

J. E. G. Downing*

Imperial College of Science, Technology and Medicine, London, UK and

M. D. Kendall

The Babraham Institute, Cambridge, UK

15.1 INTRODUCTION

Health and illness are influenced profoundly by psychosocial factors, environmental stimuli and specific behavioural states. Transduction of these factors into

---

*To whom correspondence should be addressed

Stress, Stress Hormones and the Immune System. Edited by J. C. Buckingham, G. E. Gillies and A.-M. Cowell

neural signals which can modulate immune responses relies upon central integrative pathways which regulate neurohormonal and autonomic output. In mammals, the central nervous system (CNS) regulates a wide range of auto-nomic, endocrine and behavioural responses which maintain homeostasis and confer adaptive advantage. This is achieved, for example, through the involuntary control of body temperature, cardiovascular reflexes, activity of abdominal viscera as well as the manifestation of ingestive, sexual, maternal and other behaviours which assure survival (see also Chapter 3). Over the last two decades a body of evidence has grown to support the view that immune functions are, likewise, the target of centrally-derived homeostatic regulation and that modifi-cation of neurological activities and behaviours may arise as a consequence of immune activation, infection or immune pathology.

This review attempts to provide a digest of the evidence which supports the involvement of neural networks (both central and peripheral), distinct from the neuroendocrine system, in the modulation of immune function and, conse-quently, in the maintenance of a disease-response homeostasis.

15.2 MULTIPLE LAYERS OF THE NEURAL–IMMUNE INTERFACE

The most obviously specialised tissues of immunological significance are the bone marrow and thymus (primary lymphoid tissue), the secondary lymphoid tissues (such as the spleen, the lymph nodes) and the mucosa-associated lymphoid tissues, including tonsil and Peyer's patches (see also Chapter 2). However, other diverse glands and tissues also contribute additional immunol-ogical activities. These include brown fat (pyrogenic actions), lacrimal glands (secretion of plasma cell immunoglobulins), submandibular glands (intestinal tract integrity) and liver (acute phase protein synthesis). Although disparate, all of these tissues are provided with afferent (sensory) and efferent (autonomic) nerve fibres and there are also reports of intrinsic neurones within lymphoid organs. Peripheral immune effectors are therefore considered to be "hard-wired", providing the framework for homeostatic neural regulation of adaptive immune responses (1).

In the widest sense, the autonomic innervation of all vasculature (both blood and lymphatic) provides for the regulation of lymphocytic migratory movements which underlie immune surveillance throughout the body. In addition, evidence that the innervation of parenchymatous compartments is a general feature of lymphoid tissues (see Section 15.3) has suggested that the nervous system mediates immune regulatory functions directly through cellular contacts with immunocytes, stromal cells and/or accessory cells.

The brain's involuntary control centre influences immunity through the integration of sensory inputs along with emotional, endocrinological, immunological and physical stressors (Fig. 15.1).

Alongside the neuroendocrine control axis, three generalised neural circuits are in place conveying direct neural–immune signals (2):

(a) the "axon reflex" which is responsible for local neurotransmitter release from sensory and probably autonomic nerves. This occurs as a result of antidromic activation, presumably in response to local mechanical stimulation or to activation by chemical mediators released from immune cells. It is triggered by and contributes to inflammatory processes,

(b) "spinal reflexes" which permit sensory afferents to elicit efferent reflexes through spinal loops, and

(c) ascending afferents which provide primary initiation of the central homeostatic brain circuits which preside over both neuroendocrine and autonomic outflows and thus constitute a central neural apparatus co-ordinating stress reactions (see Section 15.4).

Immunological signals, in the form of soluble cytokines and migratory immunocytes, are accessible to the central control sites important for immune regulation (Fig.15.2). This occurs by virtue of their capability to signal across the blood–brain barrier via:

(a) cellular extravasation (diapedesis),

(b) interactions at the level of the blood–brain barrier which result in the production and liberation into the CNS of chemical messengers (e.g. prostanoids), and

(c) transport of plasma-borne signals into the CNS, particularly at "fenestrated" regions, such as the organum vasculosum lamina terminalis (OVLT).

The OVLT is one of the circumventricular organs believed to facilitate access of circulating immune and endocrine signals to hypothalamic control centres. Elsewhere permeability of the blood–brain barrier is also increased during infection. These features are considered also in Chapter 11 along with the likelihood that the median eminence region of the hypothalamus may also be a target for plasma-borne immunokines as it lies largely outside the blood–brain barrier (3). In addition, there is growing evidence that the strength of transmission along the neural chain to and from peripheral immune effectors can undergo modulation (both suppression and sensitisation) in response to immunological signals.

Figs 15.1 and 15.2 schematise the rudiments of a neural system for remote sensing of peripheral immunological status which appears to be capable of co-ordinating diverse inputs, triggering appropriate neural and endocrine outputs (detailed in Sections 15.5 and 15.6) and responding with an adaptive plasticity

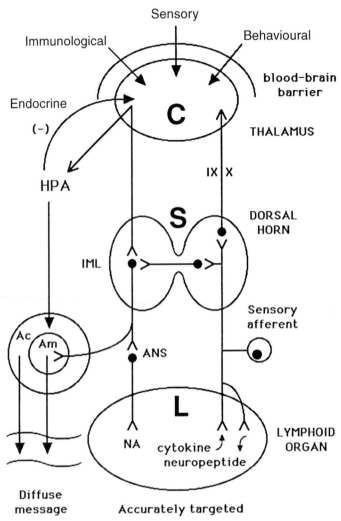

Figure 15.1 Hierarchical reflexive interface of nerves with peripheral immune sites. A neural system for remote sensing of peripheral immunological status acts both independently and together with central neural integration of emotional, endocrinological, immunological and physical stressors. Three layers of reflexive interface between peripheral immune sites and nerves are in place. L, local "axonal reflex" (also known as antidromic or anterograde); S, spinal relay of afferent nerve signals to activate efferent output; and C, centrally-derived drives for involuntary control of peripheral functions, through both autonomic and neuroendocrine channels. These higher order controls can be triggered by (i) central access of immunologically-derived cytokine signals and hormonal mediators (ii) ascending visceral afferent input, relayed via the brain-stem, and (iii) complex higher order sensory and emotional cues. Key: Ac, adrenal cortex; Am, adrenal medulla; ANS, autonomic nervous system; NA, noradrenaline; HPA, hypothalamo–pituitary axis; IML, intermediolateral cell column; IX, X, cranial nerves

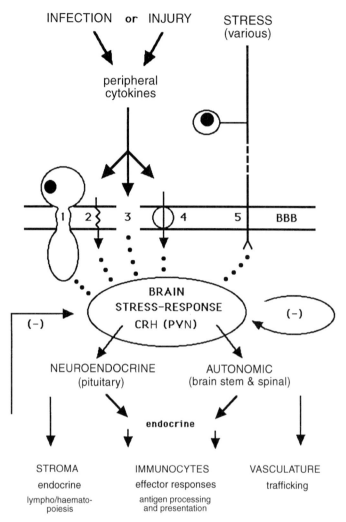

Figure 15.2 Stress-response activation and immunoregulation. Activation of neural and neuroendocrine output is achieved by various stressors, including immunologically derived signals, which gain access centrally. Five routes for immunological activation are depicted: 1, diapedesis; 2, receptor mediated transduction of cytokine signals; 3, permeability of blood brain barrier (BBB) at circumventricular organs; 4, transport of cytokines across BBB; 5, cytokine modulation of visceral afferent signals. Neurones in the hypothalamic paraventricular nucleus (PVN) producing corticotrophin releasing hormone (CRH) are central to the integration of these signals. Feedback inhibitory controls (−) also exist, not only through circulating endocrine factors (left), but also via intrinsic brain circuits (right) using other neuropeptides (AVP, αMSH and possibly IL-1 receptor antagonist). A broad range of immunological functions are affected through direct neural influences upon the vascular supply, in addition to leukocyte and stromal cell activities (see Sections 15.6 and 15.6 for details)

during the progress of an immune response. Activation of neural output is by virtue of reciprocal sensitivity to immunological cytokine signals (4, 5).

15.3   LOCAL INNERVATION OF THE LYMPHOID ORGANS

Local innervation of the lymphoid organs is derived principally from the autonomic nervous system, the major features of which are described in Chapter 2 and schematised in Fig. 15.3. Essentially, both sympathetic and parasympathetic pre-ganglionic neurones use acetylcholine as their neurotransmitter and synapse with the post-ganglionic neurones in ganglia (which in the sympathetic system lie close to the CNS and in the parasympathetic system are found near to or within the innervated effector organ). The major neurotransmitter substances released from the post-ganglionic fibres are acetylcholine, in the case of parasympathetic neurones, and generally noradrenaline for the sympathetic

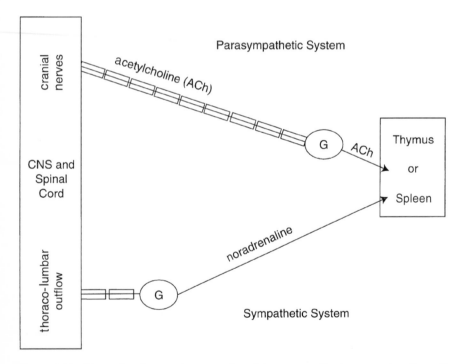

Figure 15.3   Neurochemistry and topography of the pre-ganglionic nerves (myelinated) and post-ganglionic nerves (unmyelinated) from the sympathetic and parasympathetic systems to major lymphoid organs. Not shown are the non-adrenergic, non-cholinergic (NANC) mediators (including neuropeptide, nucleotide and nitric oxide) which provide additional complexity. G, ganglion; CNS, central nervous system

nervous system. The presence of non-adrenergic, non-cholinergic (NANC) neurotransmitter systems (e.g. adenosine triphosphate, nitric oxide) within lymphoid organs remains to be fully examined.

Fig. 15.4 summarises the cranial nerves and ganglia supplying different lymphoid organs based largely on evidence from the rat. The pre-ganglionic parasympathetic fibres which supply the thymus and the spleen originate in the brain-stem and almost certainly project to their targets via the vagus (Xth) nerve. The source of parasympathetic fibres to lymph nodes or bone marrow is variable

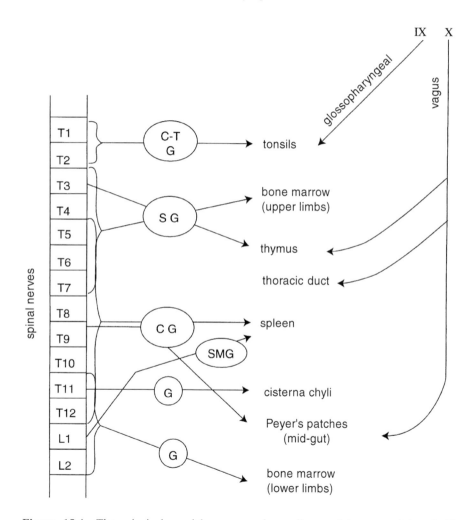

Figure 15.4 The principal cranial nerves and ganglia supplying named lymphoid structures. C-T G, cervicothoracic ganglion; SG, stellate ganglion; CG, coeliac ganglion; SMG, superior mesenteric ganglion; G, sympathetic ganglia; T, thoracic; L, lumbar

among species as, also, is the source of the sympathetic supply to both primary and secondary lymphoid tissues.

15.3.1 The Thymus

Early accounts of thymic innervation based on silver staining indicate that during development nerves enter the cervically located thymic rudiments from the vagus at the point where the corticomedullary junction will eventually form. Differentiation into cortex and medulla is a later event which occurs as blood vessels migrate into the epithelial anlage. Before this, the thymic rudiments begin to descend into the mediastinum and acquire innervation from the phrenic and recurrent laryngeal nerves which also supply the subcapsular regions. Nerves have also been traced from ganglia of the thoracic sympathetic chain, mainly from the cervicothoracic (T1–2) and stellate (T3) ganglia, to nerve nets in the subcapsular regions of the cortex and around blood vessels (see below). These observations are in accordance with an innervation by sympathetic fibres from the sympathetic chain, by parasympathetic fibres from the vagus and by sensory fibres in the phrenic nerve.

The existence of a parasympathetic supply to the thymus is however a matter of dispute, largely because of the technical difficulties involved in retrograde tracing experiments and the realisation that acetylcholinesterase, which is a commonly used marker for cholinergic fibres, may also be found in non-cholinergic nerves. Our own work (6) has demonstrated acetylcholinesterase-positive fibres and, occasionally, cell bodies in the thymic medulla, in a plexus at the corticomedullary junction, around blood vessels and a less prominent plexus in the subcapsular region. Whether this is associated with non-cholinergic nerves as well as parasympathetic fibres remains to be determined.

In contrast to the parasympathetic system, there is general agreement that the thymus is innervated by the sympathetic nervous system (7, 8). Noradrenergic fibres are first detected in the rat embryo at days 17–18 of a 21/22 day gestation period. However, the main noradrenergic innervation develops post-natally, between 7 and 14 days of age. Nerve fibres are found primarily as a plexus surrounding blood vessels and running independently in connective tissue of perivascular spaces. Such plexuses may be found associated with the capsule, subcapsular region and the corticomedullary junction. Light microscopy suggests that fine nerves enter the cortex independent of blood vessels but this has not yet been corroborated with the electron microscope.

The noradrenaline content of the rat thymus is normally maintained at a constant level (approximately 400 moles per thymus) after about three months of age despite the dramatic loss of thymic mass, although significant changes do occur in pregnancy and in the *post partum* period. It was originally considered that all of the noradrenaline was contained within the neural compartment of the thymus (9). However, recent studies suggest that the changing levels observed in pregnancy and *post partum*, which may approach those found in the circulation after stress, may reflect noradrenaline released into the vasculature (10).

Neuropeptides have also been located within thymic nerves and thymic cells (8). Among the most abundant are neuropeptide Y (NPY), which co-localises with noradrenaline fibres and with substance P, and calcitonin gene-related peptide (CGRP), both of which are found in the capsular plexus and major septa close to mast cells. Immunoreactive vasoactive intestinal peptide (VIP) is also found in nerves as well as in many cortical epithelial cells. In addition, neurokinin A and B have been identified in thymic tissue.

Investigations on the functional significance of thymic innervation are at an early stage. Several studies have shown that thymic development both pre- and post-natally is dependent on the integrity of the nerve supply. In addition, activation of the sympathetic system inhibits proliferation and promotes differentiation of thymocytes and stem cells. The functional consequences of this innervation, either directly on the thymocytes or indirectly via effects on vascular tone are discussed in Section 15.6.

15.3.2 The Bone Marrow

Fine myelinated (afferent pain) and non-myelinated (sympathetic) nerves accompany blood vessels into long bones. The autonomic nerves supplying the upper limbs emerge from the spinal column through T2–7 to enter the sympathetic trunk. Post-ganglionic fibres arise in the thoracic and stellate ganglia and travel to the brachial plexuses. The pre-ganglionic fibres innervating the lower limbs emerge from T10–12 or L1–2 and travel via the sympathetic trunk to the lower lumbar and sacral ganglia before entering bone marrow cavities. Nerves first appear in the long bones of mammals late in foetal life. These contain noradrenaline and become myelinated at the time of haemopoietic onset. It has been suggested that the development of the nerve supply to the bone marrow correlates with haemopoiesis in a manner similar to that proposed for the thymus.

Nerve fibres immunoreactive for substance P have also been detected in the bone marrow and substance P receptors are located on bone marrow stromal cells. Although substance P can stimulate the differentiation of erythroid and granulocytic progenitors *in vitro*, it remains to be determined whether the neurally derived peptide fulfils such a role in the bone marrow *in vivo*.

Stimulation of the posterior hypothalamus or of the sympathetic nerves supplying the bone marrow results in the release of reticulocytes from the marrow (11). This may be achieved either through vasomotor control of local vessels or via a direct action on the haemopoietic cells themselves. Reports of alterations on colony growth in response to manipulations of cholinergic and adrenergic receptors (12) suggest that haemopoiesis and granulocytopoiesis are responsive to neural signals.

15.3.3   The Spleen

The spleen is innervated primarily by the sympathetic system via a plexus formed from branches originating in the coeliac plexus, left coeliac ganglia (T9) and vagus nerve. In rodents there is a contribution from the superior mesenteric ganglia, with some fibres originating in the sympathetic trunk and passing through the coeliac and superior mesenteric ganglia before reaching the spleen. The noradrenergic innervation of the rat spleen has been described in detail. It first appears towards the end of gestation at embryonic day 17–19 and develops mainly post-natally. From days 1–3 after birth noradrenergic nerves are found exclusively within parenchymal compartments such as the outer periarteriolar sheath (PALS) where B lymphocytes are found; occasional branches enter the PALS to ramify amongst T cells. By 7–10 days after birth, the noradrenergic innervation is maximal with the formation of a dense plexus around the central arteriole with ramifications into the PALS of T and B cells. Noradrenergic fibres are also present in the marginal sinus where macrophages are found. As the T and B lymphocytes come to occupy their adult locations, the noradrenergic nerves surround the follicles of PALS tissue and occasional nerves are found within follicles (see also Chapter 3). It is often stated that the innervation of the spleen is related principally to the blood vessels or to splenic contraction (although the spleen can still contract in response to circulating levels of catecholamines when the nerves are ligated). However, immunocytochemistry and electron microscopic studies suggest that, in addition to the smooth muscles, the T and B lymphoid cells and the macrophages may themselves be the direct targets of noradrenergic innervation. In support of this view lymphocytes possess adrenoceptors with mature B cells having a greater density of α-adrenoceptors than T cells. Indeed, α-adrenoceptor agonists promote emigration of B cells. Between days 10 and 14, there is a two-fold increase in the density of α-adrenoceptors per cell in the spleen, while coincidentally the cell populations are changing. These observations would favour a relationship between splenic innervation and its altered colonisation during development.

Histochemical identification of acetylcholinesterase in the spleen raises the possibility that parasympathetic fibres also supply this tissue. However, as the histochemical signal is abolished in the rat by removal of the coeliac and superior mesenteric ganglia but unaffected by vagotomy, it seems more likely that any cholinergic fibres form a part of the sympathetic system.

As with the thymus, NPY (and enkephalin in some species) may be co-localised with noradrenaline. NPY may either mediate vasoconstriction directly or enhance the actions of noradrenaline. Somatostatin, substance P and VIP are also present in the spleen, mainly in association with larger blood vessels but also within the red pulp and white pulp. Some evidence suggests that the substance P nerves may be sensory.

15.3.4   The Lymphatics and Lymph Nodes

The lymphatics are supplied by both sympathetic and parasympathetic fibres which maintain lymphatic tone (13). The thoracic duct is innervated by the vagus and intercostal nerves and the cisterna chyli receives nerves from the T11 ganglion and the left splanchnic nerve. The source of the nerve supply to lymph nodes varies with node location. Almost all studies report a noradrenergic innervation which is found with the larger blood vessels at the hilus of the nodes and smaller vessels in the medullary, paracortical and cortical regions. In addition, individual fibres have been observed in similar sites but no noradrenergic fibres have been described in germinal centres. NPY and also VIP, histidine and isoleucine may be localised in noradrenergic fibres which supply the blood vessels. Dynorphin-A and cholecystokinin-immunoreactive fibres have also been identified, but only in the medulla of guinea pig lymph nodes. Acetylcholinesterase-positive fibres are restricted to the capsule and the subcapsular zone. Substance P and CGRP fibres have been observed in medullary cords, deep cortex and paracortex in association with lymphoid cells. The functional activities of these peptidergic nerves have not been examined but histological studies at the electron microscope level have revealed enlargements of unmyelinated fibres in the parenchyma which may be sensory endings. Since there is a clear relationship between the development of lymph nodes and nerves during embryogenesis, an ontogenic role for lymph node innervation seems possible.

15.3.5   Other Lymphoid Tissues

A large volume of lymphoid tissue exists in mucosal associated sites (e.g. the lungs and alimentary canal) where innervation derives from the regional nerve supply. The pharyngeal and lingual tonsils are innervated by the IXth cranial nerve (glossopharyneal nerve) which includes a large proportion of autonomic pre-ganglionic and afferent fibres. Nerves from the pharyngeal plexus and the lesser palatine nerve also contribute to nerve plexuses in the oropharynx.

   The enteric innervation is often regarded as a distinct part of the autonomic nervous system. It is well characterised and expresses a wide variety of neuropeptides and neurotransmitter substances. In particular, non-myelinated fibres have been identified between the lymphoid cells in Peyer's patches with positive staining for substance P, somatostatin, VIP and CGRP within the nerve fibres. However, little is known of the functional implications of this innervation, although it has been suggested that the maintenance of immune tolerance to neural antigens is enacted here.

15.4 CENTRAL ORIGINS OF THE AUTONOMIC CONTROL OF IMMUNITY

Linkage between stress and susceptibility to disease depends upon the translation of psychosocial factors, environmental change and behavioural activation into neural signals. Physical and emotional stressors which elicit, for example, cardiovascular changes are also coupled to the regulation of immunological functions. Thus, in a manner analogous to the central involuntary control of visceral activities (through autonomic and neuroendocrine systems), a central-ised stress-response circuitry is thought to contribute homeostatic regulatory influences upon immune function (14, 15). However, delineation of central immunoregulatory circuitry remains sketchy. In view of the innervation of both the vascular and parenchymatous compartments of peripheral immune tissues described in Section 15.3, the central pathways involved in the integration of autonomic function are those most likely to be involved in neuro-immune regulation. Three of the key structures involved in the central integration of autonomic function are:

(a) the nucleus tractus solitarius (NTS) of the brain-stem,
(b) the paraventricular nucleus (PVN) of the hypothalamus, and
(c) the central nucleus of the amygdaloid complex, which, like other limbic structures, links with cortical inputs.

Monosynaptic connections between these and other central nuclei involved in the regulation of autonomic responses are schematised in Fig. 15.5 (15, 16).

15.4.1 The Nucleus Tractus Solitarius

Brain-stem nuclei are the targets of first order afferent inputs from the viscera via cranial nerves IX and X. Most brain-stem loci send direct projections to the pre-ganglionic cells of the dorsal vagal nucleus (parasympathetic) and intermedio-lateral nucleus (sympathetic). The NTS appears to be particularly important and is capable of controlling simple reflex circuits; this control is independent of higher brain centres since cardiovascular and respiratory functions are retained following surgical transection above the pons. Catecholaminergic cell groups within the NTS, ventrolateral medulla and locus coeruleus relay sensory inputs to the hypothalamic PVN. However, it is the NTS which is pre-eminent in the co-ordination of elaborate homeostatic adjustments, through reciprocal links with higher centres and among brain-stem regions.

15.4.2　The Hypothalamic Paraventricular Nucleus

While brain-stem mechanisms demonstrate significant autonomy, the centre for control of visceral responses accompanying emotion is the hypothalamus from which both endocrine and autonomic outputs emanate. A pivotal role is ascribed to the parvocellular division of the PVN (dorsal, lateral and ventromedial portions) from whence descending fibres project to the autonomic centres, targeting not only the intermediolateral spinal column and the dorsal vagal nucleus but also most parts of the NTS (16).

Knowledge of the neurochemistry of these PVN efferents is incomplete but nine subpopulations of predominantly peptidergic neurones account for one third of the known fibres. These are oxytocin, vasopressin, dopamine, somatostatin, enkephalin, angiotensin, corticotrophin releasing hormone (CRH), thyrotrophin releasing hormone and neurotensin, with oxytocin and vasopressin accounting for 20% of these descending fibres. Of these peptides, CRH has become a major focus of attention in view of its widespread involvement in diverse stress-response activities, mediated via both autonomic and endocrine output with associated consequences on immune function (see Section 15.5 and Chapters 1, 2 and 6).

Reciprocal connections of the PVN with the limbic complex (see below) and brain-stem nuclei are the foundations for the integration of emotional drives and ascending nociceptive sensory input respectively. Interestingly, a VIP-positive projection from the suprachiasmatic nucleus to the parvocellular region of the hypothalamus appears to transmit signals from the retina and may thus contribute to the mechanisms underlying circadian rhythmicity of endocrine, autonomic and immune functions.

15.4.3　The Amygdala

The limbic structures provide the neuroanatomical substrate for emotion, motivation and reward behaviours (17). Increasing evidence indicates that the evaluation of sensory stimuli by these structures is critical to the generation of appropriate emotional responses, in the form of co-ordinated autonomic, endocrine and somatomotor activities. Indeed, the limbic structures appear to be major players in the pathogenesis of affective disorders such as schizophrenia and depression. The amygdala is particularly important for the learning of conditioning stimuli which trigger the autonomic responses observed in paradigms of aversive conditioning (a measure of fear or anxiety). In addition,

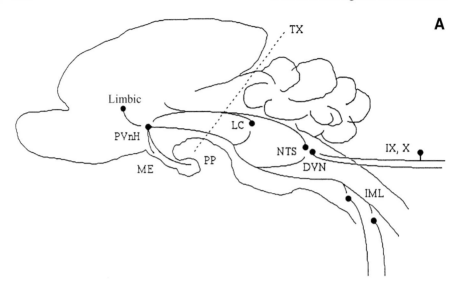

Figure 15.5 Overview of central sites involved in the integration of autonomic functions. Schematic overview of **A** central brain regions and **B** interconnections integrating diverse "stressor" signal input and supplying involuntary regulation of autonomic and endocrine outputs. Together, these brain sites represent a generalised stress-response apparatus. Reflexive control through autonomic output is emphasised. (See text for details). TX represents a line of transection of the brain-stem above the pons, which leaves the regulation of cardiovascular and respiratory functions largely intact, a finding which indicates that co-ordination of autonomic functions take place to a significant degree within the brain-stem, independent of the hypothalamus. Abbreviations: Ce, central nucleus of the amygdala; IX, 9th cranial nerve, glossopharyngeal; X, 10th cranial nerve, vagus; DVN, dorsal vagal nucleus; IML, intermediolateral sympathetic spinal zone; LC, locus coeruleus; ME, median eminence; NTS, nucleus tractus solitarius; PP, posterior pituitary; PVN, paraventricular nucleus of the hypothalamus; SCN, suprachiasmatic nucleus; BST, bed nucleus of the stria terminalis; pMg, posterior magnocellular division of DVN; mP, medial parvocellular; l, lateral; m, medial, d dorsal. Redrawn from (1) Downing and Kendall, 1996. Reproduced with permission

significant projections from the prefrontal cortex and hippocampus feed through the amygdaloid complex to regulate hypothalamic function. A clear structural basis therefore exists to substantiate reports of behavioural conditioning of immune responses and immunoregulatory effects of emotional stressors.

The neurochemical mediation of the forebrain influence over the visceral and emotional responses to stress involves excitatory and inhibitory amino acids, steroids and neuropeptides. Pharmacological manipulations, involving for example treatment with benzodiazepines (which enhance synaptic transmission by gamma-aminobutyric acid, GABA) or glucocorticoids (which accumulate in the central nucleus of the amygdala), effectively suppress the neural activity

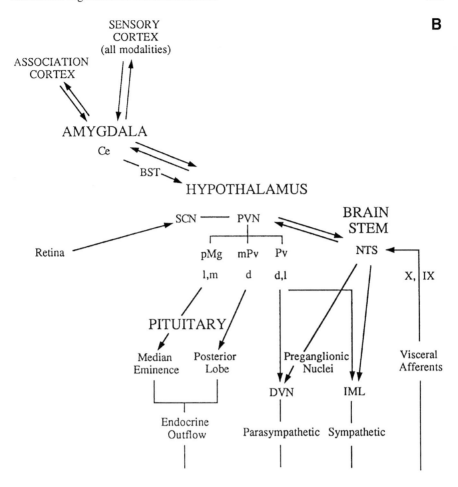

Figure 15.5 (*continued*)

triggered by adverse physical or auditory stimuli. The same treatments have also been shown to alter various indices of immune function. For example, there is evidence supporting an involvement of central benzodiazepine receptors in the suppression of natural killer (NK) cell activity (18). Interestingly, GABA receptor function can be a target for steroid modulation in an analogous way to benzodiazepines. However, it remains to be determined whether glucocorticoids can act as endogenous anxiolytics within central structures and, thus, provide a central basis through which they may influence immune function and thereby reduce somatic signs of stress.

Finally, two neuropeptides have been shown to be mutually antagonistic in animal models of anxiety, namely CRH (anxiogenic) and NPY (anxiolytic, see also Chapter 2). Delivery of CRH to the central nucleus of the amygdala enhances the behavioural responses to stressors while the CRH antagonist (α-helical CRH$_{9-41}$) elicits "anti-stress" actions. On the other hand, NPY exerts potent anxiolytic actions when injected into the amygdala; the responses to NPY, however, are blocked in animals pretreated with antisense oligonucleotides which are directed against the nucleotide encoding the type 1 NPY receptor (i.e. Y1 receptors) and which thus bring about receptor down-regulation (19). The effectiveness of the antagonist treatments implies that endogenous CRH and NPY both contribute to the expression of emotional responses. Furthermore, since the behavioural responses they elicit are independent of changes in pituitary–adrenocortical activity, it is likely that their actions are mediated via autonomic rather than endocrine outflows.

15.5   IMMUNOREGULATION THROUGH AUTONOMIC PATHWAYS

An association between the central neural mechanisms which control the stress-response and immune function has been established through studies involving brain lesioning, electrical stimulation and recording of CNS activity, behavioural stressors (ranging from restraint to sound and electric shocks), emotional acti-vation and sensory conditioning. The hypothalamo–pituitary–adrenal (HPA) axis has been the focus of many investigations into the mechanisms of communica-tion between the neural and immune systems but there is support for autonomic, as well as neuroendocrine, mediation of the effects of stress on immune function (4, 5, 20). The literature has tended also to emphasise the immunosuppressive effects of the autonomic nervous system, particularly with respect to cell-mediated immune response, but there is also evidence for immune-enhancing effects of these pathways.

15.5.1   Brain Lesioning Studies

Stereotactically localised lesions within the brain-stem, hypothalamus or cortex alter a variety of T and B cell-dependent immune measures, including the numbers of lymphocytes within the thymus and spleen, the proliferative response to mitogens, NK cell activity, antibody production, tumour suppression and allergic reactions (21). These studies support a role for the anterior hypothalamus in maintaining normal cell-mediated and humoral immune responses which could depend upon the integrity of autonomic pathways. However, a role for the neuroendocrine system cannot be excluded as removal of the pituitary or adrenal glands produces similar effects on these measures of immune function. Similarly, while findings that brain-stem specific lesions cause thymic involution favour a role for the autonomic system in the regulation of the immune system they do not rule out a role for the neuroendocrine system because the surgical procedure is likely to interrupt the ascending hypothalamic afferents as well as the descending projections to autonomic pre-ganglionic nuclei. Such studies must therefore be interpreted with caution.

15.5.2 Central Corticotrophin Releasing Hormone (CRH) and Autonomic Mediation of Immune Function

Brain signalling of the stress response, whether it is elicited by physical, behavioural, emotional or immunological stressors, hinges on the neuropeptide, CRH (22–25). Stressors which suppress cellular immune function enhance the synthesis and release of CRH centrally while, conversely, agents that block the actions of CRH in the CNS (although not in the periphery) reduce the immunosuppressive response. Thus, central administration of an antiserum which neutralises the actions of CRH inhibits the suppressive effects of foot shock treatment on NK cell activity and of tail shock on lympho-proliferative responses. By contrast, peripheral administration of the antiserum fails to influence the immunosuppressive responses to foot shock. In the same vein, central but not peripheral injections of CRH suppress NK cell activity and the IgG antibody responses to specific (T-dependent) antigens; indeed, peripheral administration of CRH may promote some immune functions, such as the secretion of interleukin-1 (IL-1) and β-endorphin from macrophages and lymphocytes respectively. Despite the importance of the HPA axis in immunomodulation (see Chapters 1, 3 and 8), these data suggest that the immunosuppressive effects of raised levels of CRH in the CNS (produced either by stress or by direct infusion of the peptide) are at least partially independent of activation of the HPA axis (25). In accord with this premise, both central and peripheral injections of CRH activate the HPA axis but only the former produces a simultaneous reduction in immune function. Moreover, peripheral administration of anti-CRH antiserum fails to modulate the stress-induced quenching of cellular immunity but it effectively impairs the rises in ACTH and glucocorticoid secretion provoked by the stress. Furthermore, the immunosuppressive responses to stress persist in adrenalectomised and hypohysectomised rats (26) and central injections of CRH antisera attenuate the stress-induced suppression of immune activity in both adrenalectomised and intact animals. Together, these results indicate that CRH released centrally in response to stress serves to activate a neural outflow which is capable of influencing peripheral immune activities via mechanisms which are independent of neuroendocrine pathways. From the discussions in Sections 15.3 and 15.4 and those detailed below, it appears that the sympathetic nervous system is likely to be the major neural pathway involved (25, 27).

Further support of the view that the sympathetic nervous system rather than the HPA axis is the effector arm of the immunosuppressive effects of central CRH is provided by studies with chlorisondamine, a ganglion-blocking drug which does not cross the blood–brain barrier. Treatment with this drug abolishes the rise in plasma noradrenaline concentration and associated reduction in NK cell activity provoked by central injection of CRH. Equally, chlorisondamine inhibits the CRH-dependent immunosuppression caused by central administration of IL-1 suggesting that a sympathetic pathway may contribute, at least in part, to the central actions of this cytokine (28). It has also been shown that chemical sympathectomy of the spleen (produced by injection of 6-hydroxydopamine, 6-OHDA) prevents the rise in plasma catecholamines and suppression of splenic NK cell activity caused by intracerebroventricular (i.c.v.) injection of CRH. Moreover, pharmacological antagonism of the β_2-adrenoceptors present on splenic lymphocytes by propranolol (a non-selective β-adrenoceptor antagonist) or butoxamine (a β_2-selective adrenoceptor antagonist) opposes the reduction of splenic NK cell activity produced by CRH (25).

15.6   NEUROMODULATION OF IMMUNITY

15.6.1   Morphological and Biochemical Evidence

Immunomodulation by neurotransmitter systems within lymphoid organs is supported by data on the four basic criteria of neurotransmission, summarised as:

(a) the presence and synthesis of the neurotransmitter substance,
(b) the release of the neurotransmitter,
(c) the expression of appropriate receptors, and
(d) effector actions of the neurotransmitter.

Synaptic Contacts

As discussed above, the innervation of lymphoid organs, particularly by the sympathetic nervous system, is targeted towards the control of vascular functions which are clearly of great significance to the processes of lymphocyte migration, namely recruitment, retention and recirculation. In addition, nerves in the parenchyma of lymphoid tissue, where the lymphocytes and stromal cells are located, have been reported to make specialised contacts especially with splenic reticular cells, immunoglobulin-secreting plasma cells, macrophages and T lymphocytes (29). Areas of B cell concentration appear to be poorly innervated but some sparse adrenergic innervation has been identified within B cell follicular zones of the spleen. Electron microscopy has shown that the "neuro-effector" contacts between the noradrenergic fibres and the lymphoid cells are the closest of all peripheral junction types (~6 nm) and that (unlike contacts between nerve terminal and smooth muscle cell) a basement membrane or interdigitating cell process does not interpose between the neural contacts with immunocytes. However, evidence of clear pre- or post-synaptic specialisations to help resolve the functional implications of these contacts in the lymphoid organs is not yet available.

Transmitter Release

Release of the sympathetic transmitters, noradrenaline and NPY, is best characterised for the spleen. It has been reported that local noradrenaline concentrations within the spleen, as measured by microdialysis, are approximately three times higher than those in the general circulation. Sympathetic nerve ablation by 6-OHDA (a treatment reported not to affect adrenal catecholamines significantly) reduces the splenic noradrenaline content by 95% and thus supports the view that the elevated levels of the catecholamine observed in the spleen originate almost entirely from nerves. Stimulation of splenic nerve terminals has also been reported to increase the release of NPY (27).

Specific Receptors

Pharmacological profiles and ligand binding studies indicate the presence of specific receptors on lymphocytes for a variety of neuropeptides (including substance P, somatostatin, VIP and opioids) and catecholamines (α_1, α_2 and β_2 adrenoceptors). Ligands for these receptors could be derived from the sensory and autonomic nerves innervating lymphoid organs; alternatively they could originate from the circulatory pools or from local or migrating immunocytes (see also Chapter 10).

Expression of β-adrenoceptors may be linked to lymphocyte sub-type. One estimate suggests that β-adrenoceptors are most abundant on NK and B cells, followed by suppressor/cytotoxic T cells (T_S/T_C) and helper T cells (T_H) in respective proportions of 2000 : 1500 : 300–500 binding sites per cell. Another estimate for β_2-adrenoceptor abundance suggests that the ratios for $T_S : T_C : T_H$ are 2900 : 1800 : 750 respectively (30). It has also been suggested that T_H1 cells, but not T_H2 cells, express β-adrenoceptors. However this result was obtained using clonal cell lines and has not been confirmed for normal circulating cells (27).

Lymphocyte responses to adrenergic signalling are far from being stereotypic and can be sensitive to the context within which the signal is delivered (2, 29, 31). While activation of T cells by one type of mitogenic treatment (concanavalin A) up-regulates β-adrenoceptor sensitivity, another treatment (phorbol ester and calcium-ionophore) decreases β-adrenoceptor binding and signal transduction. Changes in receptor expression on lymphocytes have also been associated with exposure to catecholamines, the development of the immune response and the stage of maturation of T cells.

Neuropeptide receptors on lymphocytes have been identified for substance P (B and T cells), VIP (B and T cells), somatostatin (B and T cell lines), and NPY (splenic lymphocytes). In addition, receptors for dopamine and acetylcholine (muscarinic and nicotinic) have been described on lymphocytes. Thus, there is evidence that peripheral nerves may provide a source for at least some of these ligands inside lymphatic tissues (see Section 15.3.3). It is also possible that these agents could be encountered during migration to neuropeptide producing tissues which may include immune cells and tissues, since it now appears that the production of "neuroendocrine" peptides may be switched on in lymphocytes as the immune response proceeds (see Chapters 9–11).

β-adrenoceptors are present not only on lymphocytes but also on macrophages, neutrophils and thymic epithelial cells (our own unpublished data and Mentlein, personal communication) and substance P receptors have been identified on bone marrow stromal cells. The physiological significance of these receptors remains to be determined.

Functional Evidence

There is no simple pattern or mono-functional theme in the responses of immunocytes to experimental manipulations of the neural supply to immune tissues. However, there is substantial evidence to confirm that immunocytes (effector and stromal) are responsive to neurotransmitters. For example, β-adrenoceptor agonists inhibit a range of cellular immune functions including lymphocyte and macrophage proliferation, NK cell activity (although timing of exposure to agonist is critical), macrophage cytokine production (also mediated via α-adrenoceptors) and lymphocyte expression of IL-2 receptors in response to mitogen. Some of these effects are blocked by adrenoceptor antagonists. NPY also exerts inhibitory influences on NK cell responses *in vitro* which are reversed by anti-NPY antisera, suggesting that the response is specific (32). In contrast to cell-mediated immunity, humoral immunity may be enhanced by catecholamines. Not only is the amplitude of antigen-specific IgM secretion enhanced by β_2-adrenoceptor activation but the latency of the peak antibody response is also decreased through α-adrenoceptor activation. In addition, lymphocyte-endothelial cell adhesion is decreased by β_2-adrenoceptor agonists and is therefore likely to contribute to stress-induced alterations in lymphocyte trafficking (see Section 15.6.2).

Much evidence obtained to date suggests, therefore, that the responses of the immune system to sympathetic activation (typically mediated by β_2 adrenoceptors) are suppressive with respect to cellular immune response measures but potentiating as regards antibody production. This pattern of action accords with the emergent view of endocrine-mediated stress effects which are thought to drive the balance of effector cell functions from T_H1 towards T_H2 (33). Such simplification may, however, be misleading in regard to neural actions. Further studies are needed to address the question of how the responses of isolated, discrete cell populations *in vitro* compare with those of the heterogeneous environment *in vivo*. It will also be necessary to examine the precise timing of the neural signals, to monitor in parallel the activity of multiple immunological parameters and to separate the effects of co-transmitters (peptide and catecholamine) and of multiple receptor subtypes.

15.6.2 Immunomodulatory Consequences of Innervation

Thus far discussion has been restricted to neural regulation of lymphoid organs and cells. However, evidence suggests that local interactions between nerves, foreign toxins and immune cells takes place on a wide scale at sites of injury and infection. A brief overview of immune functions believed to be regulated *in vivo* through these direct neural connections is given here (also summarised in Fig. 15.2) and this serves to emphasise the all-pervasive nature of the neural-immune interface.

Inflammation and Hyperalgesia

Peripheral nerves (sympathetic as well as sensory), immunocytes and endothelial cells act together in the local regulation of inflammation and hyperalgesia (34). The persistence of components of the "weal-and-flare" reaction in the presence of an antihistamine block of mast cell mediators suggests that alternative, probably neurogenic, mechanisms may also be involved. Indeed treatment with capsaicin (which ablates sensory nerves and hence the neural release of substance P at joints) ameliorates inflammation while exogenous substance P aggravates it. Furthermore, the local release of sensory neuropeptides by "an axon reflex" can be maintained even when the relevant nerves are transected to interrupt spinal or central reflexes.

It is known that cytokines and chemical or mechanical irritation can stimulate the release of inflammatory mediators such as prostaglandins, purines and NPY as well as noradrenaline from sympathetic nerves. Efferents may thus influence the permeability of the vasculature and sensitise afferents, thereby amplifying the neurogenic contributions to inflammation from all hierarchical levels.

Participation of higher order neural nets in the inflammatory reaction is inferred from the following findings:

(a) sympathectomy or β_2-adrenoceptor blockade alleviates arthritic symptoms,
(b) contralateral swelling has been observed in joints not subject to adjuvant treatment,
(c) severity of joint inflammation is reduced by transection of ascending spinal pathways, and
(d) central thalamic and somatosensory cortical circuits undergo increased electrical activity during an inflammatory reaction.

These examples of the tripartite mode of local, spinal and central control operating during inflammation (schematised in Fig. 15.1) offer a valuable model for neural function at lymphoid organs (2).

Leukocyte Trafficking

Circulation of leukocytes is a crucial part of immunosurveillance. The passage of lymph (serum and cells) through all tissues, including lymphoid organs, occurs as a consequence of arterial and lymphatic vasculature flow and capillary and sinus permeabilities. Immunocyte homing to a particular location in response to an immune challenge is actively controlled through adhesive reactions of the migrating cells with the endothelium and subsequent extravasation. It is now known that leukocyte trafficking (circulation and distribution in both the blood and lymph and homing at a particular site) is subject to neural controls (35) in addition to the hormonal controls described in Chapter 8.

Nerves supplying the arterial endothelium and adrenal medulla exert significant influences on the complex redistribution of immunocytes (leukocytosis) initiated by stress (e.g. acute exercise); these effects are independent of major changes in circulating glucocorticoid levels (36). Intravenous administration of catecholamines increases the numbers of circulating lymphocytes and monocytes by mechanisms which are independent of effects of the drugs on blood flow or smooth muscle contraction. Moreover, electrical stimulation of sympathetic nerves to the popliteal node promotes the release of lymphocytes and thereby contributes to the observed leukocytosis. Although the clinical implications of such phenomena need to be fully explored, it has been suggested that comparable redistributions of NK cells brought about by exercise-induced regimens may contribute to the control of tumour metastasis.

In addition to its role in blood filtration, lymphatic drainage contributes to the maintenance of the interstitial fluid volume. Lymphatic drainage of tissues is maintained by, and depends on, an intrinsic propulsive mechanism of lymphatic vessels which is regulated by hormonal and neural (principally sympathetic) processes (13). Sympathetic stimulation and the consequent changes in circulating catecholamines appear to modulate the "set point" for lymph node fluid homeostasis and an oedematous permeation of the vascular lining can result in a doubling of lymph node size within three days of an immune response (37); this is likely to lead to increased mobility and interaction among immunocytes at sites of immune responses. Tachykinins (substance P, substance K) released from afferent nerves are also likely to play a role in regulating extracellular fluid volume as they are potent vasodilators which enhance vascular permeability directly and also induce the release of potent vasodilator monoamines from mast cells (e.g. histamine).

As indicated above, electrical stimulation mobilises white cells from lymph nodes. Circulating levels of bone marrow reticulocytes and neutrophils are likewise elevated by the activation of the lumbar sympathetic trunks. High endothelial venule cells are responsive to afferent neuropeptides which serve to relax resistance to leukocytic extravasation at the endothelial junction. These peptides also regulate the expression of lymphocyte homing receptor ligands (termed the "addressins"), altering the specific adhesive properties of the apical surfaces of high endothelial venule cells (38). Consistent with this mechanism, VIP alters the binding of mucosal lymphocytes to isolated high endothelial venule cells in culture; moreover treatment of the lymphocytes with VIP *in vitro* influences the subsequent distribution of the cells when they are replaced *in vivo*.

Antigen Processing and Presentation

Lytic and phagocytotic functions of macrophages are directly enhanced by substance P, which suggests that this neuropeptide may play a role in the regulation of antigen processing (see Chapter 3). Phagocytic responses are also enhanced by mast cell mediators (monoamines and haemopoietic growth factors), the production of which may be enhanced by neuropeptides released from sensory nerves. Indeed, there is ample opportunity for such an interaction, especially in the lamina propria where intimate contact between sensory nerves and mast cells is estimated to be as high as 60–80% (39). Other peptidergic nerves present in skin which express CGRP appear to be able to down-regulate antigen presentation by epidermal Langerhans' cells (40). Dendritic cells within lymphoid organs are also important antigen presenting cells and they are innervated by CGRP-containing fibres. A functional connection, however, remains to be determined.

Diverse Organ-specific Immunological Functions

Stromal cells from lymphoid organs and cells from other tissues with less celebrated immunological roles are beginning to be recognised as targets for the autonomic and sensory nerve fibres. Our own unpublished results and personal communications with other researchers provide evidence for β-adreno-ceptors on thymic epithelial cells which, when stimulated, elicit a rise in intracellular $3'5'$-cyclic adenosine monophosphate (cAMP) and alter the electrophysiological properties and endocrine activity of these cells. Such changes are likely to have important consequences for lymphopoiesis. Other tissues with important immunological functions which are controlled, at least in part, by neural inputs include brown adipose tissue (pyrogenic activity), the liver (production of acute phase proteins), the submandibular gland (endocrine and exocrine secretions) and lacrimal gland (immunoglobulin secretions) as detailed in Section 15.2.

15.7 CONCLUSIONS

The degree to which immune cells are accessible to the neural "wing" of the immunoregulatory apparatus can be considered to be at least equal to the systemic distribution of neuroendocrine-derived messages. Germinal lymphoid tissues and other peripheral immune effector sites are each "hard-wired" with efferent (autonomic) and sensory nerve fibres. Indeed, nerves at almost any peripheral location are liable to be recruited whenever inflammatory activity arises. Within the lymphoid organs the nerves appear well-situated to influence immune function via effects on leukocyte trafficking (through regulation of blood and lymph flow and immunocyte homing properties) and antigen processing, as well as on the cellular and humoral functions of individual effector cells. In addition, stromal cells of lymphoid organs should be included among the expected targets for neural regulation, influencing immunocytes through the haematopoietic microenvironment (summarised in Fig. 15.2).

Direct neural involvement presumably provides speed and anatomical precision of signalling which are properties not easily achieved by hormonal mechanisms. Layers of complexity of the neural involvement in the affairs of immunocytes have been revealed; these range from local axon reflexes to higher order spinal reflex loops and ultimately to activation of the "stress-response" circuitry in the brain. Central integration of multiple activating cues ("stressors" featured in Fig. 15.2) and negative feedback regulatory controls are apparent (41, 42). It can also be predicted that the brain co-ordinates autonomic and endocrine outflows, thereby providing the basis for sophisticated homeostatic responsiveness of immune functions. There is not yet, however, a precise knowledge of the immunomodulatory circuitry involved and we have therefore drawn upon the organisational plan for autonomic cardiovascular control on which to model the stress-response system. The appropriateness of such an analogy for the neural supply of lymphoid organs is however implicit, since innervation of all vasculature provides regulation of the lymphocytic migratory movements which under-lay immune surveillance throughout the entire body.

The cell and molecular bases for neural–immune interaction are underpinned by:

(a) the sharing of chemical ligands and receptors by neural and immune cells,
(b) the accessibility of cells and tissues of peripheral immune effector organs to neural and endocrine mediators, and
(c) the provisions for reciprocal signalling from local to central staging posts along the length of the neural chain supplying the periphery.

However, functional coupling between the nervous and immune systems is complex. It has not been easy to resolve a clear demarcation of neural versus neurohormonal involvement, although autonomic and endocrine controls are most likely acting in concert. Nevertheless, a clear picture emerges of a familiar plan of peripheral innervation of lymphoid tissues analogous to the autonomic and sensory supply of other viscera. Evidence has built up to implicate these neural mechanisms, alongside neuroendocrine axes, as active regulators of immunological defence, the importance of which is highlighted in conditions of deficiencies of the stress system, such as those associated with ageing, depressive disorders (25), autoimmune disease (43) and a wide variety of stressors. Further work will be required, however, before the role of inter-system signalling can be clearly understood.

ACKNOWLEDGEMENTS

We are grateful for their support to the Royal Society (J. E. G. Downing) and Welton Foundation (M. D. Kendall).

REFERENCES

1. Downing J. E. G., Kendall M. D. Peripheral and central neural mechanisms for immune regulation through the innervation of immune effector sites. In J. A. Marsh, M. D. Kendall (eds) *The Physiology of Immunity*. New York, CRC Press, 1996, pp 103–26.
2. Snow E. C. Interactions among the neuroendocrine, endocrine and immune systems. In J. C. Cambier (ed) *Ligands, Receptors, and Signal Transduction in Regulation of Lymphocyte Function*. Washington, American Society for Microbiology, 1990, pp 67–95.
3. Cunningham E. T., De Souza E. B. Interleukin-1 receptors in the brain and endocrine tissues. *Immunol Today*, 1993, **14**: 171–6.
4. Besedovsky H. O., Sorkin E., Felix D., Haas H. Hypothalamic changes during the immune response. *Eur J Immunol*, 1979, **7**: 323–5.

5. Saphier D., Abramsky O., Mor G., Ovadia H. Multiunit electrical activity in conscious rats during an immune response. *Brain, Behav Immun* 1987, **1**: 40–51.
6. Al-Shawaf A., Kendall M. D., Cowen T. Identification of neural profiles containing vasoactive intestinal polypeptides, acetylcholinesterase, and catecholamines in the rat thymus. *J Anat*, 1991, **174**: 131–43.
7. Felten D. L., Felten S. Y., Bellinger D. L., Carlson S. L., Ackerman K. D., Madden K. S., Olschowki J. A., Livnat S.. Noradrenergic sympathetic neural interactions with the immune system: Structure and function. *Immunological Rev*, 1987, **100**: 225–67.
8. Felten S. Y., Felten D. L., Bellinger D. L., Olschowka J. A. Noradrenergic and peptidergic innervation of lymphoid organs. *Chem Immunol*, 1992, **52**: 25–48.
9. Bellinger D. L., Felten S. Y., Felten D. L. Maintenance of noradrenergic sympathetic innervation in the involuted thymus of the aged Fischer 344 rat. *Brain Behav Immun*, 1988, **2**: 133–50.
10. Kendall M. D., Atkinson B. A., Munoz F. J., de la Riva C., Clarke A. G., von Gaudecker B. The noradrenergic innervation of the rat thymus during pregnancy and in the post partum period. *J. Anat*, 1994, **185**: 617—25.
11. O'Flynn R. P., dePace, D. M. The effects of noradrenaline on reticulocytes of the albino rat. *J Auton Pharmacol*, 1987, **7**: 33–39.
12. Maestroni G. J., Conti A. Modulation of hematopoiesis via alpha 1-adrenergic receptors on bone marrow cells. *Exp Hematol*, 1994, **22**: 313–20.
13. McHale N. G. Role of the lymph pump and its control. *News Physiol Sci*, 1995, **10**: 112–17.
14. Cross R. J., Jackson J. C., Brooks W. H., Sparks D. L., Markesbery W. R., Roszman T. L. Neuroimmunomodulation: impairment of humoral immune responsiveness by 6-hydroxydopamine treatment. *Immunology*, 1986, **57**: 145–52.
15. Smith O. A., DeVito J. L. Central neural integration for the control of autonomic responses associated with emotion. *Ann Rev Neurosci*, 1984, **7**: 43–65.
16. Swanson L. W., Sawchenko P. E. Hypothalamic integration: Organization of the paraventricular and supraoptic nuclei. *Ann Rev Neurosci*, 1993, **6**: 269–324.
17. Price J. L., Russchen F. T., Amaral D. G. The Limbic region: II: The Amygdaloid complex in the hypothalamus. In A. Bjorklund, T. Hokfelt, L. W. Swanson (eds) *Handbook of Chemical Neuroanatomy, v 5. Integrated Systems of the CNS, Part I. Hypothalamus, Hippocampus, Amygdala, Retina.* Amsterdam, Elsevier, 1987, pp 279–388.
18. Arora P. K. Neuromodulation of natural killer cell activity. In E. J. Goetzl, N. H. Spector (eds) *Neuroimmune Networks: Physiology and Diseases.* New York, A. R. Liss, 1987, pp 39–49.
19. Heilig M., Koob G. F., Ekman R., Britton K. T. Corticotrophin-releasing factor and neuropeptide Y: role in emotional integration. *Trends Neurosci*, 1994, **17**: 80–5.
20. Carlson S. L., Felten D. L., Livnat S., Felten S. Y. Alterations of monoamines in specific central autonomic nuclei following immunization in mice. *Brain Behav Immun*, 1987, **1**: 52–63.
21. Carlson S. L., Felten, D. L. Involvement of hypothalamic and limbic structures in neural-immune communication. In E. J. Goetzl, N. H. Spector (eds) *Neuro-immune Networks: Physiology and Diseases.* New York, A. R. Liss, 1989, pp 219–26.
22. Fisher L. A . Corticotropin-releasing factor: endocrine and autonomic integration of responses to stress. *Trends Pharmacol Sci*, 1989, **10**: 189–93.
23. Owens M. J., Nemeroff C. B. Physiology and pharmacology of corticotropin-releasing factor. *Pharmacol Rev*, 1991, **43**: 425–73.

24. Fricchione G. L., Stefano G. B. The stress response and autoimmune regulation. *Adv Neuroimmunol*, 1994, **4**: 13–27.
25. Irwin M. Stress-induced immune suppression: Role of brain corticotropin releasing hormone and autonomic nervous system mechanisms. *Adv Neuroimmunol*, 1994, **4**: 29–47.
26. Weiss J. M., Sundar S. K., Becher K. J. Stress-induced immunosuppression and immunoenhancement: Cellular immune changes and mechanisms. In E. J. Goetzl, N. H. Spector (eds) *Neuroimmune Networks: Physiology and Diseases*. New York, A. R. Liss, 1987, pp 193–206.
27. Friedman E. M., Irwin M. R. Modulation of immune cell function by the autonomic nervous system. *Pharmacol and Therapeutics* (in press).
28. Sundar S. K., Cierpial M. A., Ritchie J. C., Weiss J. M. Brain IL-1-induced immunosuppression occurs through activation of both pituitary-adrenal axis and sympathetic nervous system by corticotropin-releasing factor. *J Neurosci*, 1990, **10**:3701–6.
29. Madden K. S., Felten D. L. Experimental basis for neuro-immune interactions. *Physiol Rev*, 1995, **75**: 77–106.
30. Khan M. M., Sansoni P., Silverman E. D., Engleman E. G., Melmon K. L. Beta-adrenergic receptors on human suppressor, helper and cytotoxic lymphocytes. *Biochem Pharmacol*, 1986, **35**: 1137–42.
31. Sanders V. M., Munson A. E. Role of alpha adrenoceptor activation in modulating the murine primary antibody response *in vitro*. *J Pharmacol Exp Ther*, 1985, **232**: 395–400.
32. Nair M. P. N., Schwartz S. A., Wu K., Kronfol Z. Effect of neuropeptide Y on natural killer activity of normal human lymphocytes. *Brain Behav Immun*, 1993, **7**: 70–8.
33. Rook G. A. W., Hernandez-Pando R., Lightman S. L. Hormones, peripherally activated prohormones and regulation of the T_H1/T_H2 balance. *Immunol Today*, 1994, **15**: 301–3.
34. Dray A., Bevan S. Inflammation and hyperalgesia: highlighting the team effort. *Trends Pharmacol Sci*, 1993, **14**: 287–90.
35. Ottaway C. A., Husband A. J. The influence of neuroendocrine pathways on lymphocyte migration. *Immunol Today*, 1994, **15**: 512–17.
36. Hoffman-Goetz L., Pedersen B. K. Exercise and the immune system: a model of the stress response? *Immunol Today*, 1994, **15**: 382–7.
37. Szakal A. K., Kosco M. H., Tew J. G. Microanatomy of lymphoid tissue during humoral immune responses: structure function relationships. *Ann Rev Immunol*, 1989, **7**: 91–110.
38. Duijvestijn A., Hamann A. Mechanisms and regulation of lymphocyte migration. *Immunol Today*, 1989, **10**: 23–8.
39. Bienenstock J., Tomika M., Matsuda H., Stead R. H., Quinonez G., Simon G. T., Coughlin M. D., Denburg J. A. The role of mast cells in inflammatory processes: evidence for nerve/mast cell interactions. *Int Arch Allergy Appl Immunol*, 1987, **82**: 238–43.
40. Hosoi J., Murphy, G. F., Egan C. L., Lerner E. A., Grabbe S., Asahina A., Granstein R. D. Regulation of Langerhans' cell function by nerves containing calcitonin gene-related peptide. *Nature*, 1993, **363**: 159–63.
41. Kent S., Bluthe R.-M., Kelley K. W., Dantzer R. Sickness behaviour as a new target for drug development. *Trends Pharmacol Sci*, 1992, **13**: 24–8.
42. Lipton J. M., Catania A. Pyrogenic and inflammatory actions of cytokines and their modulation by neuropeptides: Techniques and interpretations. In E. B. De Souza (ed)

Neurobiology of Cytokines, Part B. Methods in Neurosciences. Vol. 17. San Diego, Academic Press, 1993, pp 61–77.

43. Mason D. Genetic variation in the stress response: susceptibility to experimental allergic encephalomyelitis and implications for human inflammatory disease. *Immunol Today*, 1991, **12**: 57–60.

Chapter 16

Prolactin, Growth Hormone and Host Defence

Istvan Berczi

University of Manitoba, Winnipeg, Manitoba, Canada

16.1 INTRODUCTION

Growth hormone (GH) and prolactin (PRL) are secreted by the somatotroph and lactotroph cells respectively of the anterior pituitary gland while the placental lactogens (PLs) are related hormones produced in the placenta. These polypeptide hormones are now referred to collectively as the growth and lactogenic hormone (GLH) family. Both GH and PRL may be distinguished in all

Stress, Stress Hormones and the Immune System. Edited by J. C. Buckingham, G. E. Gillies and A.-M. Cowell
© 1997 John Wiley & Sons, Ltd.

vertebrates and it has been estimated that they diverged by gene duplication from a common ancestral gene about 380 million years ago. Placental lactogens emerged probably about 60 million years ago.

Until recently, the primary function of GH was regarded as the stimulation of anabolic processes and body growth, whereas the major function of PRL in higher animals was assumed to be related to reproduction. However, with recent insights, the view is emerging that the GLH family is essential for the development and the maintenance of a broad spectrum of vital bodily functions from conception until death. The mammalian fetus is constantly exposed to various members of the GLH family which are present in high concentrations in the amniotic fluid and in the circulation of the embryo where they are likely to subserve important, although not fully yet defined, functions. Post-natally, GH and PRL fulfil more diverse roles and, in some circumstances, show a considerable overlap in their biological activities. Evidence based on the distribution of specific receptors for, and measurable biological effects of, the hormones indicates that the target tissues for GH include the liver, adipose cells, intestine, heart, kidney, lung, pancreas, brain, cartilage, skeletal muscle, corpus luteum and testes; those for PRL include the reproductive organs, brain, liver, kidneys and gastrointestinal tract. Of interest here, however, is the increasing evidence that both GH and PRL influence the development and activity of the haemopoietic and immune systems. Indeed, cells of these systems not only express receptors for these polypeptides but also synthesise GH and PRL themselves (1–6). They may thus be influenced by pituitary-derived GH or PRL in an endocrine manner or by paracrine, autocrine or intracrine actions of locally-produced GH and PRL. Interestingly, the plasma levels of pituitary GH and PRL alter during physical stresses (including infection, trauma and immune and inflammatory reactions) and in emotional stress (see below and also Chapters 1, 18) and there is increasing evidence that these responses serve the defence and survival of the host (1, 2, 7, 8). In this chapter we will discuss the influences of GH and PRL on immune and inflammatory function. First, however, some features relevant to a general understanding of the subject will be presented.

In the rat there is only one GH gene but in man there is a gene cluster coding for two GH isohormones as well as for the PLs. There appears to be only one PRL gene. GH is a single chain 191 acid protein while PRL comprises 197 (rodent) or 199 (human) animo acids. However, in the circulation both GH and PRL exist in multiple forms which are produced by dimerisation and polymerisation as well as post-translational processing (e.g. glycosylation, phosphorylation and sulphation). Indeed, it has been proposed that more than 200 forms of GH may exist and, as each of the various forms of the GH or PRL molecules may exhibit a differing degree of biological activity ranging from agonist to antagonist, the net activity of the molecules present in the systemic circulation *in vivo* is difficult to predict. Indeed, although relatively few molecular forms of these hormones will predominate, these observations may explain, at least in part, some of the contradictory data regarding the effects of GLHs on immune function reported in the literature.

In the liver and many other target tissues, GH stimulates the production of insulin-like growth factor I (IGF-I), a peptide which is structurally similar to insulin and which, like insulin, cross-reacts with the insulin receptor as well as the IGF-receptor. In some, but not all circumstances, the actions of GH are mediated by IGF-I. As both IGF-I and its receptor are found in immune cells, it is possible that IGF-I may mediate at least some of the actions of GH within the immune system. PRL may also stimulate the production of secondary hormones, termed "synlactins", in the liver (2) but little is known of their biological functions.

Cloning studies have provided evidence for at least three forms of the PRL receptor (*viz.* short, intermediate and long forms) and for short and long forms of the GH receptor in various species. Most interestingly, the receptors for a number of cytokines also belong to the same family which is now termed the GLH/cytokine receptor family; members include the receptors for granulocyte colony stimulating factor (G-CSF), granulocyte macrophage colony stimulating factor (GM-CSF), erythropoietin, the β chain of interleukin 2 (IL-2) and for IL-3, IL-4, IL-5, IL-6 and IL-7. The IL-6 receptor is associated with a glycoprotein, gp130, which plays a role in signal transduction and is also a member of this family, while the receptors for interferon (IFN)-α, -β, and -γ may form a subset of the GLH/cytokine receptor family (3). Although GLHs and the cytokines have no significant sequence homology, it is evident that GH shares a certain degree of tertiary structure with IL-2, IL-4 and GM-CSF. On a molecular basis, therefore, there are striking associations between the GLHs and the principal biochemical mediators of the immune system, the cytokines.

Multiple signal transduction pathways are likely to be activated by the members of the GLH family. In the case of PRL, G proteins, tyrosine kinase and other protein kinases are strongly implicated. The possibility of direct nuclear signalling in T lymphocytes by PRL has also been proposed. Indeed protein kinase-dependent phosphorylation of transcription factors plays a major role in signal transduction by the GLH-cytokine receptor family. The IGF-I receptor belongs to the transmembrane tyrosine kinase receptor family which is characterised by a single transmembrane domain with the intracellular tyrosine kinase domain being responsible for transducing the signal. After combination of the receptor with the hormone, phospholipase C, and probably other enzymes, is activated by phosphorylation, which leads to the generation of inositol trisphosphate and diacylglycerol. These second messengers mobilise intracellular Ca^{2+} and activate protein kinase C respectively (7). Although target cells use a common set of signalling molecules to transmit receptor-generated signals, the combination of the nuclear regulatory (transacting) factors which regulates a particular promoter in a given cell type, and thus determines the biological response, is distinct. The specificity of hormone action thus depends to a large extent on the target cell's repertoire of transacting factors (9). Further information on receptors may be found in Chapter 4.

There are two distinct sites on the GH molecule which can bind to the GH receptor and, thus, one GH molecule may cross-link two GH receptor molecules on the cell surface. This cross-linking (dimerisation) is obligatory for the initiation of the signalling process. At high GH concentrations there is an increasing probability that the receptor sites will be occupied by separate molecules of GH and thus that cross-linking will not take place (Fig. 16.1). Therefore, high concentrations of GH have the potential to inhibit signalling (10, 11). The situation is likely to be similar for PRL and for all the cytokines utilising the same type of receptors. The dose–response curves to ligands of the

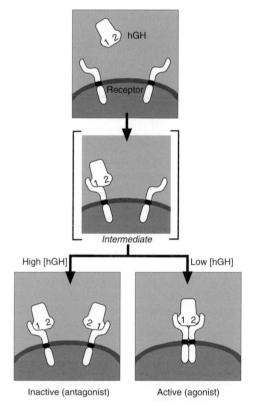

Figure 16.1 A possible mechanism of cell activation by the GLH-cytokine receptor family, using human growth hormone (hGH) as an example. In order to generate an active signal, two receptor molecules are cross-linked by a single molecule of ligand hormone-cytokine (oligomerisation). At high concentration, the ligand serves as its own antagonist. Reproduced with permission from Wells J. A., de Vos A. M. *Ann Rev Biophys Biomol Struct*, 1993, **22**, 329. © 1993 by Annual Reviews Inc

GLH/cytokine receptor family may thus be bell-shaped with self-inhibition by the hormone or cytokine occurring at high concentrations. Although additional evidence is required to substantiate this hypothesis, self-inhibition should be viewed as a key control mechanism for the prevention of excessive responses to these potent and very important regulatory hormones and cytokines. This phenomenon might also contribute to contradictory reports in the literature where a full range of concentrations of hormones has not been tested.

16.2 THE ROLE OF GROWTH AND LACTOGENIC HORMONES (GLHs) IN THE DEVELOPMENT AND FUNCTION OF THE IMMUNE SYSTEM

16.2.1 Embryonic Development

The development of the immune system in birds and mammals follows a similar but not identical course. In both cases the production of immunologically active cells is initiated in the yolk sac and is followed by the migration of embryonic stem cells to the fetal liver and spleen and, subsequently, to the bone marrow. In birds and mammals precursors of thymus-derived (T) lymphocytes migrate to the thymic rudiment, where they develop into mature T lymphocytes. In birds, the precursors of bursa-derived (B) lymphocytes migrate to the bursa of Fabricius which is attached to the rectum near the cloaca and from which mature B lymphocytes emerge. In mammals B lymphocytes develop in the bone marrow. The bone marrow, bursa and thymus are designated as primary lymphoid organs for production of mature B and T lymphocytes (12)—see also Chapter 3 for an overview of the immune system.

There is little experimental information regarding the role of GLH in the development of the immune system within the embryo, although prenatal studies suggest that the fetal pituitary gland is not important at this stage of development. This is not such a surprising result since fetal development *in utero* is dependent on placental and maternal GLHs which are present in abundance. Thus, although not proven, it is likely that embryonic development of the immune system is dependent on placental growth and lactogenic hormones. After parturition the pituitary gland subserves a vital role in the regulation of body growth, including that of bone marrow, thymus and secondary lymphoid tissues. A role for GLHs in supporting the growth and maintenance of immune tissues is suggested by demonstrations that placental GLHs promote thymus growth and bone marrow function, are mitogenic in the Nb2 rat lymphoma cell line and are capable of restoring immunocompetence in hypophysectomised rats as discussed below. In addition, pituitary dwarf animals, which are deficient in both GH and PRL, exhibit an accelerated involution of the thymus after birth together with significant deficiencies in immune function, all of which are reversed by treatment with GH or PRL. Substantial evidence suggests that some of the immune effects of GH may be mediated via the PRL receptor and interestingly pituitary dwarf humans, who exhibit deficiencies in GH but not PRL secretion, do not show severe immunological impairment (1, 2).

16.2.2   Regulation of Primary Lymphoid Organs

Bone Marrow

Current evidence indicates that the production of all subsets of leukocytes, erythrocytes and platelets is dependent on pituitary PRL and/or GH. For example, hypophysectomised rats develop anaemia and various degrees of leukocytopenia which are normalised by replacement of either GH or PRL. Moreover, PRL is capable of stimulating erythropoiesis in mice beyond the normal physiological demand. The stimulatory influence of PLs on bone marrow function may explain the increase in blood formation in mammals during pregnancy. GH has been shown recently to protect mice against the myelotoxic effect of chemotherapeutic agents used in cancer therapy. PRL also regulates the function of the bursa of Fabricius (2, 4, 8). These observations support the view that GH and PRL may act as haemopoietic growth factors and may thus be of potential value clinically to promote haematopoiesis in the face of myelotoxic therapy.

The Thymus

In dwarf, hypophysectomised and aged animals GH has a stimulatory effect on thymus growth (13) which is accompanied by an increase in the level of immunocompetence (Figs 16.2 and 16.3). GH appears to exert a direct mitogenic effect on thymocytes *in vitro* and to promote the production of thymic hormones via a mechanism which depends, at least in part, on the production of IGF-I. PRL stimulates the expression of CD3, CD4, CD8 and thymus–leukaemia surface antigens on thymocytes and the production of hormones by thymic epithelial cells. In Snell–Bagg pituitary dwarf mice, human PLs selectively stimulate the growth of the thymus without significantly affecting body growth, suggesting that the growth promoting actions of the lactogenic hormones are selective to the growth of lymphoid tissues (1, 2, 8, 14, 15).

16.2.3   Regulation of Cell-mediated Immunity

In general, GLHs promote cell-mediated immune responses such as graft rejection, contact sensitivity reaction to dinitrochlorobenzene, graft vs. host

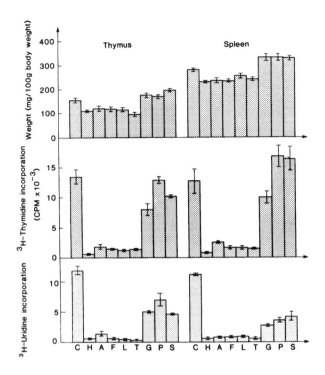

Figure 16.2 PRL or GH or both are required for the maintenance of normal thymus and spleen size and nucleic acid synthesis. Groups of five female Fischer rats weighing 150 g were used. Group designations: C, control; H, hypophysectomised; A, hypophysectomised + ACTH; F, hypophysectomised + FSH; L, hypophysectomised + LH; T, hypophysectomised + TSH; G, hypophysectomised + GH; P, hypophysectomised + PRL; S, hypophysectomised + treatment with all the above listed hormones. ACTH, FSH and LH were given at 20 μg, GH and PRL at 40 μg and TSH at 0.66 IU daily per rat, from days 12–19 after hypophysectomy. The experiment was terminated on day 20; body, thymus and spleen weights were taken and thymus and spleen cells were prepared and pooled from animals belonging to the same group. Overnight ^{3}H-thymidine and ^{3}H-uridine incorporation was measured. Mean body weights $\pm$ SE (g) of the various groups at termination were as follows: C, 174 $\pm$ 2.4; H, 126.8 $\pm$ 1.0; A, 121.6 $\pm$ 3.1; F, 127.6 $\pm$ 3.6; L, 118.2 $\pm$ 8.2; T, 129 $\pm$ 4.4; G, 134.4 $\pm$ 3.6; P, 136 $\pm$ 5.1; S, 133.2 $\pm$ 1.9 g. Statistical analysis: The two-tailed t-test was used. Thymus and spleen weights of groups H, A, F, L and T were significantly lower ($p < 0.01$) than control; for groups G, P and S, they were equal or higher than C. Thymus and spleen cells from groups with low organ weights did not synthesise nucleic acids, whereas in groups G, P, and S, normal or near normal DNA and RNA synthesis was detected. Modified from Berczi I., Nagy E., de Toledo S.M., Matusik R.J., Friesen H.G. Pituitary hormones regulate c-*myc* and DNA synthesis in lymphoid tissue. From Berczi I., Nagy E., de Toledo S. M., Matusik R. J., Friesen H. G. *J Immunol* 1991, **146**: 2201–6, reproduced with permission. Copyright 1991, The American Association of Immunologists

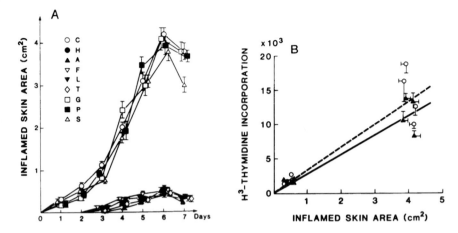

Figure 16.3 Direct correlation of contact sensitivity reaction with nucleic acid synthesis in lymphoid organs. Experimental details are the same as for Fig. 16.2. Skin painting with dinitrochlorobenzene was performed on day 12. Mean areas of inflamed skin lesions ± SE were calculated for each group and plotted against days (Panel A). The mean areas of inflamed skin were plotted against thymidine labelling (Panel B). Bars indicate SE for groups with inflamed skin area greater than 3 cm². Bars on other groups are not present because the SE was extremely small. Statistical analysis: A, Groups H, A, F, L and T had significantly lower responses ($p < 0.01$) than controls. The response of groups G, P and S was normal, with slight occasional differences. B, The correlation coefficient for DNA-labelling of spleen (○) or thymus (▲) against inflamed skin area was 93% and 96%, respectively. Reproduced by permission from Berczi I., Nagy E., de Toledo S. M., Matusik R. J., Friesen H. G. Pituitary hormones regulate c-*myc* and DNA synthesis in lymphoid tissue. From Berczi I., Nagy E., de Toledo S. M., Matusik R. J., Friesen H. G. *J Immunol*, 1991, **146**: 2201–6, reproduced with permission. Copyright 1991, The American Association of Immunologists

reactions and the mixed lymphocyte reaction *in vitro*. Suppression of PRL secretion in animals with a dopamine receptor agonist (bromocriptine) impairs cell-mediated immune reactions and augments the immunosuppressive actions of cyclosporin A. In addition, serum PRL levels are raised significantly in patients with cardiac allografts before the primary rejection episode, although such increases are not always observed during recurrent rejections.

Effects of GLHs on cell-mediated immunity have also been observed *in vitro*. For example, GH and IGF-I stimulate the growth of T lymphocytes *in vitro* and PRL stimulates the IL-2-induced proliferation of T cells at concentrations within the physiological range (1, 2, 8, 15–17). Interestingly, at supra-physiological concentrations (5–10-fold higher) PRL inhibits T cell proliferation, a finding which may reflect the bell-shaped dose-response curve often found for the GLH/cytokine family (see Section 16.1). The physiological significance of this, however, remains to be determined.

16.2.4   Regulation of Humoral Immunity

GH and PRL are essential for the maintenance of humoral immunity both in experimental animals and man. GH stimulates both the proliferation and the production of IGF-I by B lymphocytes *in vitro*. Insulin also has a stimulatory effect on lymphocytes via actions on IGF-I receptors and has been reported to increase the number of antibody forming cells and to potentiate anaphylactic reactions. Similar stimulatory effects have been ascribed to PRL. Hypophysectomised rats which lack both GH and PRL are not able to produce antibodies but their immunocompetence may be restored readily by treatment with either GH or PRL. Conversely, treatment of mice with a high dose of PRL suppresses the antibody response (1, 2, 8, 15–17).

16.2.5   Regulation of Cytokine Activity

GLHs influence cytokine production in a number of species. For example, in the mouse treatment with bromocriptine (which suppresses PRL release) produces reductions in IFN-γ production by T lymphocytes which are restored by PRL treatment. GH treatment augments the production of IL-2 by human lymphocytes and potentiates the production of IL-1 and tumour necrosis factor-α (TNFα) by rat macrophages. Cytokine receptor expression may also be modulated by GLHs and, for example, PRL increases the expression of the IL-2 receptor by rat spleen cells. Interestingly, the stimulatory effects of GLHs may be antagonised by glucocorticoids, as shown in Table 16.1, which supports the view advanced many years ago by Hans Selye (see Prologue) that these endocrine hormones may play a counter-regulatory role in the control of the immune function (2, 7, 8, 17).

16.2.6   GLHs and Innate or Natural Immunity

Several reports favour the view that PRL enhances natural killer (NK) cell-mediated cytotoxicity both in mice and in man. For example, exposure of

Table 16.1 The effects of GH, PRL and glucocorticoids on the production of major immunoregulatory cytokines

	IL-1	IL-2	IL-6	IFN-γ	TNFα
GH	↑	↑	↑		↑
PRL				↑	
GC	↓	↓	0 ↓	↓	↓

Abbreviations: GH, growth hormone; PRL, prolactin; GC, glucocorticoids; ↑, increase/potentiation of production/release; 0, no effect; ↓, decrease of production/release. Data from (2, 13, 17).

purified NK cells to PRL *in vitro* stimulates ^{3}H-thymidine uptake and cytotoxic activity. In contrast, NK cell activity, as determined in a mixed population of peripheral blood lymphocytes, is unaffected by physiological concentrations of PRL and inhibited at higher concentrations. These apparent contradictions may be accounted for by the presence of PRL-sensitive suppressor T cells in the total peripheral blood lymphocyte population as PRL enhanced the activity of purified NK cells isolated from the same donors. Pathological levels of PRL reversibly inhibit the cytotoxic activity of lymphokine-activated killer (LAK) cells triggered by low doses of IL-2 *in vitro* whereas IL-2-activated NK cells are stimulated under these conditions.

In the clinical situation, the activity of NK cells from patients with hyperprolactinaemia appears to fall within the normal range, possibly because the multiple complex homeostatic mechanisms which are likely to operate *in vivo* compensate for any inappropriately enhanced activity of the immune system. For example, high concentrations of PRL may paradoxically inhibit receptor-mediated effects (in a manner analogous to GH as discussed in Section 16.1 and depicted in Fig. 16.1, i.e. the bell-shaped curve effect); immune-enhancing activities of GLHs may be counteracted by the immunosuppressive actions of other hormones (glucocorticoids, oestradiol and testosterone under certain circumstances) or the presence of suppressor cells. Alternatively, the spectrum of PRL-like molecules produced in hypoprolactinaemic conditions may include molecules which counteract any immune-enhancing properties of PRL. Interestingly however, supra-physiological levels of GH increase both the number and the cytotoxic activity of NK cells in man (2, 8, 11, 12, 16, 17).

16.2.7   Immune Inflammatory Feedback Signals Regulating Prolactin (PRL) and Growth Hormone (GH) Secretion

As discussed elsewhere in this volume, notably in relation to the hypothalamo–pituitary–adrenal (HPA) axis (see Chapters 11, 12, 14, 15), raised levels of cytokines in the general circulation exert important actions on the endocrine system and the GH and PRL axes appear to be no exception. As shown in Table 16.2, there are many reports that cytokines influence the secretion of GH and PRL by the pituitary gland (1, 8, 18–20). Similar effects have also been noted for inflammatory mediators such as platelet activating factor, bradykinin and histamine (Table 16.2). Whether or not these immune cell-derived mediators alter GH and PRL release via influences on the secretion of the hypothalamic releasing factors (e.g. GH releasing hormone or thyrotrophin releasing hormone, respectively) and inhibitory factors (somatostatin, dopamine) or whether they act directly at the pituitary level, remains to be established. This area is under intense investigation at the present time and some of the emerging findings are

Table 16.2 Lymphoid and inflammatory feedback signals regulating GH and PRL secretion

Feedback signal	Species	Target	Effect on pituitary	
			GH	PRL
Haemorrhage (stress)	rat, swine	MBH	ND	↑
Thymosin-α_1	rat	HYP	0	↓
MB-35	rat	PIT	↑	↑
IL-1α,β	rat	HYP	↑	↑
		PIT	↑?	↑↓
IL-2	rat, mouse, man	HYP	↓	↑
		PIT?	↓	↓↑
IL-6	rat, mouse, man	HYP	↓	0
		PIT	↑	0↑
IFN-γ	rat, mouse, man	HYP	0↓↑	0
		PIT	0↓↑	0↓↑
IFN-γ	man	?	↑	ND
TNF-α	rat, calf	HYP	↓	↑
		PIT	↓↑	↑↓TRH
TGF-β, β_1	rat	PIT, PITA	↑	↓
PAF	rat	PIT	↑	↑
PDGF	rat	PITA	ND	↓
Endothelin-1	man	?	↓GH-RH	↓TRH
Bradykinin	man	PIT	ND	↑
Histamine	man	HYP	ND	↑

Abbreviations: HYP, hypothalamus; IL, interleukin; IFN, inteferon; MB-35, thymic peptide; MBH, median basal hypothalamus; ND, not done; PAF, platelet activating factor; PDGF, platelet derived growth factor; TNF-α, tumour necrosis factor α; TGF-β, β_1, transforming growth factor-β, β_1; PIT, pituitary; PITA, pituitary adenoma; ↓ GH-RH, growth hormone releasing hormone induced increase is inhibited; ↓ TRH, thyrotropin releasing hormone induced increase is inhibited; ?, site of action or nature of effect is uncertain. From (1, 11, 18–20).

contradictory. There are many important factors contributing to this controversy including the bell-shaped concentration response curves of several cytokines on pituitary hormone release (19) and the timing and nature of the immune stimulus.

16.3 THE GROWTH AND LACTOGENIC HORMONE FAMILY AND HOST DEFENCE

16.3.1 Inflammation and Infection

Insults, such as administration of sublethal doses of endotoxin or mild injury, elicit sharp, brief elevations in the serum GH and PRL concentrations which appear to contribute to efficient progress of the inflammatory response. Mild bacterial infections also cause brief but significant rises in pituitary GH and PRL in experimental animals and in man and several lines of evidence indicate that GH, IGF-I and PRL can increase host resistance. Evidence for a role for endogenous pituitary hormones has emerged from observations that hypophysectomised rats are more susceptible to the lethal effects of virulent *S. typhimurium* and that administration of GH is as effective as IFN-γ both in augmenting the bactericidal capacity of macrophages and in reducing the numbers of bacteria in spleen cells of these animals.

Mononuclear phagocytes (monocytes and macrophages) and neutrophilic polymorphonuclear leukocytes all play major roles in the pathogenesis of immune-inflammatory responses and may be activated by a variety of factors including antigen-antibody complexes (especially when complement is fixed to them), cytokines, infectious agents and foreign materials (7). Superoxide anions, IL-1 and TNFα are all essential for effective phagocytosis by mononuclear cells and production of each of these factors may be stimulated by GH. GH also primes neutrophilic granulocytes for superoxide production. In addition, it stimulates lysosomal enzyme production, oxidative metabolism and adhesiveness but inhibits chemotaxis. IGFs have effects similar to GH on phagocytic cells and may thus mediate many of the actions of GH on immune cells. Treatment of mice with PRL also results in increased phagocytosis and cytotoxicity by peritoneal macrophages as well as enhanced chemotaxis by peritoneal granulocytes. The activity of leukocytes in the general circulation is, however, not modified by PRL treatment (7, 12, 15, 21).

In vivo experiments in the rat have shown that the inflammatory response to various irritants may be potentiated by PRL, thus supporting the view that PRL is normally a pro-inflammatory hormone. On the basis of its stimulatory effects on inflammatory cells, a similar result might be expected for GH but the data are not clear-cut. Indeed, at high doses, there is evidence that GH may have anti-inflammatory actions, an effect which could be attributed to "self-inhibition" at high concentrations (see Section 16.1 and Fig. 16.1). Thus, treatment of rats with high doses (2 mg/kg) of human GH protects the gut from the inflammatory damage induced by trinitrobenzene sulphonic acid. Interestingly in the clinical situation, IGF-I levels are reported to be subnormal in children with inflammatory bowel disease (2, 7), a phenomenon which may be explained by an acquired resistance to GH which is often observed in patients with severe illness (22).

GH and PRL also potentiate the immune responses to viral antigens and can augment the response to anti-viral vaccination. However, in the case of retroviruses, including those which multiply in lymphoid cells, GH and PRL may actually promote virus production because of their general anabolic and growth stimulatory effect on the virus-producing cells (23–25). It remains to be seen whether or not the stimulation of virus production by the GLHs affects the development of immunity to these viruses.

16.3.2 The Acute Phase Response

The activation of the acute phase response (APR) during injury (infections, burns, trauma etc.) is described in Chapter 3. The associated changes in endocrine activity are complex. Characteristically the secretion of adrenocorticotrophic hormone (ACTH), glucocorticoids, catecholamines, glucagon, vasopressin and aldosterone is increased whereas the production of GH, PRL, oestrogens, androgens, insulin and thyroid hormones may be either elevated or suppressed, depending on the severity of the condition (Table 16.3). The precise role of the GLHs, therefore, remains to be determined.

16.3.3 Severe Trauma, Sepsis and Shock

The immune system is designed to act locally to contain an infection and eliminate the pathogenic agent. If this local and often specific response fails, sepsis may develop which activates a generalised, systemic response. This is a potentially hazardous situation as the excess production of cytokines such as TNF, IL-1, IFN-γ, etc. may cause severe illness and shock leading to death. Severe trauma activates the immune system nonspecifically by activating the complement cascade and by inducing the release of mediators from tissue mast cells, endothelial cells, platelets and even fibroblasts, resulting in a condition indistinguishable from sepsis. Under these conditions there is a profound glucocorticoid and catecholamine response which serves to suppress cytokine production and produce a generalised immunosuppression, leaving the patient highly vulnerable to microbes, including invasion of gram negative organisms from the gastrointestinal tract. Under these conditions the secretion of GH and PRL is suppressed (7)—see Table 16.3. Theoretically, administration of immune-enhancing GLHs, which have a beneficial effect on host defence in animal models, might aid recovery from sepsis. However, this appears not to be the case for either GH or IGF-I (22, 26–29) as, under these conditions, acquired GH

Table 16.3 GH, PRL, ACTH and glucocorticoid response to various forms of injury

Hormone	Burn	Trauma	Surgery	Infection	Endotoxin	APR
GH		↓	↑	↑↓	↑	↑↓
PRL			↑	↑↓	↑↓	
ACTH		↑	↑		↑	↑
GC	↑	↑	↑	↑	↑	↑

Abbreviations: APR, acute phase response; GH, growth hormone; PRL, prolactin; ACTH, adrenocorticotrophic hormone; GC, glucocorticoids; ↑, increase/potentiation of production/release; ↓, decrease of production/release. See (19).

resistance is present. This is characterised by reductions in serum IGF-I and IGF-I carrier binding protein (IGFBP-3) and increases in the serum concentration of the inhibitory binding protein (IGFBP-1). A greater understanding of the complex interactions between the neuroendocrine and immune systems in disease is required, therefore, before a rational hormonal therapy can be developed for the manipulation of immune functions.

16.3.4   Healing and Recovery

Host cells and tissues become damaged during an inflammatory response either by the irritant or infectious agent or by enzymes and toxins released from damaged cells and by various phagocytes. A period of wound healing is, therefore, required. Because of the ability of GH to increase both macrophage and T cell function, experimental and clinical studies are under way to examine the potential of GH treatment for the promotion of wound healing (28). Although some of the results are encouraging, other studies show little, if any, effect. Severely ill patients do not respond to GH with IGF-I production, possibly because of the presence of the IGF-I inhibitory protein IGFBP-I in their serum (22) as discussed above. This could be responsible, at least in part, for the inefficiency of GH in promoting wound healing in some patients. Once again, a further understanding of complex neuroendocrine-immune interactions might offer novel ways of improving therapy.

16.3.5   Preventive Neuroendocrine Defence Activated by Stress

Recent studies suggest that the effects of emotional stress on the neuroendocrine and immune system are simular to those of infection or trauma. The rapid elevations in GH and PRL secretion elicited by stressful stimuli, which are usually over within hours, may be viewed as endocrine responses which aim to increase the competence of all tissues and organs in the body which participate in host defence. Other hormones released during stress have a more specific role to play. For instance, it has been shown experimentally that catecholamines, in conjunction with glucocorticoids, have the ability to induce the production of acute phase proteins in the liver. These changes may prepare the body to cope more effectively with insults by increasing nonspecific resistance while suppressing the specific immune response (7). Immunosuppression may also be viewed as a preventative measure during stress since it serves to prevent the excessive production of cytokines (e.g. IL-1 and TNFα) which is triggered by injury and which may have fatal consequences if left unchecked. The relationships between stress, immune function and disease are discussed further in Chapter 19.

Conditioned immune responses may also be regarded as a preventive measure. As described in Chapter 18, conditioning may be produced in experimental animals by pairing immunisation with an antigen (e.g. cytotoxic agent or surgery) and with a sensory stimulus (e.g. taste). If the conditioned animals are subsequently exposed to the immunising antigen in association with the sensory stimulus, the secondary immune response may be either enhanced or suppressed, depending on the method of conditioning applied. Although the mechanism of conditioned immune responses has not been elucidated in full detail, there are experimental results to indicate the involvement of both endocrine and neural pathways (30).

16.3.6 GLHs and their Receptors in Cells of the Immune System

Compelling experimental evidence suggests that T and B lymphocytes themselves are capable of expressing GH and PRL together with their respective receptors (2, 6, 17). For example, PRL mRNA is found in human T and B lymphocytes, in monocytes and in the thymus and PRL binding sites are present on human NK cells and lymphocytes. It has been suggested that hypophysectomised rats depend on residual PRL for survival as treatment of these animals with PRL antiserum precipitates severe anaemia, immunological anergy and death (4). Although not proven, the lymphoid cells should be considered as a potential source of the residual PRL. It has been shown that lymphocytes secrete GH *in vitro* and that exposure of rat leukocytes from spleen, thymus and peritoneum to lipopolysaccharide results in an increased GH mRNA content. The synthesis of GH in lymphocytes is stimulated by the hypothalamic GH releasing hormone and inhibited by IGF-I in a manner analogous to the control of pituitary GH release. The transcription of the Pit-1/GHF-1 gene, the product of which regulates GH and PRL production in the pituitary gland, has also been described in the bone marrow and in other lymphoid tissues (2) but at this point little information is available regarding its regulation. Regulators of pituitary PRL secretion do not affect PRL secretion by a sub-line of human IM-9 cells (a B cell line) but dexamethasone is inhibitory as it is at the pituitary level. The PRL gene in lymphocytes is coupled with noncoding regulatory sequences which are analogous to the placental and not the pituitary gene. Therefore, the use of alternative promoters in different tissues provides a basis for tissue specificity in PRL gene expression.

Although much remains to be discovered regarding the regulation of leukocyte-derived GH and PRL, the above observations raise the possibility that the locally formed hormones may support the amplification of immune reactions in germinal centres or at sites of cell-mediated immune reactions in lymph nodes, spleen and other lymphoid tissues via an autocrine or paracrine mechanism with little, if any, systemic effect (2, 31). Interestingly, the production of leukocytes in the bone marrow is elevated during severe infection or trauma despite the fact that glucocorticoid levels are raised and the secretion of pituitary GLHs is suppressed. The apparent resistance of the bone marrow to the suppressive effect of glucocorticoids under these conditions may therefore rely on the local production of GLHs. Thus, under certain circumstances, the circulating levels of pituitary hormones may not adequately reflect the likely participation of a given hormone in regulating the immune response. However, the regular appearance of anaemia in hypophysectomised animals and hypopituitary patients indicates that bone marrow function is ultimately still dependent on pituitary GLHs (4).

16.3.7   Defective Neuroendocrine Immunoregulation and Disease

A number of investigations suggest that a deficient glucocorticoid response to immunisation, infection or inflammation can lead to increased susceptibility to infection and to the development of autoimmune disease (7, 29). A growing body of evidence also suggests that abnormalities in PRL secretion may be associated with autoimmune disease, with high levels predisposing to antibody-mediated conditions (e.g. systemic lupus erythematosus, SLE) or cell-mediated ones (e.g. encephalitis, arthritis) (32). For example, in B/W mice the progress of a spontaneous autoimmune disease resembling SLE in man may be delayed if PRL levels are reduced by treatment with bromocriptine and accelerated if female mice are grafted with syngeneic pituitaries. In the same vein, the number of PRL receptor-bearing T cells and PRL-receptor density per T cell are increased with age in the NZB mouse strain which also develops the SLE-like syndrome spontaneously, when compared to normal mice (32, 33). Pregnancy and pseudopregnancy, which are conditions characterised by high serum PRL levels, also have an aggravating effect on the disease. The development of adjuvant-induced arthritis in rats is inhibited in hypophysectomised or bromo-criptine-treated animals but this effect is reversed by treatment with either PRL or GH. The development of experimental allergic encephalomyelitis in Lewis rats, induced by immunisation with rat spinal cord in Freund's complete adjuvant, is also inhibited significantly by bromocriptine treatment and the therapeutic effectiveness of the immunosuppressant, cyclosporin A, is enhanced by additional treatment with bromocriptine (32). An important role is also played by the HPA axis in similar experimental conditions and this is discussed in Chapter 9.

In man, raised PRL levels have been described in patients with SLE, Addison's disease (a disease due to the autoimmune destruction of the adrenal cortex), autoimmune lymphocytic hypophysitis and autoimmune thyroid disease. Furthermore, hyperprolactinaemia has been implicated in the pathogenesis of some cases of iridocyclitis. In contrast, a reduction in bioactive circulating

PRL has been found in patients with rheumatoid arthritis, which is also thought of as an autoimmune condition. Moreover, rheumatoid patients frequently exhibit a blunted nocturnal increase in PRL and GH levels together with an altered circadian rhythm of cortisol, resulting in a generally increased blood level (33). These apparent anomalies emphasise the complexity of neuroendocrine influences on immune function and emphasise the need for further understanding.

16.4   SUMMARY AND CONCLUSIONS

The development of the immune system *in utero* is likely to be dependent on placental growth and lactogenic hormones. After birth the function of lymphoid tissues and cells is dependent, to a large extent, on pituitary GH and PRL, which maintain and amplify immunocompetence both by stimulating lymphocyte production and growth and by promoting the function of mature lymphocytes and other leukocytes (1)—see Figs 16.2 and 16.3. In addition to the influence of nutritional factors, the development and growth of vertebrates is regulated by:

(a) systemically acting hormones belonging to the GLH family,
(b) locally acting stromal and adherence signals delivered by adhesion molecules and membrane- or matrix-fixed growth factors, and
(c) cytokines (2).

The immune system obeys the general rules for growth control and GLH actions are critical to all stages mentioned above. Thus, GLHs supply the competence signal which is essential for lymphocytes to develop and to respond appropriately to antigen or to inflammatory stimuli. The expression both of cytokines and of cell surface receptors is also potentiated by GLHs, thus facilitating primary and secondary signalling by GLHs, antigens and adhesion molecules and possibly also IGF-I and insulin within lymphoid cells (2).

In terms of the whole body response, the brief rise in pituitary-derived GH and PRL observed in response to many stresses, including injury and immune challenges, may be critical to host defence mechanisms. However, if the stimulus persists, the continued potentiation of immune reactions, cytokine production or inflammation in general may be disastrous, as is the case in trauma, sepsis or shock. Indeed, under these conditions the level of GLHs tends to be subnormal and a significant decrease in bioactivity of GLH molecules may also occur. In all probability this represents an adaptive neuroendocrine response to feedback signals which are mediated, at least in part, by immune and inflammatory cytokines. As immune or inflammatory responses proceed, glucocorticoids and catecholamines are elevated and serve the interest of host defence by curbing excess cytokine production and increasing nonspecific host defence mechanisms. Thus, the effects of GH or PRL and of glucocorticoids on immune and inflammatory reactions are antagonistic in nature. Indeed, there is evidence to suggest that serum glucocorticoid levels are raised in response to high PRL or GH levels and this may therefore be regarded as a compensatory reaction within the endocrine system (2). Conversely glucocorticoids suppress PRL secretion. Additional non-endocrine feedback signals concerning the state of immune activation may also be delivered by the nervous system which can relay signals from the site of injury to the central nervous system which may ultimately be integrated at hypothalamic level, thereby modifying pituitary hormone secretion (7). There is, in fact some evidence for cross-talk between HPA stress axis and GH and PRL but the precise mechanisms remain to be fully elucidated.

In conclusion, GLHs clearly play a basic physiological role in regulating immune and inflammatory responses. The immune system also plays an important role in recovery from severe trauma, sepsis and shock and contributes to healing processes. It remains to be established, however, whether or not host resistance or recovery can be influenced favourably by treatment with GH and PRL. As the effects on immune and inflammatory reactions of GH and PRL, on the one hand, and glucocorticoids, on the other, are generally antagonistic in nature, it may be possible to induce changes in immune activity by altering the ratio of these hormones (1). Whether this represents a potential novel therapy for immune disorders is an interesting question for the future. Abnormalities of PRL or GH secretion, as well as an insufficient ACTH-glucocorticoid response to immunisation or inflammation, have been associated with autoimmune disease; self-recognition by lymphocytes may evolve into self-reactivity if the endocrine milieu or regulation becomes abnormal (29, 32, 33). A greater understanding of the processes involved in the interrelationships of the immune and neuroendocrine systems, therefore, is needed as it may offer new therapeutic strategies for certain diseases.

REFERENCES

1. Berczi I. (ed). *Pituitary Function and Immunity.* Boca Raton, CRC Press, 1986.
2. Berczi I. The role of the growth and lactogenic hormone family in immune function. *Neuroimmunomodulation*, 1994, **1**: 201–16.
3. Kelly P. A., Djiane J., Postel-Vinay M. C., Edery M. The prolactin/growth hormone receptor family. *Endocr Rev*, 1991, **12**: 235–51.
4. Berczi I., Nagy E. Effects of hypophysectomy on immune function. In R. Ader, D. L. Felten, N. Cohen (eds) *Psychoneuroimmunology (2nd ed).* London, Academic Press, 1991, pp 339–75.
5. Sabbadini E., Berczi I. The submandibular gland: a key organ in the neuro-immunoregulatory network? *Neuroimmunomodulation*, 1995, **2**: 184–202.
6. Weigent D. A., Immunoregulatory properties of growth hormone and prolactin. *Pharmacol Therapeutics*, 1996, **69**: 237–57.

7. Berczi I., Nagy E. Neurohormonal control of cytokines during injury. In N. J. Rothwell, F. Berkenbosch (eds) *Brain Control of Responses to Trauma*. Cambridge, Cambridge University Press, 1994, pp 32–107.
8. Berczi I. The immunology of prolactin. *Sem Reprod Endocrinol*, 1992, **10**: 196–219.
9. Horseman N. D., Yu-Lee L. Y. Transcriptional regulation by the helix bundle peptide hormones: growth hormone, prolactin, and hematopoietic cytokines. *Endocr Rev*, 1994, **15**: 627–49.
10. Fuh G., Cunningham B. C., Fukunaga R., Nagata S., Goeddel D. V., Well J. A. Rational design of potent antagonists to the human growth hormone receptor. *Science*, 1992, **256**: 1677–80.
11. Wells J. A., de Vos A. M. Structure and function of human growth hormone: implications for the hematopoietins. *Ann Rev Biophys Biomolec Struct*, 1993, **22**: 329–51.
12. Paul W. E. The immune system. An introduction. In W. E. Paul (ed) *Fundamental Immunology (3rd ed)*. New York, Raven Press, 1993.
13. Berczi I., Nagy E., de Toledo S. M., Matusik R. J., Friesen H. G. Pituitary hormones regulate c-myc and DNA synthesis in lymphoid tissue. *J Immunol*, 1991, **146**: 2201–6.
14. Savino W., Mello-Coelho V., Dardenne M. Neuroendocrine control of the thymic microenvironment: role of pituitary hormones. In I. Berczi, J. Szelenyi (eds) *Advances in Psychoneuroimmunology*. New York, Plenum Press, 1994, pp 75–82.
15. Kelley K. W. Growth hormone in immunobiology. In R. Ader, D. L. Felten, N. Cohen (eds) *Psychoneuroimmunology (2nd ed)*. San Diego, Academic Press, 1991, pp 377–402.
16. Matera L., Bellone G., Cesano A. Prolactin and the immune network. *Adv Neuroimmunol*, 1991, **1**: 158–72.
17. Berczi I., Chalmers I. M., Nagy E., Warrington R. J. The immune effects of neuropeptides. *Clin Rheumatol*, 1996, **10**: 227–57.
18. Besedovsky H. O., del Rey A. Immune-neuroendocrine circuits: integrative role of cytokines. *Frontiers Neuroendocrinol*, 1992, **13**: 61–94.
19. McCann S., Karanth S., Kamat A., Dees W. L., Lyson K., Gimeno M., Rettori V. Induction by cytokines of the pattern of pituitary hormone secretion in infection. *Neuroimmunomodulation*, 1994, **1**: 2–13.
20. Berczi I. Hormonal interactions between the pituitary and immune system. In C. J. Grossman (ed) *Bilateral Communication Between the Endocrine and Immune Systems*. New York, Springer-Verlag, 1994, pp 96–144.
21. McKay D. M., Bienenstock J. The interaction between mast cells and nerves in the gastrointestinal tract. *Immunol Today*, 1994, **15**: 533–8.
22. Bentham J., Rodriguez-Arnao J., Ross R. J. M. Acquired growth hormone resistance in patients with hypercatabolism. *Horm Res*, 1993, **40**: 87–91.
23. Berczi I., Szentivanyi A. The pituitary gland, psychoneuroimmunology and infectious disease. In H. Friedman, T. Klein, A. L. Friedman (eds) *Psychoneuroimmunology, Stress and Infectious Disease*. Boca Raton, CRC Press, 1996, pp 79–109.
24. Laurence J., Grimison B., Gonenne A. Effect of recombinant human growth hormone on acute and chronic human immunodeficiency virus infection *in vitro*. *Blood*, 1992, **79**: 467–72.
25. Chen H. W., Meier H., Heiminger H. J., Huebner R. J. Tumorigenesis in strain BW/J mice and induction by prolactin of the group specific antigen of C-type RNA tumor virus. *J Nat Cancer Inst*, 1972, **49**: 1145–53.
26. Inoue T., Saito H., Fukushima R., Inaba T., Lin M.-T., Fukatsu K., Muto T. Growth hormone and insulin like growth factor I enhance host defense in a murine sepsis model. *Arch Surg*, 1995, **130**: 1115–22.

27. Gottardis M., Benzer A., Koller W., Luger T. J., Phringer F., Hackl J. Improvement of septic syndrome after administration of recombinant human growth hormone (rhGH)? *J Trauma*, 1991, **31**: 81–6.
28. Lippe B. M., Nakamoto J. M. Conventional and nonconventional uses of growth hormone. *Recent Progr Horm Res*, 1993, **48**: 179–235.
29. Wick G., Hu Y., Scwarz S., Kroemer G. Immunoendocrine communication via the hypothalamo–pituitary–adrenal axis in autoimmune disease. *Endocr Rev*, 1993, **14**: 539–63.
30. Ader R., Cohen N. The influence of conditioning on immune responses. In R. Ader, D. L. Felten, N. Cohen (eds) *Psychoneuroimmunology (2nd ed)*. San Diego, Academic Press, 1991, pp 611–46.
31. Weigent D. A., Blalock J. E. Effect of the administration of growth-hormone-producing lymphocytes on weight gain and immune function in dwarf mice. *Neuroimmunomodulation*, 1994, **1**: 50–8.
32. Berczi I. The role of prolactin in the pathogenesis of autoimmune disease. *Endocr Pathol*, 1994, **4**: 178–95.
33. Berczi I., Baragar F. D., Chalmers I. M., Keystone E. C., Nagy E., Warrington R. J. Hormones in self tolerance and autoimmunity: a role in the pathogenesis of rheumatoid arthritis? *Autoimmunity*, 1993, **16**: 45–56.

Chapter 17

Thymic Polypeptides and their Role as Mediators in Neuroendocrine– Immune Communication

Bryan L. Spangelo*

University of Nevada Las Vegas, Las Vegas, Nevada, USA

William C. Gorospe

Medical University of South Carolina, Charleston, South Carolina, USA

17.1 INTRODUCTION

The thymus gland is the primary lymphatic tissue effecting cell-mediated immunity. In the neonate it represents a substantial tissue mass within the thorax. However, although the thymus is functional throughout life, both its activity and its mass decline markedly with age. The main role of the thymus is to provide the microenvironment for thymopoiesis, i.e. the development of prothymocytes

---

*To whom correspondence should be addressed

Stress, Stress Hormones and the Immune System. Edited by J. C. Buckingham, G. E. Gillies and A.-M. Cowell
© 1997 John Wiley & Sons, Ltd.

into mature T lymphocytes. In addition, all mature T lymphocytes reside in this tissue for some period of time. The first step in thymopoiesis involves the entry into the thymus of prothymocytes which are devoid of the cluster differentiation (CD) antigens, CD4 and CD8, which are exposed on the cell surface. These cells, which are described as CD4⁻/CD8⁻ or "double negative", enter the thymus at the subcapsular cortex and traverse the cortex to the corticomedullary region. During their transit the cortical thymocytes express either CD4 or CD8 before the greater proportion becomes positive for both surface antigens (i.e. CD4⁺/ CD8⁺ or double positive). A further critical stage in thymocyte development is the appearance, at the double negative stage, of the polypeptide chains of the T cell receptors which enable the thymocytes to recognise many different antigens. Many of the developing thymocytes, which could potentially become autoreactive clones, undergo apoptosis and are phagocytosed by resident macrophages or epithelial cells. This elimination is termed negative selection and follows on from the positive selection of cells with increased T cell receptor expression and down-regulation of either CD4 or CD8 expression. These positively selected cells emigrate via the corticomedullary venules or lymphatics and are mature T cells which are self-tolerant and recognise foreign antigens only in the context of the major histocompatibility complex (MHC) class I or II antigens. The cells which are generally classified as T helper cells (CD4⁺ cells) recognise antigens in the MHC class II context whereas T suppressor/cytotoxic cells (CD8⁺ cells) require MHC class I expression for activation (1, 2)—for further details see Chapter 3.

The events underlying the differentiation of the thymocyte are controlled by the thymic microenvironment, an important component of which is the body of epithelial cells lying within the cortex (1). At least six subtypes of thymic epithelial cells have been defined on the basis of differences in ultrastructural morphology. These cells express MHC antigens and secrete a variety of cytokines and polypeptide hormones (the thymic peptides or thymic hormones).

The thymic hormones represent a large heterogeneous group of polypeptides which includes the thymosins (e.g. thymosin $\alpha 1$, Tα1), thymulin, thymopoietin, MB-35 and a number of less well characterised peptides (see Table 17.1). The role of these peptides is poorly defined but several lines of evidence suggest that together with cytokines they exert significant actions within the thymus and in the periphery which influence T lymphocyte differentiation and, hence, immune function (1).

Increasing evidence suggests that hormones derived from the anterior pituitary gland and peripheral endocrine organs are critically important to the regulation of thymic function and, hence, the control of the T cell repertoire. In particular, these hormones play a key role in the regulation of the synthesis and release of the thymic peptides; in addition, hormones such as the corticosteroids also influence other important aspects of thymic function. Data accumulated largely in the last decade also advocate the existence of an intricate feedback mechanism

Table 17.1 Thymic hormone preparations. Relative molecular weights are shown in parentheses. NB several other peptides have been partially purified including thymosin $\alpha 5$ (mol wt ~ 2200 Da), thymosin $\alpha 11$ (as thymosin $\alpha 1$, plus an additional seven amino acids at the C-terminus), thymopoietin 1 (differs from thymopoietin II by two amino acids)

Preparation	Chemistry	Sequenced
Thymosin fraction 5	Partially purified extract of calf thymus; 30–40 peptides	–
Thymosin $\alpha 1$	28 amino acids (3108)	+
Thymosin $\beta 4$	43 amino acids (4982)	+
Thymulin	9 amino acids (847)	+
Thymopoietin II	49 amino acids (5562)	+
MB-35	35 amino acids (3756)	+
Thymus fraction	(28 000)	–
Thymus polypeptide hypocholesterol-aemic factor (TphF)	(17 000)	–

which enables the neuroendocrine system to detect and respond to alterations in thymic function; important candidate mediators are the thymic peptides which provide opportunity for a humoral link between the thymus and the neuroendocrine system. This chapter will review the evidence for reciprocal communication between the thymus and the neuroendocrine system with specific reference to the thymic peptides.

17.2 THE INFLUENCE OF THE NEUROENDOCRINE SYSTEM ON THE THYMUS

17.2.1 The Anterior Pituitary Gland and Immunomodulation: Influence of Prolactin and Growth Hormone

Following the pioneering studies of Smith (3), which showed that hypophysectomy causes thymic involution and atrophy in the rat, ample evidence has accumulated which strongly supports a role for the neuroendocrine system in the regulation of the structure and function of the thymus. For example, the mass of the thymus, bone marrow and lymphoid tissues is impaired in two strains of hypopituitary mice (Snell-Bagg and Ames dwarf) which lack the growth hormone (GH) and prolactin (PRL) secreting pituitary acidophilic cells (4). In the Ames mouse, transplantation of ectopic pituitary tissue under the kidney capsule increases thymic weight and thymic lymphocyte number (5). A similar functional dependency of the thymus and the immune response on the pituitary gland has been reported in hypophysectomised rats and mice (6)—see also

Chapter 16. A role for the neuroendocrine axis in the control of thymic function is also supported by the observations that the age-dependent decline in thymulin secretion occurs prematurely in the dwarf mouse (7) and that injection of hypothalamic extracts into aged mice restores the serum thymulin concentration to levels normally observed only in young animals (8). Collectively, these data support the existence of a hormonally-mediated link between the hypothalamo–pituitary axis and the thymus.

Credence in the above notion has been further enhanced by the demonstration that the pituitary hormones, PRL and GH, can both exert direct actions on the thymus (9). For example, PRL stimulates the release of thymulin from the thymic epithelium *in vivo* or *in vitro* while suppression of PRL secretion *in vivo* by treatment with bromocriptine (an agonist of D_2 dopamine receptors) reduces the circulating levels of thymulin (10). In the same manner, administration of PRL antisera to neonatal mice disrupts the pattern of lymphocyte development in the thymus, implying a role for PRL in thymocyte differentiation. In addition, PRL induces the proliferation of thymic cells *in vitro*. Finally, the expression of several mRNAs in thymic epithelial cells, including cytokeratin and c-*myc* proto-oncogene, have been attributed to the direct effects of PRL on the cells as also has the increase in DNA synthesis (10).

There is also evidence for an important link between GH and the thymus. For example, GH has been shown to exert a thymopoietic effect *in vivo* by influencing the development and differentiation of certain classes of T lymphocytes (11). Moreover, administration of GH increases circulating levels of thymulin in the dog (12). GH also stimulates the release of thymulin from thymic epithelial cells *in vitro* (19), possibly by inducing the local production of insulin-like growth factor-I (13). Clinical studies have indicated that the elevated GH levels evident in acromegalic patients are accompanied by increased levels of thymulin (14). Furthermore, GH therapy prevents the abnormal thymic development and associated wasting syndrome evident in dwarf puppies (14, 15). The roles of PRL and GH as immunomodulators of thymic function have been further substantiated by the elegant demonstration of Kelly *et al.* (16) that implantation of GH_3 cells (pituitary adenoma cells which produce PRL and GH) into ageing rats reverses thymic degeneration and the decline in thymic function. Finally, the impairment of antibody production and the development of delayed-type hypersensitivity induced by hypophysectomy (6, 17) is corrected by daily treatment with either PRL or GH (6).

The phenomenological correlates between inadequate pituitary production of PRL and/or GH and impaired thymic function are well recognised. However, the respective regulatory actions of these hormones at the cellular and molecular levels remain enigmatic. Nevertheless, all events triggered by either PRL or GH are thought to be mediated via specific receptors (see also Chapter 4) which have been biochemically identified for both hormones on thymocytes and thymic epithelial cells (9, 18, 19).

17.2.2   Role of the Hypothalamo–Pituitary–Adrenal Axis

Since the early studies of Selye, which are highlighted in the prologue, it has been recognised that the adrenal gland exerts a profound influence over lymphoid tissue. More specifically, glucocorticoids are mediators of immunosuppression and, potentially, lymphoinvolution (21). Indeed, adrenalectomised animals treated with the glucocorticoid, dexamethasone, exhibit a significant (50%) reduction in the weight of the thymus and an 80% reduction in thymocyte number (22). These morphological changes and the associated disruption in thymic function may be directly related to the ability of glucocorticoids to evoke apoptosis in thymocytes (23, 24). This process is a form of "physiological" cell death which permits selective cell deletion involving the activation of an endogenous endonuclease (25, 26). The mechanism underlying glucocorticoid-induced apoptosis in thymocytes is complex and still remains to be elucidated. However, it is recognised that it occurs predominantly in $CD4^+/CD8^+$ cells and that it requires new mRNA and protein synthesis (23). For detailed descriptions of thymocyte apoptosis the reader is referred to a number of excellent reviews (23, 24).

Interestingly, while glucocorticoids clearly evoke apoptotic death in thymocytes, increasing evidence suggests that acute activation of the hypothalamo–pituitary–adrenocortical (HPA) axis may enhance other aspects of thymic function, in particular the secretion of the thymic hormones—reviewed in (27). For example, in both the rat and man, thymulin exhibits a circadian periodicity which closely parallels the rhythmic activity of the HPA axis. Moreover, thymulin, like ACTH and the glucocorticoids, is released in conditions of acute stress. *In vivo* and *in vitro* studies suggest that the main driving factor is of pituitary origin. Thus, chronic adrenalectomy, which effectively elevates the plasma concentration of adrenocorticotrophic hormone (ACTH), and other peptides derived from the ACTH precursor, pro-opiomelanocortin (POMC)—see also Chapter 1—precipitates a pronounced increase in thymulin release which is readily reversed by treatment with dexamethasone (28). Furthermore, both ACTH and β-endorphin (which is co-released with ACTH) elicit concentration-dependent increases in the release of thymulin from thymic tissue *in vitro*. Although these results would favour an action of the POMC-derived peptides, other data suggest that glucocorticoids themselves may also exert direct effects on the thymic epithelial cells. For example, injection of hydrocortisone into young adult mice causes proliferation of a subset $(KL1^+)$ of thymic epithelial cells (29). Moreover, treatment of thymic epithelial cells *in vitro* with adrenal steroids promotes the secretion of thymulin (10) and increases cytokeratin expression (16). It is also interesting to note that the thymulin releasing activity of dexamethasone *in vitro* is potentiated markedly by ACTH although the underlying mechanism is obscure (28).

The stimulatory influence of the hormones of the HPA axis on the thymic epithelium appear to be in direct opposition to the well documented inhibitory actions of endogenous and exogenous glucocorticoids on thymocyte and systemic immune function (21)—see also Chapters 1, 8, 12 and 13. The physiological importance of these paradoxical actions is unknown but clearly they must be considered in the context of the much more complex scenario manifest *in vivo* which encompasses the numerous factors (e.g. cytokines, neurotransmitters and neuropeptides) now implicated in the regulation of thymic function and immunoactivity.

17.2.3   Influence of the Thyroid Gland

Several lines of evidence suggest that thymulin secretion is sensitive to alterations in thyroid status. For example, the hypothyroidism which follows surgical thyroidectomy is associated with a consistent reduction in serum thymulin concentrations. By contrast, serum thymulin is elevated in hyperthyroidism due to diffuse goitre, particularly in elderly subjects in whom the resting secretion of thymulin is characteristically low. Similar conclusions have been drawn from *in vitro* studies which have demonstrated the ability of thyroid hormones, in particular tri-iodothyronine, to stimulate the synthesis and release of thymulin and to induce epithelial cell proliferation—reviewed in (27).

17.2.4   Influence of the Hypothalamo–Pituitary–Gonadal Axis

The hypothalamo–pituitary–gonadal (HPG) axis exerts profound effects on immune function which include modulation of the secretion of the thymic peptides—for review see (29). For example, ovariectomy produces a transient fall in serum thymulin levels together with an increase in the intracellular content of the peptide (10). Furthermore, exogenous oestrogen stimulates thymulin release, probably via an action on the oestrogen receptors located in the thymic epithelial cells (30). While a detailed discussion of this aspect of thymic physiology is beyond the scope of this chapter, it is worth noting that the alterations in gonadal function induced by stress (see Chapter 1) may be expected to contribute to associated changes in immune function.

17.2.5   Presence of Neuroendocrine Hormones in the Thymus

The already complex regulation of the thymus by the neuroendocrine axes is further complicated by the presence of "classical" neuroendocrine peptides in thymic cells themselves. Immunohistochemical studies have identified follicle stimulating hormone (FSH), luteinising hormone (LH), POMC-derived peptides (ACTH and β-endorphin), GH, PRL, somatostatin, gonadotrophin releasing hormone (GnRH), corticotrophin releasing hormone (CRH) and metenkephalin in human or rat thymus (31). In addition, neurohypophysial-like peptides including arginine vasopressin, oxytocin and the neurophysins have also been identified in the thymic epithelium, medulla and subcapsular cortex. In many cases the immunological properties of these polypeptides have been shown to be essentially identical to those produced within the hypothalamo–pituitary axis. In fact, recent studies showed that the cDNA cloning and expression of PRL from normal human thymocytes produced a protein identical to the 23 kDa form of the pituitary hormone (32).

The physiological role of the neuroendocrine peptides produced within the thymus is uncertain. It is unlikely that the peptides are involved in the manifestation of systemic effects but, since receptors for at least some of them (e.g. ACTH, oxytocin, opioid peptides, GnRH) are expressed within the thymus, it is possible that they fulfil significant roles in the local control of thymic function through autocrine or paracrine mechanisms (33). In accord with this premise, Geenen *et al.* (33) have proposed that the thymus-derived neuroendocrine peptides contribute to the development of a specialised microenvironment in which cell-to-cell interactions (cryptocrine communication) allow for induction of immune tolerance to the peptides of the hypothalamo–neurohypophysial system.

17.3 THE INFLUENCE OF THE THYMUS ON THE NEUROENDOCRINE SYSTEM

17.3.1 Studies in Congenitally Athymic Mice and Surgically Thymectomised Animals

The first evidence of a role for the thymus in the regulation of hypothalamo–pituitary function emerged from the work by Pierpaoli and co-workers (34, 35) who used the classical approach of endocrine ablation. Their data showed that in male and female mice, removal of the thymus within 12 hours of birth results over the next month in a marked, age-dependent degranulation of the acidophilic cells in the anterior pituitary gland (i.e. the PRL and GH secreting cells). Similarly, in congenitally athymic nude mice the size and number of granules in pituitary acidophilic cells are both substantially reduced (35). Subsequent studies showed that athymic nude mice also exhibit reduced plasma PRL concentrations which are "normalised" by implantation at birth of thymic tissue obtained from new-born normal littermates (36). Several other endocrinopathies have been observed in thymus deficient animals. For example, the pituitary concentrations of LH and FSH are reduced in athymic nude mice but raised to control levels by neonatal transplantation of thymus tissue (37). Congenitally athymic mice also exhibit low plasma concentrations of LH and FSH while neonatally thymectomised mice show impairments in the secretion of GH as well as the gonadotrophins (29, 38). In primates, prepubertal thymectomy is associated with decreases in plasma ACTH and cortisol (39) while fetal thymectomy performed *in utero* results in a reduction in plasma PRL and concomitant rise in FSH in the rhesus monkey at birth (40).

Taken together, these studies provide circumstantial evidence for the existence of thymic hormonal factors which regulate neuroendocrine function. The chemical identification of these factors and the elucidation of their roles in the regulation of the hypothalamo–pituitary axis have since provided an important focus for research.

17.3.2   Modulation of Neuroendocrine Function by Thymic Peptides *In Vivo* and *In Vitro*

As indicated in Section 17.1, few thymic peptides have been fully characterised and made available in a pure form for pharmacological study. Accordingly, much of the work concerning the influence of these peptides on neuroendocrine function has been performed using a protein extract of the thymus, termed thymosin fraction 5 (TF5). This material is derived from the bovine thymus and contains at least 40–60 heat stable polypeptides including thymosins $\alpha 1$ (T$\alpha 1$) and $\beta 4$ (T$\beta 4$). TF5 has numerous biological activities including induction of T lymphocyte markers, enhanced lymphocyte responses to mitogen, increased antibody production and mixed lymphocyte reactivity (41) and increased production of interleukin 6 (IL-6) by mitogen stimulated splenocytes (42); it thus enhances both T lymphocyte differentiation and cytokine production.

With respect to the neuroendocrine system, TF5 has been shown to increase the secretion of ACTH and corticosterone or cortisol when given peripherally to rats, mice (43) or prepubertal monkeys (39) and to reduce thyrotrophin secretion in young but not aged rats of either sex (44, 45). Others have reported that TF5 stimulates the release of GnRH from perifused medial basal hypothalami derived from female rats as also does one of its component peptides, T$\beta 4$ (46). Similarly, injection of synthetic T$\beta 4$ into the lateral cerebroventricle of mice (where it would be expected to gain ready access to the GnRH cell bodies) increases the serum concentrations of LH but not corticosterone (47). On the other hand, T$\alpha 1$ produces prompt reductions in the plasma concentrations of thyrotrophin (TSH), PRL and ACTH, but not GH, within 1 hour of injection into the third ventricle (48). These actions appear to be mediated in part at the hypothalamic level for, at nanomolar concentrations, T$\alpha 1$ inhibits the release of thyrotrophin releasing hormone (TRH), CRH and somatostatin from rat medial basal hypothalami *in vitro* (49).

Several groups have exploited *in vitro* methods to investigate the possibility that TF5 and its component peptides exert direct actions at the anterior pituitary level. In a preliminary report, Spangelo *et al.* (50) showed that TF5 (but not Tα1 or Tβ4) stimulates PRL release from GH$_3$ cells. In a further study TF5 was shown to elicit the release of PRL and GH but not LH from cultured rat anterior pituitary cells (51). TF5 also stimulates the release of β-endorphin/ACTH in three different pituitary preparations by actions which are Ca^{2+}-dependent, glucocorticoid reversible and, like those of vasopressin, potentiated by CRH (27, 52, 53). The molecular mechanisms underlying the effects of TF5 on pituitary hormone release are poorly understood; they appear to be independent of changes in intracellular cyclic adenosine monophosphate (cAMP) or inositol polyphosphate concentrations but may be linked to a rapid mobilisation of arachidonic acid (51). Studies with purified Tα1 on pituitary hormone release have generated conflicting data. This peptide has no discernible effects on pituitary hormone release from cultured pituitary cells *in vitro*. However, according to Milenkovic and McCann it increases the release of TSH, ACTH and especially LH from hemipituitary tissue *in vitro* without affecting the secretion of PRL, GH or FSH (48). By contrast, others have observed that Tα1 inhibits the neurochemically evoked release of ACTH from rat pituitary quarters *in vitro* (54). The reasons for these discrepant results are not known but they may relate to the preparations used and in particular to the diverse paracrine communications inherent to tissue pieces.

In view of its heterogeneous nature, it seems unlikely that Tα1 and Tβ4 are the sole factors effecting modulation of pituitary hormone release by TF5 and, accordingly, several recent studies have focused on the isolation of further neuroendocrine regulating principles in this thymic preparation. These studies have led to the identification of a highly basic (pI 9.3) peptide which comprises 35 amino acids and is termed MB-35 (55). The natural and synthetic forms of MB-35 readily elicit the secretion of PRL and GH by rat anterior pituitary cells *in vitro* and both are more potent than the parent preparation (i.e. TF5) in this regard (55). Considerable attention has focused on the observation that the amino acid sequence of MB-35 is identical to a section of histone H2A (residues 86–120), a component of nuclear protein A24 (55). Although production of MB-35 from histone H2A has not yet been demonstrated, this observation raises the novel possibility that proteolysis of histone nucleoproteins during cell activation may produce peptides (e.g. MB-35) which migrate to the cytoplasm where they may exert local (intracrine) actions or be secreted and thereby exert biological actions via autocrine, paracrine or systemic (endocrine) mechanisms. In this event, MB-35 may act locally to modulate thymocyte differentiation as well as exerting actions on distant target cells such as the pituitary gland.

Several other thymic peptides have also been shown to influence neuroendo-crine function. For example, thymulin, thymopoietin and thymopentin (the active moiety of thymopoietin) have each been shown to stimulate the secretion of

ACTH and β-endorphin from pituitary tissue *in vitro*. These effects appear to be specific to the POMC derived peptides and, thus, they are not associated with concomitant hypersecretions of PRL, LH, FSH, GH or TSH (56). The actions of thymulin appear to be dependent on the generation of cAMP; they are thus accompanied by significant increases in the tissue cAMP content and are potentiated markedly by drugs which inhibit the degradation of this cyclic nucleotide (54). Another thymic factor implicated in the regulation of the hypothalamo–pituitary axis is the so called thymic neuroendocrine releasing factor (TNRF) which is derived from rat thymic reticular monolayers which stain positively for keratin filaments, a marker for epithelial cells (57). TNRF, which has a relative molecular weight of 10–20 kDa and is probably unrelated to the thymosin peptides, stimulates the release of PRL, GH and LH *in vitro* in a time- and concentration-dependent manner. Finally, two further thymic peptides have been shown to modulate pituitary hormone secretion, namely thymus polypeptide hypocholesterolaemic factor (TphF), a 17 kDa calf thymus protein which increases the catabolism of low density lipoproteins, and thymus fraction (TF), a 28 kDa protein isolated by acetone extraction of thymic tissue from male rats. These peptides are particularly interesting as they appear not to evoke hormone release directly but to "prime" the pituitary tissue for subsequent stimulation. Thus, pre-incubation of pituitary tissue with TphF augments the subsequent PRL response to neurochemical stimulation while TF potentiates GnRH-induced LH and FSH secretion without affecting the basal release of either peptide (58, 59).

17.4 CONCLUSIONS AND OVERVIEW

In addition to being the primary lymphoid organ effecting cell-mediated immunity, the thymus is an endocrine organ that is responsible for the secretion of a heterogeneous family of polypeptide hormones. Evidence from a number of studies suggests that these peptides not only exert significant effects within the immune system but that they also provide an interface between the immune and the neuroendocrine system; for schematic diagram see Fig. 17.1. Importantly, their synthesis and release is controlled at least in part by hormones from the pituitary gland and peripheral endocrine organs. Moreover, several of the thymic peptides themselves have been shown to modulate neuroendocrine function in experimental models *in vivo* and *in vitro*. Their actions in this regard are highly complex. Some (e.g. TF5, TNRF) stimulate the release of several anterior pituitary hormones whereas others appear to exert more selective actions either at the level of the anterior pituitary gland (e.g. TphF, thymulin, thymopoietin) or the hypothalamus (e.g. Tα1 and Tβ4). Although most of the thymic factors examined to date appear to initiate robust prosecretory actions on hypothalamic and pituitary hormone release, some (e.g. TF, TphF) appear to induce hormone

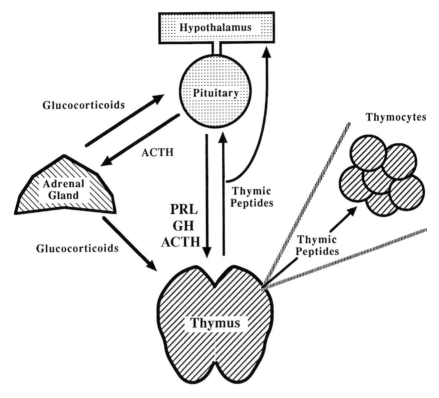

Figure 17.1 Schematic presentation of the proposed relationship between the endocrine thymus and the neuroendocrine system. Thymic peptides include, but are not restricted to, thymosin, thymulin, and thymopoietin. PRL, prolactin; GH, growth hormone; ACTH, adrenocorticotrophin

release only after a priming period while others (e.g. Tα1) may exert inhibitory actions (54). In principle, the battery of thymic peptides capable of modulating neuroendocrine function provides opportunity for a complex control mechanism, with the overall response depending on the complement of thymic peptides released as well as on the status of the other homeostatic mechanisms which serve to regulate neuroendocrine function.

It is important to note that the regulatory influence of the thymus on anterior pituitary function is most pronounced in the neonatal period, coincident with the phase of intense T lymphocyte differentiation. The significance of this is unclear although it should be noted that many of the pre-programmed changes in hormone secretion which occur in adult life are determined by subtle events in the perinatal phase. It is also poignant that activation of the HPA axis during inflammation, endotoxaemia or stress may lead to enhanced secretion of thymic hormones which not only target the immune system but may also exert significant effects on neuroendocrine tissues. Similar arguments apply to PRL which is also released in conditions of stress (see Chapter 1).

A substantial body of evidence supports the view that the anterior pituitary gland and peripheral endocrine organs fulfil a significant role in the regulation of thymic function. However, although the data cited above point to a reciprocal role for the thymic peptides in the control of the neuroendocrine system, firm evidence for a such a mechanism is lacking. Much of the evidence available at present is based on data from *in vitro* studies and cannot necessarily be translated to the situation *in vivo*. Recent work indicates that at least some of the thymic peptides are present in neuroendocrine cells; for example, the precursor of $T\alpha1$, prothymosin-α, is expressed in GH1 pituitary tumour cells, $T\beta4$ has been identified in the hypothalamus and immunoreactive thymulin is present in protein extracts of both the pituitary gland and the hypothalamus (27, 60). It is thus possible that the responses observed *in vitro* reflect those normally effected *in vivo* by locally produced "thymic peptides" rather than by peptides derived from the thymus. The hypothesis that the thymic polypeptides exert feedback actions within a hypothalamic–pituitary–thymic axis thus requires further investigation (61). Alterations in hormone secretion following thymectomy or thymic polypeptide administration (e.g. TF5) have been shown only for TSH and the glucocorticoid stress axis and, in most instances, the active thymic hormones effecting these responses have not yet been identified. Similarly, while the morphological changes in the anterior pituitary acidophilic cells noted in athymic mice have been reversed by implantation of thymic tissue, the effects of thymic peptide administration have not been studied. Interestingly, a recent study has provided novel evidence that mice thymectomised at four weeks exhibit significant impairments in learning and memory. These data support a role for thymic hormones in the regulation of central nervous system function and suggest that their realm may stretch beyond the neuroendocrine system to the modulation of learned behaviours (62). Future studies are urgently needed not only to elucidate the direct or indirect feedback loops of the various thymic polypeptides on neuroendocrine function but also to investigate the potential role of these peptides in the regulation of other aspects of brain function. With the advent of further characterisation of and the development of good assays for the thymic polypeptides, it will be of fundamental importance to determine to what extent their actions are local or systemic and how they respond to immunological challenge and manipulations of the neuroendocrine axes.

ACKNOWLEDGEMENTS

This work was supported by NIH grants DK-42059, to B. L. Spangelo, and HD-25262, to W. C. Gorospe.

REFERENCES

1. Kendall M. D. Functional anatomy of the thymic microenvironment. *J Anat*, 1991, **177**: 1–29.
2. Boyd R. L., Tucek C. L., Godfrey D. I., Izon D. J., Wilson T. J., Davidson N. J., *et al.* The thymic microenvironment. *Immunol Today*, 1993, **14**: 445–59.
3. Smith P. E. Effect of hypophysectomy on the involution of the thymus in the rat. *Anat Rec*, 1930, **47**: 119–29.
4. Bartke A. Histology of the anterior hypophysis, thyroid and gonads of two types of dwarf mice. *Anat Rec*, 1964, **149**: 225–36.
5. Esquifino A. I., Villanua M. A., Szary A., Yau J., Bartke A. Ectopic pituitary transplants restore immunocompetence in Ames dwarf mice. *Acta Endocrinol*, 1991, **125**: 67–72.
6. Nagy E., Berczi I., Friesen H. G. Regulation of immunity in rats by lactogenic and growth hormones. *Acta Endocrinol (Copenh)*, 1983, **102**: 351–7.
7. Pelletier M., Montplaisir S., Dardenne M., Bach J. F. Thymic hormone activity and spontaneous autoimmunity in dwarf mice and their littermates. *Immunology*, 1976, **30**: 783–8.
8. Folch H., Eller G., Mena M., Esquivel P. Neuroendocrine regulation of thymus hormones: hypothalamic dependence of "facteur thymique serique" level. *Cell Immunol*, 1986, **102**: 211–7.
9. Gala R. R. PRL and GH in the regulation of the immune system. *Proc Soc Exp Biol Med*, 1991, **198**: 513–27.
10. Dardenne M., Savino W. Neuroendocrine control of the thymic epithelium: modulation of thymic function, cytokeratin expression and cell proliferation by hormones and neuropeptides. *Prog Neuro Endocrin Immunol (PNEI)*, 1990, **3**: 18–25.
11. Murphy W. J., Durum S. K., Longo D. L. Role of neuroendocrine hormones in murine T cell development: growth hormone exerts thymopoietic effects *in vivo*. *J Immunol*, 1992, **149**: 3851–7.
12. Goff B. L., Roth J. A., Arp L. H., Incefy G. S. Growth hormone treatment stimulates thymulin production in aged dogs. *Clin Exp Immunol*, 1987, **68**: 580–7.
13. Timsit J., Savino W., Safieh B., Chanson P., Gagnerault C., Bach J.-F., *et al.* Growth hormone and insulin-like growth factor-I stimulate hormonal function and proliferation of thymic epithelial cells. *J Clin Endocrinol*, 1992, **75**: 183–8.
14. Mocchegiani E., Paolucci P., Balsamo A., Cacciari E., Fabris N. Influence of growth hormone on thymic endocrine activity in humans. *Horm Res*, 1990, **33**: 248–55.
15. Roth J. A., Kaeberle M. L., Grier R. L., Hopper S. G., Spiegel H. E., McAllister H. A. Improvement in clinical condition and thymus morphological features associated with growth hormone treatment in immunodeficient dwarf dogs. *Am J Vet Res*, 1984, **45**: 1151–4.
16. Kelley K. W., Brief S., Westly H. J., Novakofski J., Bechtel P. J., Simon J., *et al.* GH3 pituitary adenoma cells can reverse thymic aging in rats. *Immunology* 1986, **83**: 5663–7.
17. Berczi I., Nagy E., Asa S. L., Kovacs K. Pituitary hormones and contact sensitivity in rats. *Allergy*, 1983, **38**: 325–30.
18. Dardenne M., Kelly P. A., Bach J.-F., Savino W. Identification and functional activity of PRL receptors in thymic epithelial cells. *Proc Natl Acad Sci USA*, 1991, **88**: 9700–4.
19. Ban E., Gagnerault M.-C., Jammes H., Postel-Vinay M.-C., Haour F., Dardenne M. Specific binding sites for growth hormone in cultured mouse thymic epithelial cells. *Life Sci*, 1991, **48**: 2141–8.

20. Selye H. Thymus and adrenals in the response of the organisms to injuries and intoxications. *Br J Exp Pathol*, 1936, **17**: 234–8.
21. Munck A., Guyre P. A., Holbrook N. Physiological functions of glucocorticoids in stress and their relation to pharmacological actions. *Endocr Rev*, 1984, **5**: 25–44.
22. Compton M. M., Cidlowski J. A. Identification of a glucocorticoid-induced nuclease in thymocytes: a potential "lysis gene" product. *J Biol Chem*, 1987, **262**: 8288–97.
23. Schwartzman R. A., Cidlowski J. A. Apoptosis: the biochemistry and molecular biology of programmed cell death. *Endocr Rev*, 1993, **14**: 133–51.
24. Cohen J. J. Programmed cell death in the immune system. *Adv Immunol*, 1991, **50**: 55–85.
25. Waring P., Kos F. J., Mullbacher A. Apoptosis or programmed cell death. *Med Res Rev*, 1991, **11**: 219–36.
26. Wyllie A. H. Glucocorticoid-induced thymocyte apoptosis is associated with endogenous endonuclease activation. *Nature*, 1980, **284**: 555–6.
27. Millington G., Buckingham J. C. Thymic peptides and neuroendocrine-immune communication. *J Endocrinol*, 1992, **133**: 163–8.
28. Buckingham J. C., Safieh B., Singh S., Arduino L., Cover P. O., Kendall M. Interactions between the hypothalamo–pituitary adrenal axis and the thymus in the rat: A role for corticotrophin in the control of thymulin release. *J Neuroendocrinology*, 1992, **4**: 295–301.
29. Savino W., Cirne-Lima E. O., Teixeira-Soares J. F., Leitede-Moraes M. C., Ono I. P. C., Dardenne M. Hydrocortisone increases the number of KL1+ cells, a thymic epithelial cell subset characterized by high molecular weight cytokeratin expression. *Endocrinology*, 1988, **123**: 2557–64.
30. Chapman C., Despande R., Michael S. Estrogen-mediated interactions between the immune and female reproductive systems. In J. A. Marsh, M. D. Kendall (eds) *The Physiology of Immunity*. New York, CRC Press, 1996: pp 239–61.
31. Batanero E., DeLeeuw F.-E., Jansen G. H., van Wichen D. F., Huber J., Schuurman H.-J. The neural and neuro-endocrine component of the human thymus: II hormone immunoreactivity. *Brain Behav Immun*, 1992, **6**: 249–64.
32. O'Neal K. D., Montgomery D. W., Truong T. M., Yu-Lee L. Prolactin gene expression in human thymocytes. *Mol Cell Endocrinol*, 1992, **87**: 19–23.
33. Geenen V., Martens H., Robert F., Legros J.-J., Defresne M.-P., Bonvier J., *et al.* Thymic cryptocrine signaling and the immune recognition of self neuroendocrine functions. *Prog NeuroEndocrinImmunol (PNEI)*, 1991,**4**: 135–42.
34. Bianchi E., Pierpaoli W., Sorkin E. Cytological changes in the mouse anterior pituitary after neonatal thymectomy: a light and electron microscopical study. *J Endocrinol*, 1971, **51**: 1–6.
35. Ruitenberg E. J., Berkvens J. M. The morphology of the endocrine system in congenitally athymic (nude) mice. *J Path*, 1977, **121**: 225–31.
36. Pierpaoli W., Kopp H. G., Bianchi E. Interdependence of thymic and neuroendocrine functions in ontogeny. *Clin Exp Immunol*, 1976, **24**: 501–6.
37. Rebar R. W., Morandini I. C., Erickson G. F., Petze J. E. The hormonal basis of reproductive defects in athymic mice: diminished gonadotropin concentrations in prepubertal females. *Endocrinology*, 1981, **108**: 120–6.
38. Michael S. D., Taguchi O., Nishizuka Y. Effect of neonatal thymectomy on ovarian development and plasma LH, FSH, GH and PRL in the mouse. *Biol Reprod*, 1980, **22**: 343–50.
39. Healy D. L., Hodgen G. D., Schulte H. M., Chrousos G. P., Loriaux D. L., Hale N. R., *et al.* The thymus–adrenal connection: thymosin has corticotropin-releasing activity in primates. *Science*, 1983, **222**: 1353–5.

40. Healy D. L., Bacher J., Hodgen G. D. Thymic regulation of primate fetal ovarian adrenal differentiation. *Biol Reprod*, 1985, **32**: 1127–33.
41. Spangelo B. L., Hall N. R., Goldstein A. L. Biology and chemistry of thymosin peptides: modulators of immunity and neuroendocrine circuits. *Ann NY Acad Sci*, 1987, **496**: 196–204.
42. Attia W. Y., Badamchian M., Goldstein A. L., Spangelo B. L. Thymosin stimulates interleukin-6 production from rat spleen cells *in vitro. Immunopharmacol*, 1993, **26**: 171–9.
43. McGillis J. P., Hall N. R., Vahouny G. V., Goldstein A. L. Thymosin fraction 5 causes increased serum corticosterone in rodents *in vivo. J Immunol*, 1985, **134**: 3952–5.
44. Goya R. G., Takahashi S., Quigley K. L., Sosa Y. E., Goldstein A. L., Meites J. Immune-neuroendocrine interactions during aging: age-dependent thyrotropin-inhibiting activity of thymosin peptides. *Mech Ageing Dev*, 1987, **41**: 219–27.
45. Goya R. G., Sosa Y. E., Quigley K. L., Gottschall P. E., Goldstein A. L., Meites J. Differential activity of thymosin peptides (thymosin fraction 5) on plasma thyrotropin in female rats of different ages. *Neuroendocrinology*, 1988, **47**: 379–83.
46. Rebar R. W., Miyake A., Low T. L. K., Goldstein A. L. Thymosin stimulates secretion of luteinizing hormone-releasing factor. *Science*, 1981, **214**: 669–71.
47. Hall N. R., Spangelo B. L., Farah Jr J. M., O'Donohue T. L., Goldstein A. L. Regulation of neuroendocrine pathways by thymosins. In T. W. Moody (ed) *Neural and Endocrine Peptides and Receptors*. New York, Plenum, 1986, pp 683–94.
48. Milenkovic L., McCann S. M. Effects of thymosin α-1 on pituitary hormone release. *Neuroendocrinology*, 1992, **55**: 14–9.
49. Milenkovic L., Lyson K., Aguila M. C., McCann S. M. Effect of thymosin α-1 on hypothalamic hormone release. *Neuroendocrinology*, 1992, **56**: 674–9.
50. Spangelo B. L., Hall N. R., Dunn A. J., Goldstein A. L. Thymosin fraction 5 stimulates the release of PRL from cultured GH3 cells. *Life Sci*, 1987, **40**: 283–8.
51. Spangelo B. L., Judd A. M., Ross P. C., Login I. S., Jarvis W. D., Badamchian M., *et al.* Thymosin fraction 5 stimulates prolactin and growth hormone release from anterior pituitary cells *in vitro. Endocrinology*, 1987, **121**: 2035–43.
52. Farah J. M. Jr., Hall N. R., Bishop J. F., Goldstein A. L., O'Donohue T. L. Thymosin fraction 5 stimulates secretion of immunoreactive β-endorphin in mouse corticotropic tumor cells. *J Neurosci Res*, 1987, **18**: 140–6.
53. McGillis J. P., Hall N. R., Goldstein A. L. Thymosin fraction 5 (TF5) stimulates secretion of adrenocorticotropic hormone (ACTH) from cultured rat pituitaries. *Life Sci*, 1988, **42**: 2259–68.
54. Hadley A. J., Rantle C., Buckingham J. C. Thymic peptides selectively influence the release of pituitary hormones from rat adenohypophysial tissue *in vitro* by cyclic nucleotide dependent mechanisms. *J Endocrinol*, 1994, **143**: P89.
55. Badamachian M., Wang S.-S., Spangelo B. L., Damavandy T., Goldstein A. L. Chemical and biological characterization of MB-35: a thymic-derived peptide that stimulates the release of growth hormone and prolactin from rat anterior pituitary cells. *Prog Neuro Endocrin Immunol (PNEI)*, 1990, **3**: 258–65.
56. Malaise M. G., Hazee-Hagelstein M. T., Reuter A. M., Vrinds-Gevaert Y., Goldstein G., Franchimont P. Thymopoietin and thymopentin enhance the levels of ACTH, β-endorphin and β-lipotropin from rat pituitary cells *in vitro. Acta Endocrinol*, 1987, **115**: 455–60.
57. Spangelo B. L., Ross P. C., Judd A. M., MacLeod R. M. Thymic stromal elements contain an anterior pituitary hormone-stimulating activity. *J Neuroimmunol*, 1989, **25**: 37–46.
58. Santangelo F., Grimaldi M., Landolfi E., Ventra C., Belfiore A., Meucci O., *et al.*

Effect of calf thymus protein on prolactin release and second messenger systems in rat pituitary cells. *Prog Neuro Endocrin Immunol (PNEI)*, 1992, **5**: 172–8.

59. Mendoza M. E., Romano M. C. Prepubertal rat thymus secretes a factor that modulates gonadotropin secretion in cultured rat pituitary cells. *Thymus*, 1989, **14**: 233–42.

60. Alvarez C. V., Zalvide J. B., Cancio E., Dieguez C., Regueiro B. J., Vega F. V., Dominguez F. Regulation of prothymosin alpha mRNA levels in rat pituitary tumor cells. *Neuroendocrinology*, 1993, **57**: 1048–56.

61. Spangelo B. L. The thymic-endocrine connection. *J Endocrinol*, 1995, **147**: 5–10.

62. Zhang Y., Saito H., Nishiyama N. Thymectomy-induced deterioration of learning and memory in mice. *Brain Res*, 1994, **658**: 127–34.

Chapter 18

Behaviour, Stress and Immune Function

Pierre J. Neveu

INSERM, Bordeaux, France

18.1   INTRODUCTION

Concepts in neuroimmunomodulation have emerged from clinical observations of the relationship between emotions, stress and physical illness and have progressed towards experimental research. Since ancient times, people have believed that psychological factors, such as emotional experience, personality and coping strategy can affect susceptibility to disease or its course. "Joyful people always recover from illness," said Rabelais, a 16th century French author. Recent years have seen a resurgence of interest in the influence of psychological factors on immunologically mediated illness, including cancer and autoimmune disorders as well as infectious diseases.

18.2   STRESS AND IMMUNITY

18.2.1   Human Studies

Data from human studies have been extensively reviewed elsewhere (1–3). The majority of psychoimmunology studies have focused on the effects of acute short-term stress on immunity. Increasing evidence suggests that stress resulting from

Stress, Stress Hormones and the Immune System. Edited by J. C. Buckingham, G. E. Gillies and A.-M. Cowell
© 1997 John Wiley & Sons, Ltd.

drastic changes in the life of an individual, such as the death of a spouse or unemployment, may induce a spectrum of unfortunate medical consequences that may be related to dysfunction of the immune system. For example, the stress caused by academic examinations has been shown to depress various immune parameters including the numbers of helper and suppressor or cytotoxic T cells, the lymphocyte response to mitogens, natural killer (NK) cell activity and the cellular immune response to latent herpes virus. Likewise, sleep deprivation, considered as a stressor, diminishes the response of lymphocytes to mitogens and the phagocytic capacity of leukocytes in healthy subjects. Thus far, relatively little research has taken account of the effects of chronic stress on immune function. Some studies have reported alterations of immune reactivity in people living near a nuclear power station which had been the site of a serious accident. These alterations include higher levels of neutrophils and lower levels of B and T lymphocytes and NK cells. In people taking care of relatives afflicted with Alzheimer's disease, the numbers of T lymphocytes as well as the T4:T8 ratio are depressed. Prolonged stress may result in sustained immunosuppression, the consequences of which could conceivably be severe, although a degree of intermittent mild stress may have an immune-enhancing effect. Although the adaptive responses of the hypothalamo–pituitary–adrenal (HPA) axis to repeated or chronic stress have been demonstrated (see Chapter 9), a possible adaptation or compensation by the immune system during chronic stress remains to be fully investigated.

Epidemiological studies in humans are often difficult to interpret because of methodological problems. Indeed, the choice of controls for stressed populations may introduce some bias and the influence of one or several pertinent psychological factors involved in a complex situation of stress on immune functioning is difficult to delineate. Furthermore, in most of the paradigms used, the respective roles of psychological and physiological effects are often confounded. Finally, the functioning of the immune system is usually assessed by tests (such as cellular counts, levels of serum immunoglobulins or mitogen-induced lymphoproliferation) which are easy to perform but are of limited biological significance (see also Chapter 3). These methodological problems are particularly difficult to solve in humans, rendering it necessary to perform experiments on laboratory animals where the variables involved in the stress-immunity relationship may be better controlled.

18.2.2   Animal Studies

Exposure of laboratory animals to a variety of stressful stimuli induces profound changes in cellular and humoral immune functions (4, 5). For example, rodents subjected to electric shock or restraint usually exhibit a depressed T lymphocyte mitogenesis. Likewise, exposure to experimental stress generally decreases host resistance. Thus, mice subjected to experimental stress by physical restraint or crowding are more susceptible to a variety of infectious diseases. In a few cases, however, stress has been demonstrated to protect against infection. For example, excessive social interactions reduced the susceptibility of chickens to *S. aureus* and *E. coli*. Cause and effect relationships between stress and susceptibility to infection may be demonstrated in adequately controlled experiments. However, the nature of the stress, the time at which the infective agent is introduced in relation to the stress applied, housing and social conditions of the animals (which can vary between institutions) as well as the nature of the cellular interactions involved in the immune response to the pathogen are all critical factors affecting the outcome. Moreover, the immune reactivity of animals to stress depends on their sex, genetic background and neuroendocrine status (see also Chapter 9). At the present time, the respective roles of all of these variables, as well as their possible interactions in stress-induced alterations of immune responses, are not known. More interestingly, it has been demonstrated clearly that a stressor should be characterised on the basis of the way the individual experiences it rather than on that of the physical properties of the stressor (see also Chapter 2). The ability to control and predict the occurrence of stressors is a critical factor in the influence of stress on immunity. A single session of inescapable electric shock enhances tumour growth in rats compared with rats given the opportunity to escape the shock. Inescapable but not escapable shock also significantly impairs lymphoproliferative responses to lectins. The effects of antici-pation on cellular immune responses have also been studied with and without prior signalling of inescapable electric shocks. Mitogen-induced proliferation of T lymphocytes is reduced in rats subjected to unsignalled shock but not in rats subjected to signalled shock. Predictability and the ability to control or cope with stressful situations thus appear to be major factors in neuroimmunomodulation.

Most of our knowledge of the immunomodulating effects of stress comes from studies using acute stress. However, the ethological relevance of acute stress is questionable. Chronic stress such as social stress, including for example housing males with females and relocation of an animal to a new grouping, should be extensively studied in neuroimmunomodulation since it appears to be more relevant from a pathophysiological point of view and may represent a better model for human situations. Animal studies relating to chronic stress in the form of experimentally induced chronic inflammatory conditions and the effects of such stresses on the HPA axis and the reciprocal effect of HPA status on the development and progress of such conditions are discussed in Chapter 9.

18.3   BEHAVIOURAL CONDITIONING OF IMMUNE RESPONSES

Behavioural conditioning of immune responsiveness represents another para-digm useful for neuroimmunomodulation studies (6)—see also Chapter 2. In classical experiments adapted from Pavlov's work on the conditioning of physiological responses, rats are given an appetitive drinking solution (usually saccharin) as a conditioned stimulus just before they are injected with an immunosuppressive substance as an unconditioned stimulus. Re-exposure to saccharin alone is followed by depressed immune responses (Fig. 18.1), thus suggesting that immune responses may be conditioned. Such a conditioned immunosuppression was reported to prolong the life of mice which spontane-ously develop an autoimmune disease. However, the link between the aversive effects of a drug and conditioned immunosuppression has not always been found. The physiological mechanism of conditioned alterations in immune function is not yet known. Conditioned changes may involve those neural and endocrine systems which can modulate lymphocyte activity. Conversely, conditioning may alter the release of immune products in the periphery which are able to alter brain functioning. Furthermore, some people have claimed that depression of immune responses is not really due to conditioning but rather it results from the stress induced by the conditioning procedure. Interestingly, antibody production to an antigen, haemocyanin, has been shown to be conditionally enhanced when a repeated immunisation is used as the unconditioned stimulus. Enhanced immune reactivity as measured by NK cell activity can also be conditioned when an immunostimulating substance such as polyinosinic:polycytidylic acid, which induces interferon production, is used as the unconditioned stimulus. In such experiments, the unconditioned stimulus has been supposed to act directly at the brain level where it interferes with the conditioned stimulus.

18.4   GENETIC ASSOCIATION BETWEEN BEHAVIOUR AND IMMUNITY

A study of the links between behaviour and immune reactivity in intact, unstressed animals provides further insight into neuroimmunomodulation. Animals can be genetically selected on the basis of their behavioural and neuro-endocrine response to environmental stimulation (7). In such animals, immune functions may be tested to establish links between stress, behaviour and immunity and also to study the possible role of intermediary mechanisms. For example, domestic chickens have been bred selectively according to their response to a social stress, as measured by plasma levels of corticosterone. Interestingly, this selection, based on divergent neuroendocrine reactivity, is associated with a peculiar pattern of immune reactivity. Chickens were housed in an environment promoting considerable social interaction. The line that had high levels of plasma corticosterone was more resistant to bacterial infections but was more susceptible to viral infections and tumours and produced fewer antibodies in response to an antigen than those selected for low levels of plasma cortico-

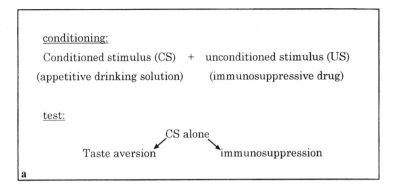

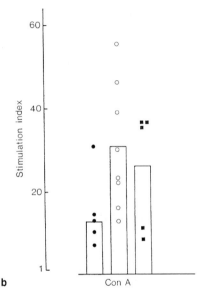

Figure 18.1 Conditioned immunosuppression. **a** Experimental procedure. During the conditioning session, animals were given an attractive drinking solution as a conditioned stimulus (usually saccharin) and injected the same day with an immunosuppressive drug as an unconditioned stimulus. The time interval between conditioned and unconditioned stimuli is critical to good conditioning. During the test session, animals were given the conditioned stimulus alone. This was followed by a taste aversion and immunosuppression. The test session must be performed shortly after the conditioning because of attenuation of the phenomenon with time. **b** Concanavalin A (Con A)-induced *in vitro* proliferation of T lymphocytes (stimulation index) from mice subjected to a conditioning procedure. In a first step, mice were given cyclophosphamide paired with saccharin and in a second step, animals received saccharin alone. Proliferation of T lymphocytes from animals subjected to conditioning ● was depressed when compared to animals which were given saccharin alone ○ or to animals which received cyclophosphamide not paired with saccharin ■. Adapted from P. J. Neveu *et al.*, *Neurosci Lett*, 1986, **65**: 293–8 (13)

sterone. A correlation between HPA axis activity and susceptibility to experimentally-induced inflammatory disease in various strains of rat has also been
reported and is discussed in Chapter 9. Immune reactivity has also been shown
to differ in two lines of rats genetically selected on the basis of their performance
in two-way, active avoidance behaviour. The Roman high avoidance (RHA) rats
quickly acquire the active avoidance response, whereas Roman low avoidance
rats (RLA) fail to acquire this response, mostly showing escape or freezing
behaviour upon shock presentation. A clear-cut dissociation of the two lines is
achieved within a few generations (8). NK cell activity and mitogen-induced
proliferation of T lymphocytes were both lower in the high avoidance line (Fig.
18.2). Prolactin, which appears to be an important variable for differentiating the
Roman lines, may play a role in the differences observed between these two lines
of rats regarding their immune reactivity. (Further discussion of the roles played
by prolactin in the regulation of immune function will be found in Chapter 16.)
The study of genetic factors involved in individual characteristics of reactivity
may help to elucidate the biological mechanisms which couple behaviour and
immune reactivity. However, these experiments have not yet established a direct
association between behaviour and immunity and it should be appreciated that
differences in immune reactivity may be related to genetic factors which are co-
selected and not necessarily involved in behaviour.

18.5   EPIGENETIC ASSOCIATION BETWEEN BEHAVIOUR AND IMMUNITY

Immune reactivity may be related to a particular brain organisation which is not
directly associated with genetic but rather with epigenetic factors. Within an
animal population differences in brain organisation, as defined behaviourally,
may be experimentally induced or directly observed (9). Post-natal stress applied
during a critical stage of brain development induces permanent changes in brain
organisation as demonstrated by a depression of emotional reactivity and an
alteration of the mesolimbic dopaminergic response to stress in adult life (see
also Chapter 2). In the adult animal stressed during the post-natal period,
responsiveness of the HPA axis to stress was reduced while NK cell activity and
mitogen-induced proliferation of T lymphocytes were enhanced.

Likewise, spontaneous behavioural and functional lateralisation, supposed to
reflect asymmetrical brain organisation, has been associated with a particular
pattern of immune reactivity in humans and in mice. For example, humans may
be classified as left- or right-handed according to their hand preference in usual
tasks and an association has been described between left-handedness and the
incidence of immune disorders including allergy and autoimmune diseases.

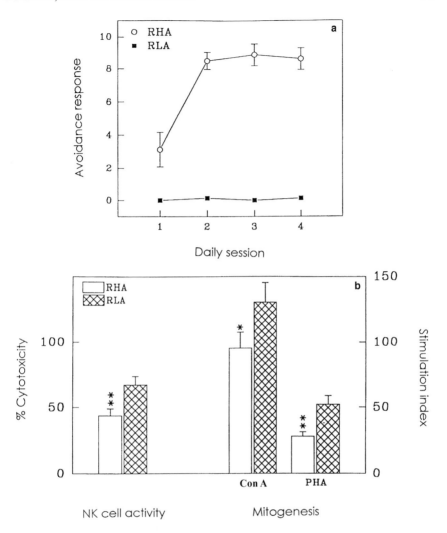

Figure 18.2 **a** Avoidance responses of Roman high avoidance (RHA) and Roman low avoidance (RLA) rats monitored over a four day period and **b** natural killer (NK) cell activity (% cytotoxicity) and proliferation of T lymphocytes (stimulation index) induced by concanavalin A (Con A) or phytohaemagglutinin (PHA) in the spleen from RHA and RLA rats. * p < 0.05; ** p < 0.01. Adapted from Sandi *et al.*, *J. Neuroimmunol*, 1991, **31**: 27–33) (14)

However, these observations remain controversial. The discrepancies in different human studies probably result from differences between patient populations. Furthermore, in these studies only the clinical signs of immune disorders were taken into account while the immune status of patients was not established.

These contradictions are difficult to resolve because of both theoretical and methodological problems and certainly require further research.

To overcome difficulties in demonstrating an association between an asymmetrical brain and immune responses in humans, an experimental approach in laboratory animals has been set up (10). Mice can be selected for right- or left-pawedness by measuring paw preference in a food reaching task. Paw preference is stable with time and each animal can be characterised by a paw preference score. In females, left-pawed mice exhibit higher mitogen-induced T lymphocyte proliferation but showed the same level of NK cell activity as right-pawed animals. In contrast, no association between paw preference and T cell mitogenesis was found in males but left-pawed male mice showed lower NK cell activity in comparison to right-pawed animals. Thus, mitogenesis and NK cell activity have been shown to be directly or inversely correlated with paw preference scores in females and males respectively. In both sexes, B lymphocyte mitogenesis was not related to paw preference (Fig. 18.3). These results indicate that the association between functional brain asymmetry and the modulation of the immune system is not an "all or nothing" phenomenon but appears to involve particular components of the immune system and varies according to the sex, as well as the strain, of animals tested. Indeed, differences in immune functions between left- and right-pawed mice, when present, were shown to vary in direction, according to the strains studied, or in intensity, according to the sub-strains tested, the association being stronger in CH3/He mice than in C3H/OuJ Ico. The association between paw preference and immune responsiveness has been extended to autoimmunity in a murine systemic lupus erythematosus model. New Zealand Black mice are known to develop spontaneously autoimmune diseases such as lupus-like glomerulonephritis and haemolytic anaemia, related to anti-DNA and anti-erythrocyte antibodies respectively. In left-pawed females, both anti-DNA and anti-erythrocyte antibodies appeared earlier than in right-pawed mice. Interestingly, only IgG but not IgM production against DNA was associated with paw preference. This suggests that paw preference may be related to lupus pathogenesis because pathogenic anti-DNA antibodies belong to the IgG isotype. No association between paw preference and autoimmunity was observed in males.

The mechanisms involved in the association between functional brain asymmetry and immune reactivity are not yet known. However, it has been shown recently that the regional expression of monoamines in various brain structures differs in left- and right-pawed animals, as does the activity of the HPA axis in response to an immune challenge by lipopolysaccharide, which is supposed to be a stress inducer (11). Inter-individual differences in immune reactivity associated with brain asymmetry result in a polymorphic response to various insults involving the immune system by which a species may thus survive more readily (12). Animal studies on the asymmetrical brain modulation of immune reactivity show that individual differences may be introduced in the relationship between

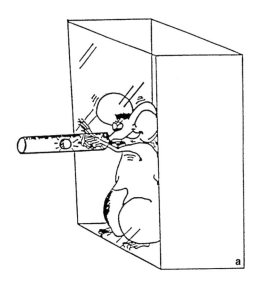

Strain	Mitogen-induced proliferation of T-lymphocytes	Natural killer cell activity	T Lymphocyte subsets (T4,T8)	Auto antibody production
C3H/He				
Females	L > R	L = R	L = R	
Males	L = R	L < R	n.d.	
C3H/Ou JIco				
Females	L > R	L = R	L = R	
Males	L = R	L < R	L = R	
NZB				
Females	n.d.	n.d.	n.d.	L > R
Males	n.d.	n.d.	n.d.	L = R

b

Figure 18.3 a Experimental design for paw preference in mice. Mice are deprived of food for 12–24 hr and then placed in a testing cubicle with a central feeding tube containing a pellet of food. The sequence in which the right or left paws are used to reach food is scored. In a testing session, 50 paw reaches are observed for each mouse. Individual mice are classified as right-pawed when the number of right paw entries (RPE) is greater than 30 and left-pawed when RPE is less than 20. **b** Differences in immune reactivity between left (L)- and right (R)-pawed mice from different strains of experimental animals; n.d., not determined

behaviour and immune responsiveness and may give new insights into neuro-immunomodulation.

18.6   CONCLUSION

The experimental models currently used in neuroimmunomodulation studies demonstrate the immunomodulatory functions of brain and behaviour using a correlative approach. These models may be improved by the choice of pertinent behavioural and immunological parameters in order to delineate the respective roles of the various mediators (hormones, neurotransmitters, neuropeptides, immunopeptides) known to be involved in brain–neuroendocrine–immune inter-actions.

REFERENCES

1. Evans D. L., Leserman J., Pedersen C. A., Golden R. N., Lewis M. H., Folds J. A., Ozer H. Immune correlates of stress and depression. *Psychopharmacol Bull*, 1989, **25**: 319–24.
2. O'Leary A. Stress, emotion, and human immune function. *Psychol Bull*, 1990, **108**: 363–82.
3. Walker L. G., Eremin O. Psychoneuroimmunology: A new fad of the fifth cancer treatment modality? *Am J Surg*, 1995, **170**: 2–4.
4. Borysenko M., Borysenko J. Stress, behavior, and immunity: Animal models and mediating mechanisms. *Gen Hosp Psychiat*, 1982, **4**: 59–67.
5. Dantzer R., Kelley K. W. Stress and immunity: An integrated view of relationships between the brain and the immune system. *Life Sci*, 1989, **44**: 1995–2008.
6. Ader R., Cohen N. CNS-immune system interactions: Conditioning phenomena. *Behav Brain Sci*, 1985, **8**: 379–94.
7. Castanon N., Mormède P. Psychobiogenetics: Adapted tools for the study of the coupling between behavioral and neuroendocrine traits of emotional reactivity. *Psychoneuroimmunology*, 1994, **19**: 257–82.
8. Castanon N., Perez-Diaz F., Mormède P. Genetic analysis of the relationships between behavioral and neuroendocrine traits in Roman high and low avoidance rat lines. *Behav Genet*, 1995, **25**: 371–84.
9. Neveu P. J., Delrue C., Deleplanque B., D'Amato F. R., Puglisi-Allegra S., Cabib S. The influence of brain and behavioral lateralization in brain monoaminergic, neuroendocrine, and immune stress responses. *Ann NY Acad Sci*, 1994, **741**: 271–82.
10. Neveu P. J. Asymmetrical brain modulation of the immune response. *Brain Res Rev*, 1992, **17**: 101–7.
11. Delrue C., Deleplanque B., Rouge-Pont F., Vitiello S., Neveu P. J. Brain monoaminergic, neuroendocrine, and immune responses to an immune challenge in relation to brain and behavioral lateralization. *Brain Behav Immun*, 1994, **8**: 137–52.
12. Neveu P. J. Asymmetrical brain modulation of immune reactivity in mice: A model for studying interindividual differences and physiological population heterogeneity? *Life Sci*, 1992, **50**: 1–6.

13. Neveu P. J., Dantzer R., Le Moal M. Behavioually conditioned suppression of mitogen-induced lymphoproliferation and antibody production in mice. *Neurosci Letts*, 1986, **65**: 293–8.
14. Sandi C., Castanon N., Vitiello S., Neveu P. J., Mormade P. Different responsiveness of spleen lymphocytes from two lines of psychogenetically selected rats (Roman high and low avoidance). *J Neuroimmunol*, 1991, **31**: 27–33.

Chapter 19

Clinical and Social Implications of Stress-induced Neuroendocrine–Immune Interactions

George Freeman Solomon

University of California, Los Angeles, California, USA

19.1 INTRODUCTION

From the previous chapters, the stalwart reader will by now have learned much about stressful influences upon and neuroendocrine interactions with the immune system. In addition to providing basic scientific knowledge, this research raises other important issues. Do experiential events, including the impact of external factors (e.g. social support) and psychological behavioural factors (e.g. coping) and their neuroendocrine sequelae have health implications? If neuroendocrine–

Stress, Stress Hormones and the Immune System. Edited by J. C. Buckingham, G. E. Gillies and A.-M. Cowell
© 1997 John Wiley & Sons, Ltd.

immune interactions are clinically relevant, what are the implications for the practice of modern medicine and, as a consequence, should the practice of medicine be altered? If so, what are the socio-economic implications? If psychosocial factors, by means of extraordinarily complex neuroendocrine-immune mechanisms, affect health, are existing models of the body, of health and of disease adequate, or must we challenge some basic biomedical concepts and models? The close bidirectional communication links between the nervous system (central and autonomic) and the immune system tempt teleological and analogical thinking about both systems acting as one integrated system to serve functions of adaptation, defence and regulation, with both having a sense of "self" and a capacity for memory (1).

19.1.1 Old Wisdom

A recognition of the interactions between the nervous, endocrine and immune systems and their clinical and bioregulatory implications has spawned the exciting field of psychoneuroimmunology (PNI), also variously called neuroim-munomodulation, neuroendocrine immunology or behavioural neuroimmunol-ogy. Studies in this now burgeoning field are unravelling underlying biological mechanisms of phenomena recognised by wise philosophers, healers, and physicians for centuries. Aristotle, for example, clearly showed foresight of PNI when he said, "Soul and body, I suggest, react sympathetically upon each other: A change in the state of the soul produces a change in the shape of the body and, conversely, a change in the shape of the body produces a change in the state of the soul". The importance of the interactions between the brain and the peripheral systems was also recognised by the seventeenth century Transylvanian physician, Papai Pariz Ferenc, who said, "When the parts of the body and its humours are not in harmony, then the mind is unbalanced and melancholy ensues but, on the other hand, a quiet and happy mind makes the whole body healthy". Indeed, the celebrated second century Greek physician Galen observed that melancholy women were more prone to develop cancer, while Lorenzo Sassoli wrote to a patient in 1402, "To get angry and shout pleases me, for this will keep up your natural heat, but what displeases me is your being grieved and taking all matters to heart. For it is this, as the whole of physic teaches, which destroys our body more than any other cause".

Many ancient Eastern traditions of medicine share concepts of energetic life forces at work within the body. For example, Indian (Ayurveda, yoga), Chinese (acupuncture, herbal medicine) and Tibetan traditions have realised a subtle mental sovereignty over bodily processes and have treated mind and body as an indivisible unit (2); hence, these treatments are often concerned more with promoting life and health than in just dealing with disease (3). This thinking also encompasses concepts of natural and acquired immunity and the beliefs that the highest levels of spiritual development require a fit body; disease results from imbalances of forces within the body; correction of imbalances, whether by material, mental or spiritual means, allows healing to take place. At a biochemical level, the practice of yoga has been shown to have beneficial effects on levels of stress hormones, cholesterol and blood pressure and has been used with some success in the relief of stress-related diseases such as peptic ulcer, asthma, headache and hypertension.

The pre-modern nineteenth and early to mid twentieth century physician was able to place an emphasis (probably more than today's physician) on talking to and getting to know his patient as a whole person, including personality patterns, habits and stresses at work and in the family. As early as 1836 a notable physician wrote that a judicious practitioner never gives attention to either the organic or the mental to the exclusion of the other because they are perpetually acting and inseparably linked together. The pre-antibiotic era physician still had much to offer patients with infectious diseases. In the 1890s, tuberculosis was treated with sleep, appetite restoration and methods to reduce cough and pain on the basis that ". . . by modifying the terrain, I encourage the forces of resistance against the invading microbe". In 1910 Sir William Osler, arguably the "father" of modern medicine, said that it is just as important to know what is going on in a man's head as in his chest in order to predict the outcome of pulmonary tuberculosis. Indeed, in the 1930s it was claimed that a subject must be exposed to an event, such as clinical depression, which acts as a co-factor, along with the specific bacterium and susceptible lungs, before active pulmonary tuberculosis can develop.

19.1.2 "Classical" Psychosomatic Observations on Immunologically Resisted and Mediated Diseases

For a number of years many immunologists remained convinced that the immune system was "autonomous" and self-regulatory. Anecdotal and systematic observations, however, were made on psychological factors which either predispose an individual to develop certain diseases or affect the course of diseases which are normally resisted by the immune system (infections and at least some cancers) or result from aberrations of immune function (e.g. the autoimmune diseases and allergies). This field of psychosomatic medicine began to develop in the late 1930s and included diseases such as rheumatoid arthritis, diabetes and allergies (4). It encompasses the view that psychosomatic pathology is the consequence of physiological concomitants of emotion (5) and, by 1960, George Engel clearly expressed the emerging multifactoral model of disease as having biopsychosocial antecedents (6).

Infectious Diseases

As already pointed out, some of the best early psychosomatic observations were made in regard to tuberculosis in the first half of the twentieth century. It was realised by many physicians that the helpful influence of the sanatorium in recovery from tuberculosis was based on the isolation of the patient from the stresses of everyday life, the caring atmosphere and the fresh air and sunlight as well as the medical procedures available (e.g. pneumothorax). A number of pre-PNI clinical studies, reviewed in (7), investigated the influence of psychological factors, such as stress and depression, on the susceptibility to, progression of and recovery from infectious diseases including infectious mononucleosis, brucellosis, influenza and herpes simplex (a latent virus normally kept in check by means of cellular immunity). Indeed, it does not necessarily take a PNI researcher to recognise the relationship between stress and clinical susceptibility to common infectious diseases. This is amply illustrated by the heroine of the musical *Guys and Dolls* who, in her song, *A person can develop a cold*, was expressing her view that the recurrent upper respiratory infections from which she suffered were caused by the failure of her long-time boyfriend to propose marriage!

Autoimmune Diseases

A number of studies on the influence of emotional and personality factors on the onset and course of autoimmune diseases, particularly rheumatoid arthritis, have been published and reviewed (8). It emerges that arthritics are generally described as quiet, introverted, reliable, conscientious, restricted in the expression of emotion (especially anger), conforming, self-sacrificing, tending to allow themselves to be imposed upon, sensitive to criticism, distant, overactive and busy, pseudo-independent, stubborn, rigid and controlling. The onset of disease often follows either a period of psychological stress or interruption of established patterns of defence and adaptation. Moreover, failure of prior adaptations and inability to cope with new stresses are related to the rate of disease progression, degree of incapacitation and poor response to medical treatment in rheumatoid arthritis. When making psychological comparisons, it emerged that healthy relatives of rheumatoid arthritics whose sera showed the characteristic autoantibody of that disease (rheumatoid factor, FII, an anti-IgG) as well as those healthy relatives who were FII seronegative, lacked the dysphoria (anxiety, depression, alienation, resentment, etc.) and dissatisfaction with occupations and relationships often reported in the arthritics. This observation suggests that mental well-being may contribute a protective influence to those with a probable genetically-determined immunologic predisposing factor from overt disease. Psychological findings similar to those in rheumatoid arthritis have been reported in patients with other diseases probably of an autoimmune nature, such as Graves' disease, multiple sclerosis, systemic lupus erythematosus, ulcerative colitis and psoriasis.

Allergic Diseases

In regard to allergic diseases, personality and stress factors have been related to atopic dermatitis, urticaria, allergic rhinitis and asthma. One study found 75% of persons with allergic disorders showed both immunological (post-histamine eosinophilia and positive skin tests for allergens) and psychological disturbances (by history and psychological tests) compared to 25% of controls (9).

Cancer

There is a large, controversial literature on the relationships between psychosocial factors (both life stress and personality pattern predisposition) and cancer. In their 1956 review of the old cancer psychosomatic literature, Leshan and Worthington (10) found four consistent factors:

(a) loss of an important relationship prior to development of a tumour,
(b) inability to express hostile feelings and emotions,
(c) unresolved conflict regarding a parent figure, and
(d) sexual difficulties.

Klopfer related long survival with metastatic disease either to successful mechanisms of denial or to a mature, calm acceptance of reality; by contrast he related rapid death to malfunctioning ego defensiveness with a high degree of poorly communicated subjective distress—poor repression, high suppression (11). The so-called "Type C" or cancer-prone behaviour pattern is characterised by unexpressiveness, even unawareness of emotions (alexithymia), particularly anger; lack of "fighting spirit", unassertiveness; self-sacrificing behaviours and martyr-like uncomplaining attitudes; conventionality, compliance and lack of a sense of control—resignation, pessimism or fatalism (12).

19.2 PSYCHONEUROIMMUNOLOGICAL STUDIES WITH HEALTH OUTCOME DATA

There are far too few studies which directly correlate psychoneuroimmunological changes with effects on the health of the individual. Hopefully, this deficit will be remedied before long. There is, however, a long tradition of clinical research on the influence of psychosocial factors on health and the progress of disease. This may be described as A → C research with A being psychosocial factors, B immunological change and C disease outcome. There is also animal work demonstrating effects of stress on susceptibility to infectious diseases (particularly viral) and on the course of tumours and of experimental autoimmune disease such as adjuvant induced arthritis and experimental allergic encephalomyelitis (not always in the direction of exacerbation). As the reader of this volume by now fully realises, particularly from Chapters 3, 9 and 18, there has been much animal and human work on experimental and naturally-occurring stresses and other experiential influences on various aspects of immunity, thus covering the A and B phases of research. What is now needed is A → B → C research which demonstrates that psychosocial or experimental influences on immune function have consequences for health. Measurable changes or even "abnormalities" in immune function do not necessarily lead to disease or to demonstrable increases in susceptibility to disease. This non-linear relationship is well illustrated in patients infected with the human immunodeficiency virus (HIV) who do not usually develop opportunistic infections and neoplasms until the number of CD4$^+$ helper or inducer T cells falls below 200/ml, and sometimes as low as 50/ml, i.e. well below the normal range of 800–1200/ml. Persons with CD4$^+$ cell counts above 500/ml generally appear to be perfectly healthy and to recover normally from, for example, ordinary upper respiratory infections. However, we must remember the complexity of the immune system, its numerous interacting cell types, cytokines and feedback loops and redundancies and, of course, its modulation by neurohormones, neuropeptides and neurotransmitters which, themselves, may be influenced by extrinsic as well as intrinsic factors. Single measurements are, therefore, unlikely to provide us with the whole picture.

19.2.1 Stress and the Development of Immunologically Resisted Diseases

In one example of an "outcome" study, it was found that the incidence of infection (clinical colds or increase in virus-specific antibody) induced by intranasal administration of fixed doses of five rhinoviruses correlated in a dose-dependent manner with stress (amount and perception) experienced in the previous year (13). Although it seems highly likely that the findings are the result of effects on immunity, no measures of immunity (e.g. salivary or nasal secretory IgA) were made and other factors could have been involved. Another study found that psychosocial factors correlate both with severity of infectious mononucleosis associated with Epstein–Barr virus (EBV) and with the titres of antibody to EBV in subjects who had seroconverted during the four year study period (14). Stresses, such as medical school examinations, marital strife and caring for patients with Alzheimer's disease can also produce changes in immune function of potential clinical importance (15, 16). For example, stress has been shown to activate herpes group virus, including HSV-1 ("cold sore" virus) and EBV, although the activation is generally at a sub-clinical level. Carers of Alzheimer's patients show decrements in several measures of immunity which are coupled with an increased experience of infectious diseases. Similarly, students self-report more upper respiratory tract symptoms during examination periods. The findings that students who failed to seroconvert when immunised with hepatitis B vaccine during examinations were more stressed and anxious are likely to be of clinical importance as also are reports that the antibody titres and blastogenic responses induced by three inoculations of hepatitis antigen are reduced in subjects with less social support. A major review of psychosocial factors and recurrent genital herpes (HSV-2) also concludes that psychosocial variables are important elements in the prediction maintenance and management of that disease (17).

19.2.2 Depression and Immunologically Resisted Diseases

In studies of minor depression, a longitudinal PNI study of inner city adolescents showed that those with depressed mood or syndromal depression at a given time experienced more physical illnesses subsequently (18). Susceptibility to illness correlated with reductions in B cell number and mitogen responses and with the presence of activated T-cells at the time of the initial depression (18). In a rare $A \rightarrow B \rightarrow C$ type of prospective study of ostensibly normal young adults, investigators found that a sub-group persistently presented with low levels of natural killer (NK) cell activity and that this was associated subsequently with an increased incidence of higher upper respiratory illness (19). In addition, this sub-group exhibited lower levels of β-endorphin, an endogenously produced opioid peptide known to stimulate NK cell cytotoxicity.

There are many studies on the relationships between major depressive disorders and immunity. The results are often somewhat contradictory but the general consensus is that depression is associated with reductions in T cell immunity, especially in older depressed patients, and NK cell activity irrespective of age. Both the duration and the severity of depression are relevant and there are reports of immune activation as well as suppression (20). There are also several epidemiological studies showing increased mortality in depressed patients, especially the elderly (21). A number of studies have shown immunosuppression following bereavement (22); there is an increase in morbidity following sudden and unexpected bereavement and increased mortality among bereaved parents (23).

19.2.3 Significance of Attitudes, Coping and Relationships on Immune Function

In an interesting prospective study of Harvard students who had been the subjects of an intense psychological assessment 35 years earlier, it was found that good physical health at mid-life was best predicted by reports of a caring and loving relationship with parents at age 20 (24). This study concluded that successful adaptation to stress is essential for survival while another study proposed that pessimism in early adult life also appears to be a risk factor for poor health in middle and late adulthood (25). Although these reports suggest that attitudes, coping and relationships in "normal" subjects influence the health of the individual, such claims require further scientific evaluation. For example, it needs to be established whether relatively low immunologic measures (e.g. T cell, NK cell and B cell function), which could possibly be within normal limits, have significant correlations with less adaptive behaviours and could thus be predictive measures of health status.

19.2.4   Psychoneuroimmunological Approaches to Human Immunodeficiency States

There is a fair amount of PNI research underway in HIV infection and AIDS, particularly in regard to psychosocial influences as co-factors in the rate of progression of the disease. Kemeny and co-workers found that both chronically depressed mood and an attitude of fatalism were associated with an increased rate of decline in $CD4^+$ helper or inducer T cells in asymptomatic HIV seropositive subjects (26). My collaborators and I have consistently found highly adaptive coping skills, especially assertiveness, ability to find meaningfulness in life and ability to attend to their own needs both in long-term survivors with AIDS and, more recently, in those infrequent individuals who remain asymptomatic for prolonged periods of time in the face of very low levels of $CD4^+$ T cells (27, 28). The latter subjects also show intact NK cytotoxic activity which is normally rare in late-stage HIV infection and is particularly interesting because of the "psychosocial sensitivity" of NK cell activity. A prospective study of HIV positive subjects in Stage II (asymptomatic) and Stage III (lymphoadenopathy) found that progression to Stage IV was negatively associated with "fighting spirit" and positively with a coping style of denial and repression (29).

19.2.5   Psychoneuroimmunological Studies and Ageing

An appealing alternative to considering the potential role of psychoneuro-immunological factors in disease onset and progression is to look at such factors in health maintenance. Obviously, there is a high frequency of morbidity and mortality in old people. Moreover, although there is much inter-individual variability, most ageing humans, like other mammals, show a senescence of the immune system which is characterised mainly by defects in cell-mediated immunity. We have studied longitudinally a group of apparently very healthy old people in their 70s, 80s and 90s who live independently (30). In these people, unlike a more general elderly population, T cell function, as determined by mitogenesis, is intact and NK cell activity is normal to high. The strong immunological profile is accompanied by lack of dysphoria although an increased incidence of depression, characteristic of the elderly, is apparent. Furthermore, both immunological and psychological measures have remained remarkably stable over a period of five years. Another study showed that a group of healthy, independently living Italian centenarians had high NK cell activity and a normal T cell mitogenic response to concanavalin A. Members of the group were also psychologically resilient following bereavement and continued to be optimistic, actively engaged in life and future orientated (31). Clearly, it appears that psychological and physical well-being are closely intertwined in the elderly. Our studies should eventually provide scientific evidence as to whether stressful life events, failure of coping and consequent distress in the elderly precede immunologic changes which, in turn, precede illness and death.

19.2.6 Psychological Intervention Studies in Immunity and Disease

Psychological interventions in disease are as old as shamanism—but Shamans did not measure immunity! There have been numbers of studies on the effects of psychological interventions on various aspects of immunity in healthy volunteers which show some post-intervention changes. These have included hypnosis in highly hypnotisable subjects (32), humour-induced laughter (33) and "method" acting of despair vs. elation (34). Brief experimental mental stress caused NK cell activity and numbers, but not T cell mitogenesis, to increase (35). Similarly brief maximal (aerobic) exercise induces transient increases in NK cell activity in both young and old subjects. Evidence suggests that this phenomenon may be mediated by endogenous opioids and continuing research suggests that regular physical conditioning may enhance measures of cellular immunity in the elderly (36, 37). Both exercise and active stress management buffer distress responses and immunologic changes following notification of HIV seropositively (38). A convincing therapeutic intervention in disease, presumably but not demonstrably based on local immune changes, has been hypnotherapy for common warts (39). There are also many reports of "spontaneous" remissions of advanced cancer and other usually irreversible diseases, preceded by experiences such as worship at the shrine at Lourdes (40). Whether such tumour regressions are immunologically-mediated remains unknown.

One prospective PNI study on cancer by Fawzy et al. stands out as a model for future research by virtue of its longitudinal design, psychosocial and immune variables and mortality outcomes (41–43). This study offered patients with malignant melanoma a 6-week post-surgical group therapy for enhancement of problem-solving skills, stress-management and social support. Active coping skills increased and distress decreased. At six months (but not six weeks) following the intervention, there were higher numbers of lymphocytes with markers associated with NK cell activity and increased NK cytotoxicity. A six year follow-up revealed that intervention patients had lower rates of recurrence and greater survival, although the alteration in immune function did not persist; controls were like national norms. Both higher baseline coping and enhanced active coping were predictive of lower rates of recurrence and death, as was baseline affective distress (non-repressive coping). Clearly further outcome studies are needed in this area.

19.3 THE "OVERSELLING" OF PSYCHONEUROIMMUNOLOGY IN THE POPULAR LITERATURE

It should be clear that convincing scientific evidence that psychosocial factors and behavioural interventions modulate the recovery from immunologically-related diseases is modest, as too is our knowledge of the putative intervening neuroendocrine–immune mechanisms. Much more truly objective, clinically-based research is urgently required, including both outcome and psychobiological variables. Additionally, as this publication more than amply illustrates, the bulk of research on neuroendocrine–immune interactions has aimed to elucidate the regulatory mechanisms which, although ultimately are likely to be of vital clinical relevance, are not clinical studies *per se*. The likely interactions between the immune system and the brain are, however, immensely appealing to the general public who have been exposed to exaggerated claims for PNI as being the answer for conditions as varied as cardiac arrhythmias and digestive abnormalities. The grounds presented for such claims include, for example, the view that conscious thought processes might induce specific molecular changes on the cell surface membrane to resist viral and bacterial invasions and cancer and that certain diets aid recovery from illness by enhancing immune activity. Although some recommendations may be helpful, for example, antioxidants such as vitamins C, E and beta-carotene may help block free-radical damage of immune and other cells, others may be harmful. Indeed, a suggestion that the immune system can be "strengthened by natural energies such as sunlight" contradicts the evidence of reduced immunity and of increased incidence of skin carcinogenesis by exposure to ultraviolet light. Furthermore, current medical opinion recommends that HIV-positive individuals should avoid excessive exposure to sunlight. However, we must keep open minds about unproven claims;

as the Prologue highlighting Hans Selye's work reminds us, the view that stress can be immunosuppressive was once thought unorthodox.

In the face of the hardships accompanying the popularisation and often the misrepresentation of new ideas which challenge scientific dogma (which itself has no place in real science), PNI is attempting to explain mechanisms underlying some valid observations of the effects of traditional and unorthodox medicine on immunologically-related diseases. The work of Robert Ader and others on the classical conditioning of immunity (both suppression and enhancement) may, indeed, lead to a greater understanding of the active nature of the placebo than immunity. At present the US National Institute of Health has an initiative to provide funding for scientific evaluation of non-traditional techniques which, hopefully, will include some with immunologic variables. Most importantly, such studies should control for psychosocial and/or stress effects on immunity which may vary considerably from individual to individual, depending on coping ability.

19.4 IMPLICATIONS OF PSYCHONEUROIMMUNOLOGY FOR MEDICAL PRACTICE, MEDICAL ECONOMICS AND PUBLIC HEALTH

In many respects the remarkable recent discoveries concerning the role of the brain in the regulation of the immune system have reintroduced us to the values of the practice of medicine in the nineteenth century, when the physician really knew his patient and his or her personal habits, the family and work stress. With automated laboratory testing, batteries of blood chemistry analyses are readily performed and, excluding the constraints of cost, considered choices need not be made. Unless caution is exercised, various forms of highly technological imaging from computer assisted tomography (CT), magnetic resonance imaging (MRI) and positron emission tomography (PET) scans to echocardiograms and electro-encephalogram (EEG) brain mapping could be in danger of making obsolete the discerning eye, the sensitive finger, the keen ear and the traditional aids, the stethoscope and reflex hammer. Equally, appreciation of the importance of the time spent on the long and detailed (non-automated) history, the careful complete physical examination, the sensitive follow-up interviews, is in danger of becoming completely lost. Powerful economic and social forces drive medical practice and, at least in the United States, "cognitive" services (talking) to patients do not have mandatory reimbursement. Such a system thus redirects medical students to the now-lucrative areas of orthopaedics, invasive cardiology, plastic surgery and ophthalmology whereas family practice, internal medicine, paediatrics, obstetrics and psychiatry may be in danger of losing them. Perhaps emphasis in pre-medical studies on the humanities, social sciences and even economics will turn out to be as relevant to medical practice as chemistry and physics. Indeed, as great an appreciation should go to the medical student's humanistic character-istics and ability to reason and think originally as to their test-taking abilities in quantitative subjects. Some training in PNI might thus help a medical student understand that extreme sadness, for example, might be relevant to cancer prognosis.

19.4.1 The Practice of Family Medicine

PNI has implications for the practice of family medicine, in which the under-standing of family dynamics may have great relevance to the health of family members (44). In the family context, gender as well as the social and cultural perspective has been found to be relevant to physical and mental well-being and to health-related behaviours, such as smoking and drinking and preventive activities. We therefore need a greater understanding of the associations between disruption of immune function and any significant clinical consequences. Inter-ventions such as distress reduction may then be found to be cost-effective not only in terms of health service provision but possibly even in terms of days lost from work, disability payments, etc. with important implications for the com-munity as a whole.

19.4.2 Relevance to Public Health

Since mental and physical well being are so intertwined, the study of PNI would suggest that stresses within society may well have relevance to public health. The higher morbidity and mortality associated with very low socioeconomic status and the accompanying stresses of providing daily sustenance while living in inadequate housing in unsafe, possibly violent neighbourhoods may provide a good example. Indeed, it is of note that all the healthy old people we have studied (see Section 19.2.5) had incomes adequate to meet their basic needs and to provide primary preventative health care, thus freeing them from the stress mentioned above. Epidemiological studies of individuals' responses to public disasters also provide further evidence for a relevance to PNI to public health. One such disaster, which has been the subject of much scrutiny, is the nuclear accident in the USA at Three Mile Island. Not surprisingly, post-accident anxiety (e.g. perceived threat, demoralisation, psychological symptoms) was directly correlated with proximity to the plant. In the year following the accident, the incid-ence of cancer, particularly non-Hodgkin's lymphoma (known to be immunologically resistant), increased in subjects living closest to the plant (45); those living further away, but still within a 10 mile radius, showed no change in the incidence of cancer. These observations are interesting because calculations involving the radiation released (which was, in fact, very little), the wind direction and the geographical features of the terrain suggest that the increased incidence of cancer in the relatively restricted region could not correlate with the intensity of radiation. It did, however, correlate with anxiety, thus placing distress as a significant factor in pathogenesis of the disease. This view is further strengthened by the work of Glaser and associates who suggested that naturalistic stress in man not only reduces aspects of immunity but can also increase proto-oncogene expression and reduce DNA repair, a "triple threat" for carcino-genesis.

Common life stressors, not only disasters, may well also turn out to be public health threats. A very healthy 93 year-old, whose NK and T cell function were like those of a younger healthy subject, said, "Nothing bothers me anymore. I can't understand why most people get so up-tight about trivia."

19.4.3 Psychoneuroimmunology, Stress and Litigation

The past decade has seen an explosion of cases claiming compensation for psychological damage (post-traumatic stress disorder) following culpable stress in civil litigation, at least in the United States. Increasingly, therefore, the courts have need of expert witnesses in relevant medical disciplines which have become "established by scientific method" in order to evaluate scientifically the arguments presented by the defence or prosecution. The following is an example of some questions which might arise in such a case. Did repeated sexual harassment at work, subsequent unjustified firing, unemployment and consequent despair and resentment contribute: (a) 10% (or 20% or 30% etc.) to the development of breast cancer four months after discharge from work, or (b) to metastasis of a cancer that had been surgically removed two years previously without prior evidence of recurrence, or (c) to the permanent neurological impairment consequent to the development of bacterial meningitis two weeks after dis-charge?

Such questions will clearly be difficult to resolve but, with growing scientific evidence to establish further the clinical relevance of PNI, experts in that discipline may be much in demand. Indeed, there is a popular conception, arising possibly as a result of overstatement of facts in the media, that stress is an aetiological factor in diseases such as cancer. Inevitably, therefore, juries will tend to be influenced by popular preconceptions in addition to the presentations of the prosecutors, so the question arises, "Will PNI open a Pandora's box of already extensive stress-related litigation?" As "hard" evidence for the clinical relevance of stress-related effects on neuroendocrine–immune interactions grows, the answer may well be "yes".

19.5 TOWARDS NEW MODELS OF THE BODY, OF HEALTH AND OF DISEASE

Collaborative studies with the philosopher, David Levin, have led us to the view that the body itself is more than an evolutionary biological entity; it is a result of processes that communicatively interact with its biological nature, to develop and transform it (46). Humans are sociable from their beginning with bodies organised biologically for communication, both via the senses and the immune system. Thus, it is hard to draw a line between the body of nature and the body of experience (nature). The history of medicine has presented many different, often conflicting, representations of the human body. The advancement of medicine depends, now more than ever, on breaking free of schemata which are incomplete and no longer work. The ancients placed what went on within the body in communication with natural and supernatural forces without the body. However, medicine in the Middle Ages and the Renaissance went from abstraction to concreteness and a fascination with internal structures with the beginnings of dissection by Da Vinci and Vessalius. Viewing the body as a machine with, for example, the central nervous system (CNS) being analogous to a telephone switchboard in the late nineteenth century or to a computer in the mid-twentieth century, led to linear concepts of causality of disease, namely the malfunctioning of the machine. Early modern medicine was concerned with structures and how they worked. Late modern medicine, with more complexity, has been concerned with functions and processes, culminating in a commitment to understanding systems. Significantly, an understanding of the endocrine system set the stage for a blurring of the distinction between the inner (homeostasis) and the outer (adaptation). Now we can come to the point of systemic integration, as exemplified by PNI with its nervous, neuroendocrine and immune components. The shift from the structural to the functional has thus been useful, yet still mechanistic. Although the complexity of systems and processes has been recognised, we need now to develop new, non-linear, non-mechanistic understandings based on systems, chaos and informational theories. Extremely complex feedback loops interact with other complex loops and, as non-linear mathematics points out, small perturbations can change sine waves to bimodal or trimodal waves and then chaotic fluctuations and back again. There are systems which are so complex and so interrelated that the conditions of the whole are not predictable on the basis of its elements. The body is more than anatomy, physiology and biochemistry or even psychosomatics and molecular biology. Disease may be more complex than even a multifactorial model can adequately describe. Is chronic fatigue immunodeficiency fibromyalgia syndrome a result of depression-induced low NK cell activity and activation of latent virus or does a viral infection release cytokines which induce fatigue? Is it a sleep disorder which results in immune dysregulation or immune dysregulation which results in sleep disturbance? In any of these situations inappropriate CNS-induced immune or neuroendocrine activation may well be involved.

PNI, increasingly, is dissolving dualisms of mind–body, body–environment and individual–population. In realising that states of the medical body are correlated with the individual's bodily experience, Levin and I expressed the hope that patients themselves will begin to understand their bodies in new ways. For some time, I have felt that somatic awareness is akin to psychological insight and that the former has a similar relationship to physical health as the latter has to psychological well-being. Patients may begin to realise the extent to which the body that he or she presents to medicinal practitioners for diagnosis and treatment is a body of meaningful experience, of significant intelligence, which is informed about itself and its environment and is influenced by his or her own sensitivity and embodied awareness. The degree to which the patient is skilled at sensing the body's diseases and its health are also conditions of meaning, as integrated through interpretations of life experienced by the mind–brain–immune system.

We anticipate that an understanding of the interactions between the nervous, endocrine and immune systems and their importance in the balance between states of health and disease, as embodied by PNI, will not only contribute to the clinical understanding and treatment of disease but also to valuing the doctor–patient relationship, to redefining the nature of pathophysiology and of health and to changing the nature of the patient's own role in recovery. Arising from antecedents in immunology, endocrinology, psychosomatic medicine and neuroscience, PNI, hopefully, will promote a new, more integrated, productive and clinically helpful era (47).

REFERENCES

1. Booth R. J., Ashbridge K. R. A fresh look at the relationship between the psyche and the immune system: Teleological coherence and harmony of purpose. *Advances*, 1993, **9**: 4–23.
2. Sheikh A. A., Sheikh K. S. *Eastern and Western Approaches to Healing. Ancient Wisdom and Modern Knowledge*. New York, John Wiley, 1989.
3. Shukla H. C., Solomon G. F., Doshi R. S. The relevance of some Ayurvedic (traditional Indian) medical concepts to modern holistic health. *J Holistic Health*, 1981, **4**: 125–31.
4. Dunbar F. *Psychosomatic Diagnosis*. New York, Paul B. Hoeber, 1943.
5. Alexander F., French T. M. (eds) *Studies in Psychosomatic Medicine*. New York, Ronald Press, 1948.
6. Engel G. L. A unified concept of health and disease. *Perspect Biol Med*, 1960, **3**: 459–85.
7. Solomon G. F., Amkraut A.A. Psychoneuroendocrinological effects on the immune response. *Ann Rev Microbiol*, 1981, **35**: 155–84.
8. Solomon G. F. Emotional and personality factors in the onset and course of

autoimmune disease, particular rheumatoid arthritis. In R. Ader (ed.) *Psychoneuroimmunology*. New York, Academic Press, 1981.

9. Jacobs M. A., Friedman S., Franklin M. J., Anderson L. S., Muller J. J., Eisman H. D. Incidence of psychosomatic predisposing factors in allergic disease. *Psychosom Med*, 1966, **28**: 679–95.

10. Leshan L. L., Worthington R. E. Personality as a factor in pathogenesis of cancer; review of literature. *Brit J Med Psychol*, 1956, **29**: 49–56.

11. Klopfer B. Psychological variables in human cancer. *J Proj Techn*, 1957, **21**: 331–9.

12. Temoshok L., Dreher H. *The Type C Connection*. New York, Random House, 1992.

13. Cohen S., Tyrrell D. A. J., Smith A. P. Psychological stress and susceptibility to the common cold. *New Eng J Med*, 1991, **325**: 606–12.

14. Kasl S. V., Neiderman J. C., Evans A. A. Psychosocial risk factors in the development of infectious mononucleosis. *Psychosom Med*, 1979, **41**: 445–66.

15. Kiecolt-Glaser J., Cacioppo J. T., Malarkey W. G., Glaser R. Acute psychological stressors and short-term immune changes: what, why, for whom, and to what extent? *Psychosom Med*, 1992, **54**: 680–5.

16. Kiecolt-Glaser J., Dura J. R., Speicher C. E., Trask O. J., Glaser R. Spousal caregivers of dementia victims: Longitudinal changes in immunity and health. *Psychosom Med*, 1991, **53**: 345–62.

17. Longo D., Koehn K. Psychosocial factors and recurrent genital herpes: a review of prediction and psychiatric treatment studies. *Intl J Psychiat in Med*, 1993, **23**: 99–117.

18. Keller S. E., Schleifer S. J., Bartlett J. A., Eckholdt H. Affective processes and immune dysfunction have health consequences. *Biol Psychiat*, 1992, **31**: 236A.

19. Levy S. M., Femstrom J., Herberman R. B., Whiteside T., Lee J., Ward M., Massoudi M. Persistently low natural killer cell activity and circulating levels of plasma beta endorphin: risk factors for infectious disease. *Life Sci*, 1991, **48**: 107–16.

20. Schleifer S. J., Keller S. E., Sirios S. G. Depression and immunity. *Arch Gen Psychiat*, 1985, **42**: 129–33.

21. Murphy E., Smith R., Lindesay J., Slattery J. Increased mortality rates in late-life depression. *Brit J Psychiat*, 1988, **152**: 347–53.

22. Schleifer S. J., Keller S. E., Camarino M., Thomton J. C., Stein M. Suppression of lymphocyte stimulation following bereavement. *JAMA*, 1983, **250**: 374–7.

23. Lundin T. Morbidity following sudden and unexpected bereavement. *Brit J Psychiat*, 1984, **144**: 84–8.

24. Russek L. G., Schwartz G. E. Perceptions of parental caring predict health status in mid-life: a 35 year follow up of the Harvard Mastery of Stress Study. *Psychosom Med*, 1992, **59**; 144–9.

25. Taylor S. E. *Positive Illusions*. New York, Basic Books, 1989.

26. Reed G. M., Kemeny M. E., Taylor S. E., Wang H.-Y. J., Visscher B. R. "Realistic acceptance" as a predictor of psychological adjustment and survival time in gay men with AIDS. *Health Psychol*, 1994, **13**: 299–307.

27. Solomon G. F., Temoshok L., O'Leary A., Zich J. An intensive psychoimmunologic study of long-surviving persons with AIDS: Pilot work, background studies, hypotheses, and methods. *Ann NY Acad Sci*, 1988, **496**: 647–55.

28. Solomon G. F., Benton D., Harker J. O., Bonavida B., Fletcher M. A. Prolonged asymptomatic states in HIV seropositive persons with fewer than 50 CD4+ cells/mm³: Psychoneuroimmunologic findings. *J Acquir Immune Defic Syndr*, 1993, **6**: 1172–3.

29. Solano L., Costa M., Salvati S., Coda R., Aiuti F., Mezzaroma I., Bertini M. Psychosocial factors and clinical evolution in HIV-1 infection: a longitudinal study. *J Psychosom Res*, 1993, **37**: 39–51.

30. Solomon G. F., Fiatarone M. A., Benton D., Morley J. E, Bloom E, Makinodan T.

Psychoimmunologic and endorphin function in the aged. *Ann NY Acad Sci*, 1988, **521**: 43–57.

31. Sansoni P., Brianti V., Fagnoni F., Snelli G., Marcato A., Passeri G., Monti P., Cossarizza A., Franceschi C. NK cell activity and T-lymphocyte proliferation in healthy centenarians. *Ann NY Acad Sci*, 1992, **663**: 505–7.

32. Hall H. R. Hypnosis and the immune system: A review with implications for cancer and the psychology of healing. *Am J Clin Hypnosis*, 1983, **25**: 92–103.

33. Berk L. S., Tan S. A., Berk D. B., Eby W. C. Immune changes during humor associated laughter. *Clin Res*, 1991, **39**: 124A (abstract).

34. Futterman A. D. Positive and negative mood states: immune and nervous system responses *(dissertation)*. Los Angeles, Dept of Psychology, UCLA, 1990.

35. Naliboff B. D., Benton D., Solomon G. F., Morley J. E., Bloom E. T., Fahey J. L., Makinodan T. Psychological, psychophysiological, and immunological changes in young and old during brief laboratory stress. *Psychosom Med*, 1991, **53**: 121–32.

36. Fiatarone M. A., Morley J. E., Bloom E. T., Benton D., Solomon G. F., Makinodan T. The effect of exercise on natural killer cell activity in young and old subjects. *J Gerontol*, 1989, **44**: M37–M45.

37. Fiatarone M. A., Morley J. E., Bloom E. T., Benton D., Makinodan T., Solomon G. F. Endogenous opioids and the exercise-induced augmentation of natural killer cell activity. *J Lab Clin Med*, 1988, **112**: 544–52.

38. Antoni M. H., Baggett L., Ironson G., LaPerriere A., August S., Schneiderman N., Fletcher M. A. Cognitive-behavioral stress management intervention buffers distress responses and immunologic changes following notification of HIV-1 seropositivity. *J Cons Clin Psych*, 1991, **59**: 906–15.

39. Spanos N. P., Williams V., Gwynn M. I. Effects of hypnotic, placebo, and salicylic acid treatments on wart regression. *Psychosom Med*, 1990, **52**: 109–14.

40. O'Regan B., Hirshberg C. *Spontaneous Remission. An Annotated Bibliography.* Sausalito, Institute of Noetic Sciences, 1993.

41. Fawzy F. I., Cousins N., Fawzy N. W., Kemeny M. E., Elashoff R., Morton D. A structured psychiatric intervention for cancer. I. Changes over time in methods of coping and affective disturbance. *Arch Gen Psychiat*, 1990, **47**: 720–5.

42. Fawzy F. I., Kemeny M. E., Fawzy N. W., Elashoff R., Morton D., Cousins N., Fahey J. A structured psychiatric intervention for cancer patients. II. Changes over time in immunological measures. *Arch Gen Psychiat*, 1990, **47**: 729–35.

43. Fawzy F. I., Fawzy N. W., Hyun C. S., Elashoff R., Guthrie D., Fahey J., Morton D. L. Malignant melanoma: effects of an early structured psychiatric intervention, coping, and affective state on recurrence and survival 6 years later. *Arch Gen Psychiat*, 1993, **50**: 681–9.

44. Fisher L., Ransom D. C., Terry H. E. The California family health project. VII. Summary and integration of findings. *Fam Proc*, 1993, **32**: 69–86.

45. Hatch M. C., Wallerstein S., Beyea J., Nieves J. W., Susser M. Cancer rates after the Three Mile Island nuclear accident and proximity to residence to the plant. *Am J Pub Health*, 1991, **81**: 719–24.

46. Levin D. M., Solomon G. F. The discursive formation of the body in the history of medicine. *J Med Philos*, 1990, **15**: 515–37.

47. Solomon G. F. Whither psychoneuroimmunology? A new era of immunology, of psychosomatic medicine, and of neuroscience. *Brain Behav Immun*, 1993, **7**: 352–66.

Index

Index compiled by Liz Granger